Aphasia and
Related Neurogenic
Language Disorders

CURRENT THERAPY OF COMMUNICATION DISORDERS

Series Editor
William H. Perkins, Ph.D.

Aphasia and Related Neurogenic Language Disorders

Leonard L. LaPointe, Ph.D.

Professor and Chair
Department of Speech and Hearing Science
Arizona State University
Tempe, Arizona

Consultant
VA Medical Center, Phoenix
VA Outpatient Clinic, Los Angeles

1990
THIEME MEDICAL PUBLISHERS, INC.   New York
GEORG THIEME VERLAG   Stuttgart · New York

Thieme Medical Publishers, Inc.
381 Park Avenue South
New York, New York 10016

APHASIA AND RELATED NEUROGENIC LANGUAGE DISORDERS
Leonard L. LaPointe

Library of Congress Cataloging-in-Publication Data

Aphasia and related neurogenic language disorders / [edited by]
    Leonard L. LaPointe
        p.   cm. — (Current therapy of communication disorders)
    Includes bibliographical references.
    ISBN 0-86577-314-9 (TMP)
    1. Aphasia.   2. Language disorders.   3. Central nervous system —
Diseases — Complications and sequelae.   I. LaPointe, Leonard L.
II. Series.
    [DNLM: 1. Aphasia.   2. Central Nervous System Diseases —
complications.   3. Language Disorders.   WL 340.5 A6405]
RC425.A615   1990
616.85′52 — dc20
DNLM/DLC
for Library of Congress   90-10721
                                                                                CIP

Important note: Medicine is an ever-changing science. Research and clinical experience are continually broadening our knowledge, in particular our knowledge of proper treatment and drug therapy. Insofar as this book mentions any dosage or applications, readers may rest assured that the authors, editors, and publishers have made every effort to ensure that such references are strictly in accordance with the state of knowledge at the time of production of the book. Nevertheless, every user is requested to carefully examine the manufacturers' leaflets accompanying each drug to check on his own responsibility whether the dosage schedules recommended therein or the contraindications stated by the manufacturers differ from the statements made in the present book. Such examination is particularly important with drugs that are either rarely used or have been newly released on the market.

Some of the product names, patents, and registered designs referred to in this book are in fact registered trademarks or proprietary names even though specific reference to this fact is not always made in the text. Therefore, the appearance of a name without designation as proprietary is not to be construed as a representation by the publisher that it is in the public domain.

Printed in the United States of America.

5   4   3   2

TMP ISBN 0-86577-314-9
GTV ISBN 3-13-747702-6

To the kids raised in that tall house in the little railroad town
in the Upper Peninsula of Michigan
(Sally, Tom, Marybeth, and Renee).
We share struggles and love

and

To the spirit of the Champagne Cowboy Breakfasts
and all of my jokester friends who appreciate
the oasis of laughter and fun.

Other Volumes in the Series

Contents

Contributors

Brenda L.B. Adamovich, Ph.D.
Administrative Director of Rehabilitation Services
Albany Medical Center
Albany, New York

Kenn Apel, Ph.D.
Assistant Professor
Department of Speech Pathology and Audiology
Western Washington University
Bellingham, Washington

Michael James Collins, Ph.D.
Director of Speech and Language Pathology
Dean Medical Center and Clinics, and
Adjunct Associate Professor
Department of Communication Disorders
University of Wisconsin-Madison
Madison, Wisconsin

Leslie J. Gonzalez Rothi, Ph.D.
Clinician
Audiology and Speech Pathology Service
VA Medical Center
Gainesville, Florida

Lisa Graham, M.S.
Department of Speech and Hearing Science
Arizona State University
Tempe, Arizona

Jennifer A. Henderson, M.S.
Director of Speech Pathology and Audiology
Morton Hospital
Taunton, Massachusetts

Kevin P. Kearns, Ph.D.
Chief of Audiology and
Speech Pathology
Veterans Administration

Medical Center
North Chicago, Illinois, and
Associate Professor
Department of Communication Disorders
and Sciences
Northwestern University
Evanston, Illinois

Leonard L. LaPointe, Ph.D.
Professor and Chair
Department of Speech and Hearing Science
Arizona State University
Tempe, Arizona, and
Consultant
Veterans Administration Medical
Centers, Phoenix and Los Angeles

Craig W. Linebaugh, Ph.D.
Research Professor and Chair
Department of Speech and Hearing
The George Washington University
Washington, D.C.

E. Louise Mackisack, M.A.
Director
Department of Speech Pathology and Audiology
Riverside Rehabilitation Institute
Newport News, Virginia

Malcolm R. McNeil, Ph.D.
Professor
Department of Communicative Disorders
University of Wisconsin-Madison, and
Consultant
Department of Speech Pathology and Audiology
Veterans Administration Hospital
Madison, Wisconsin

ix

Penelope S. Myers, M.A.
Department of Communication Disorders
University of Minnesota
Minneapolis, Minnesota

Marilyn Newhoff, Ph.D.
Associate Professor
Department of Communication Sciences
    and Disorders
The University of Georgia
Athens, Georgia

William H. Perkins, Ph.D.
Emeritus Professor
Department of Communications and Arts and
    Sciences
University of Southern California
Los Angeles, California

Nina N. Simmons, M.S.
Director of Speech Pathology
Touro Infirmary
New Orleans, Louisiana

Lana O. Shekim, Ph.D.
Clinician
Speech Pathology and Audiology Service
The George Washington University Medical
    Center, and
Clinical Assistant Professor
Department of Speech and Hearing
George Washington University
Washington, D.C.

Chin-Hsing Tseng, M.S.
Department of Communicative Disorders
University of Wisconsin-Madison
Madison, Wisconsin

Wanda G. Webb, Ph.D.
Division of Hearing and
    Speech Sciences, and
Department of Neurology
Vanderbilt University Medical Center
Nashville, Tennessee

Foreword

Not many years ago, one could be expected to be an expert in all aspects of neurological disorders. But knowledge of brain function and effects of impairing these functions has expanded rapidly in the last decade. Now, the challenge is to be expert in the individual manifestations of neurogenic language disorders. To prepare this text, an editor who knows the experts in all of the areas was needed. At the top of our list of candidates was Leonard LaPointe, Ph.D., Professor and Chair, Department of Speech and Hearing Science, Arizona State University. In addition to his knowledge of the types of neurogenic impairments of language and those who are working on the frontiers of these impairments, his own long record of scholarship and clinical skill is outstanding.

The text he and his authors have prepared is not only current, it is also remarkably well organized. After each type of disorder is introduced, it is discussed in terms of its pathophysiology, its nature and differentiating features, methods of evaluating it, and methods of treating it. The result is a presentation that is optimally useful clinically.

William H. Perkins

Preface
Roots, Routes, Chants, and Reasons

In the house made of evening twilight.
In the house made of dark cloud.
In the house made of rain and mist.
Where the dark mist curtains the doorway.
The path is on the rainbow. . . .

Happily I recover.
My eyes regain their power.
My head cools.
My limbs regain their strength.
I hear again.
My voice restore for me.

In the white of the wings are the footsteps of
morning.
Wandering on a trail of beauty.
Living again.
May I walk.
May I talk.

A selection of Navajo chants from Cronyn.[1]

The Navajo people, in the American Southwest, live in a land that some have said is barren and sparse; cruel and chilled in the winter and dry-parched in the summer. Yet they have found beauty in this land. They have found a way not only to survive but to reveal their optimism about life and their appreciation of the butter-orange sunsets and the subtle earth tones of a hundred shades of brown and coral. This optimism and appreciation is apparent not only in the delicately crafted patterns of their unique weavings, but also in the chants and songs and prayers that shape their relationship to the world and their reactions to the adversities that are inevitable in the course of living. From the chants and songs above we discern not so thinly-veiled themes. Dark clouds. Mist curtains. Adversity. Trouble. But also hope. Paths. Recovery. Restoration.

In my view, the metaphor is not stretched too far to reveal some of these same themes and lessons in the harsh reality and eventual restoration of function and attitude that accompanies those struck down with disorders of speech and under-standing and writing and reading and memory and perception due to a shattered nervous system. And that is an underlying theme of this book. While one may be dealt a harsh existence by nature or events, there exists always the possibility of hope and effort and restoration. The contributors of the chapters of this book have retained these themes. In fact the very heart of rehabilitation relies on retention of optimism, appropriate objectives, and the application of studied and enlightened strategies for overcoming significant barriers.

Surfacing in this book are several interwoven and interrelated matters of language, brain, loss, and restoration or adjustment. Foremost among these is the process of human communication, that life's-blood process that allows living and learning and loving. As Colin Cherry has stated, "human language is vastly more than a complicated system of cluckings."[2] It allows us the means of transacting daily business and getting on with the exchanges necessary to get through a day. Cursing the alarm, calming the parrot, scanning the *Enquirer*, planning the day, calling in late for work, greeting, reviewing, phoning, writing, thanking, arguing, requesting, arranging, studying, listening, waving, ordering, buying, correcting, revealing, begging, soothing, praising, cooing — all require the subtle manipulations necessary for social interaction. These are taken for granted by most of us because we have lost the memory of the struggle of acquisition. But once this medium of human contact is compromised, by stroke or disease or accident, it is taken for granted no longer and instead is sorely missed. In most cases a monumental struggle ensues to regain the gift. The science and art of that struggle has been the focus of investigation and clinical effort for generations, and recently it has seemed as though thin rays of light have become apparent in the efforts to understand and do something about these complex and variegated disorders.

Primary among the neurogenic disorders that affect language are the aphasias, that group of disruptions that result in convoluted syntax and meaning. More than a million people suffer from aphasia in the United States alone, and each day almost 300 new cases are added to the list. As with so many communication disorders, this condition is ill-recognized and ill-understood by the general public as well as by some professional groups. It is ironic that the public has a greater recognition of Froot Loops, panty hose, and the horrors of pet-induced carpet odor than it does of aphasia. To counter this, an excellent new organization, the National Aphasia Association (P.O. Box 1887, Murray Hill Station, New York, NY 10156-0611) has been formed to stimulate and encourage the development and utilization of resources to better serve the needs of individuals and families who have to cope with aphasia.

A rich array of related disorders that may or may not coexist with aphasia also can result from damage to the delicate neurological network that subserves communication function. Increasingly, the communication deficits that result from traumatically induced brain injury, the strange mix of perceptual–linguistic problems that accompany nondominant hemisphere damage, and the clouding of cognition and words created by abnormal aging and dementia have become recognized as equally or sometimes even more devastating than the traditionally recognized forms of aphasia. Traumatic brain injury has been called the "silent epidemic," particularly in the 15 to 24 year age category, and it has been estimated that between 30,000 and 50,000 people per year in the United States sustain a head injury severe enough to impede a return to a normal lifestyle.[3] Nearly 20% of the elderly population is estimated to suffer from some form of dementia, which almost always affects communication in some way. Against the backdrop of the well-recognized population explosion in this age group, this problem will do nothing but increase in terms of societal cost and human suffering.[4]

These are not insignificant disorders or issues, and their management is becoming increasingly crucial. This book presents a dozen chapters that deal with these issues and should provide enlightenment and direction to students, to practicing clinicians, to professionals in the health care system, and to anyone interested in learning more about the nature and management of those disorders of language created by a nervous system gone awry. In Chapter 1 Kevin Kearns writes about one of the most frequently occurring and frustrating types of aphasia, Broca's Aphasia. Kearns provides a sound foundation for chapters that follow since he traces a bit of history, outlines principles of both evaluation and treatment that are applicable to more than just one type of aphasia, and in his usual cautious fashion, dictates an approach to customizing treatment that always has an eye on the functionality, generality, and good sense of therapeutic strategies.

In Chapter 2 Lisa Graham undertakes the difficult task of explaining Wernicke's Aphasia, one of the most puzzling and frustrating of the aphasic disorders. Graham extracts the best from a scanty literature on the disorder, infuses it with her clinical experience, and creates a chapter that makes sense out of disorder. Chapter 3, on Conduction Aphasia, is written by Nina Simmons. This controversial aphasia type is treated with objectivity and care, and Simmons is up to her usual excellence in writing style as she generates a chapter that is accurate, smooth, and easy on the eyes. Chapter 4, on the Transcortical Aphasias, is written by Leslie Gonzalez-Rothi of the Gainesville Veterans Administration Medical Center. Gonzalez-Rothi's work is thorough and well-researched, and she represents an imitable fusion of principles and ideas from the orientations of behavioral neurology, neuropsychology, and speech–language pathology.

Chapter 5 deals with more than a type of aphasia. Lexical–retrieval and misnaming problems are dramatic and ubiquitous in aphasia, and Craig Linebaugh has provided a scholarly and clinically useful compilation of the subject. Chapter 6, Global Aphasia, is written by Michael Collins, a clinician who has had a good deal of experience in attempting to do something about the devastation of the near totality of language loss. He finds more optimism about the disorder than many writers; in fact has written a book on it, and fashions a chapter that should guide well our understanding as well as our attitudes about this condition.

Chapter 7 is on those crippling reading problems that accompany aphasia, the acquired dyslexias, and Wanda Webb is a most qualified author. She has generated scholarly articles, creative evaluation materials, and excellent review summaries on the topic, and this chapter is both current and clinically relevant. Chapter 8, on a related topic, the Acquired Dysgraphias, is a much needed scholarly synthesis of neurogenic writing disorders. Malcolm McNeil and Chin-Hsing Tseng of the University of Wisconsin–Madison have crafted this excellent piece. McNeil's thoughtfulness is evident throughout the work; clearly it is one of the most thorough syntheses of the topic in the literature.

The next chapter, on Right Hemisphere Syndrome, is written by two clinicians who know of what they write. Penelope Myers and Louise Mackisack are not cowed by the task of bringing a semblance of order to this topic, which has been neglected and has appeared in somewhat chaotic form in some writings. The authors are sought-after speakers on the subject and have created innovative systems of both evaluation and treatment of right hemisphere dysfunction. Chapter 10, Traumatic Brain Injury, was written by Brenda Adamovich and Jennifer Henderson, two of the country's experts on the communication disorders that accompany this diffuse and difficult-to-manage condition. Adamovich has written books, chapters, and has lectured extensively on this silent epidemic condition, and this chapter veritably dances with organization and clinical utility.

Chapter 11 was written by Lana Shekim, whose career I have followed since her days as a doctoral student at the University of Florida. Shekim has always exhibited the qualities of incisive intelligence and persistence in her work, and this chapter on Dementia is a good example. Her care and humanity are as obvious in her writing as they are in her clinical work. The final compilation, Chapter 12, Impairments in Pragmatics was written by Marilyn Newhoff and Kenn Apel. This chapter is a bit of a deviation in format from the others because it deals with an important issue that crosses all of the other types of disorders. Functionality, pragmatics, and ecological validity of our clinical work has captured the attention of several enlightened investigators, and Newhoff and her colleagues have been responsible for generating much of that refreshing breeze that has blown across language disorders. Newhoff and Apel's chapter reflects that freshness.

Although these contributors bring diversity and a variety of approaches to these topics, as editor I have attempted to exert some degree of format standardization in the hope that the book would be smooth and perhaps less disjointed across chapters. We have asked everyone to discuss their topic from the perspective of Introduction, Pathophysiology, Nature and Differentiating Features, Evaluation, Treatment, Specific Treatment Tasks, and finally Suggested Readings and References. I think this format has worked well, and we have a creative and scholarly work that is long on both understanding of these disorders as well as on specific suggestions as to how to treat them. If we can capture some of the dust of the optimism about restoration and recovery inherent in the chants and songs of the Navajo and transfer these attitudes and applications to the mist curtains and clouds of these people afflicted with neurogenic disorders of language, we will have good reason to look forward to the footsteps of morning.

Leonard L. LaPointe

References

1. Cronyn GW: *The Path on the Rainbow.* New York: Boni and Leverright, 1918.
2. Cherry C: *On Human Communication,* 2nd ed. Cambridge, Massachusetts: MIT Press, 1968.
3. Schwartz R: Early rehabilitation in trauma centers: Have speech–language pathology services progressed? *ASHA* 1989; August, 91–94.
4. Albert PC, Albert ML: History and scope of the geriatric neurology. In Albert ML (ed): *Clinical Neurology of Aging.* New York: Oxford University Press, 1984, pp 3–8.

Aphasia and
Related Neurogenic
Language Disorders

Broca's Aphasia

Kevin P. Kearns

Introduction

Although a variety of language disorders had been recognized prior to the mid-nineteenth century,[1] the study of aphasia can be directly traced to the work of a 37-year-old surgeon and anthropologist Paul Pierre Broca.[2,3] Ironically, the first patient described by Broca did not appear to have the syndrome that bears his name.[4,5] Broca was primarily interested in localizing the faculty of articulate speech (i.e., motor aspects of speech production) and not the "general faculty of language."[6]

The core features of Broca's aphasia include a nonfluent, halting verbal output that is characterized by a reduced phrase length, a prosodic disturbance, and awkward articulation. The verbal output problems of Broca's patients often reflect a concomitant apraxia of speech, and agrammatism is also a frequent, although not invariant feature. When agrammatism is present, patients often omit function words (i.e., articles, conjunctions, pronouns, auxiliary verbs, and prepositions) and grammatical morphemes from their speech while retaining a relatively greater proportion of content words (i.e., nouns, verbs, and adverbs). Auditory comprehension ability, although impaired, is relatively spared and often is functional for everyday conversation. Repetition of spoken words and phrases and confrontation naming ability are also impaired in this syndrome. Writing is also impaired in Broca's aphasia, and written errors may resemble verbal production errors qualitatively. Similarly, reading comprehension is deficient to a degree that generally parallels auditory comprehension.[7-10]

It is both interesting and informative to trace Broca's seminal role in the history of aphasia. At the time of Broca's rise to prominence, phrenologists such as Gall and Bouillaud claimed that specific character traits and mental functions, such as speech ability, emotional feelings, and spirituality, resided in specialized areas of the brain. The phrenologists believed that there was a direct relationship between the size of a given area of the brain responsible for a mental function and an individual's ability, skill, or development in that area. Furthermore, they claimed that they could predict an individual's ability or character traits by examination of various portions of the skull. That is, they believed that there was a direct relationship between the size of a particular portion of the skull and the underlying cerebral organs that controlled specific psychological and behavioral functions. This position was highly controversial at the time, and it was vehemently opposed by proponents of a more holistic view of brain function. It was, however, Bouillaud's notion that the brain's center for the "faculty of speech" could be localized in the frontal lobes that set the stage for Broca's historic discoveries.

There was an ongoing debate about localization of cerebral functions during the meetings of the French Anthropology Society in 1861.[6] Unfortunately, the debate consisted mostly of logical arguments and rigid opinions rather than data-based presentations. While immersed in this professional atmosphere, Broca had the opportunity to examine a patient who presented with loss of speech and other clinical signs of frontal lobe damage. He viewed this patient as a possible test case of the theory of localization of the faculty of speech to the frontal lobes. The patient, Leborgne, had been an epileptic throughout his life, but he had functioned quite well prior to being hospitalized after he had lost the use of his speech. He had been in the hospital for more then twenty years prior to his referral to Broca. Head[6] notes that Broca could not determine whether the patient's speechlessness had occurred suddenly or gradually. However, the patient appeared to have normal hearing and could understand almost all that was said to him. He could not speak or write. Fortunately for science, but unfortunately for Leborgne, he died several days after Broca's clinical examination.

Broca was reportedly a superb anatomist with the foresight to perform an autopsy on his patient, and he presented his observations to the Anthropology Society the day after his postmortem examination. Broca concluded that his case supported the claim that the frontal lobes were indeed responsible for the "faculty of articulate language." Despite the fact that Broca provided the first objective findings to support the localizationist position, the response to his conclusions were underwhelming. As Head[6] reports, "It is customary to speak of Broca's discovery as if it came like a clap of thunder from a clear sky; this was by no means the case" (p. 17).

In August 1861, Broca subsequently presented a precise anatomical description of his autopsy findings on Leborgne to the French Anatomical Society and he labeled the loss of the "special faculty for articulated language" as "aphemia." (The term "aphasia," coined by Trousseau in 1864, was adopted in place of "aphemia" despite Broca's objections.) Later that year Broca had the good fortune to examine a second patient who, years earlier, had collapsed and "lost the power of speech." Similar to Leborgne, this patient appeared to be intelligent and could understand most or all of what was said to him. His verbal output was restricted to a limited vocabulary of poorly articulated words.

This second patient also died while under Broca's care and was subsequently autopsied. Despite rather extensive and diffuse damage, Broca relied on neuroanatomical concepts of the day to conclude that "the aphemia was the result of a profound, but accurately circumscribed lesion of the posterior third of second and third frontal convolutions"[6] (p. 25). Thus, post-mortem examination of his two patients led to Broca's now famous conclusion that the faculty for articulate speech could be localized to the third frontal convolution. The posterior-inferior frontal gyrus of the left cerebral hemisphere continues to be referred to as "Broca's area."

Broca's contributions to aphasiology were not confined to the discovery that speech production capabilities were localizable to the posterior portion of the frontal lobes. Broca's neurological postulations were also remarkable in that he rejected the phrenologists approach to cerebral localization which relied on absolute measurements from landmarks of the skull and brain. Instead, he postulated that convolutions are relatively constant and are, therefore, a more appropriate site for localization of psychological functions.[6,11,12] In addition, following analysis of eight consecutive cases of aphasia, Broca[13] observed that the left cerebral hemisphere appeared to be specialized for subserving expressive language functions. (Although Dax discussed hemispheric specialization 30 years prior to Broca, his observations were unpublished and relatively unknown; see refs. 6, 14.)

Broca[13] is also credited with linking left hemisphere dominance for language with handedness, in commenting on embryological differences between the hemispheres, and for noting that the right hemisphere has receptive language capabilities. From a clinical perspective, it is remarkable that Broca also observed that the right hemisphere could subsume left hemisphere functions and that language rehabilitation could benefit aphasic patients.[11,12] As Caplan[11] notes "(Broca) concluded that the failure of most patients with aphasia to recover was due to inadequate rehabilitative efforts: he thought that adequate rehabilitation would have to consist of as much exposure to language as a child learning his first language . . ." (p. 47).

It seems impossible to overestimate Paul Pierre Broca's influence on aphasiology. He provided the first principled account of localization of speech and language abilities and his observations provided the impetus for subsequent debate and investigation. He also laid the cornerstone for the classical taxonomy of the aphasias that guided principled investigations of aphasia for more than a century later.[15,16,41] As Benton[17] observed, Broca was largely responsible for elevating the study of aphasia from a minor curiosity to its current position as a disorder with diagnostic implications for identifying focal brain damage and cerebral localization.

Pathophysiology

Extensive reviews of the early aphasia literature document the proliferation of interest in localization and aphasia following Broca's discoveries.[18] Although there was a shift away from the localizationist position during the early part of this century, the issue of whether language functions could be localized to specific regions of the brain remained an area of intense interest.[19,20] Unfortunately, despite the shifting tides of popular opinion, early clinical–anatomical correlations of the localizationists and holists alike provided limited insight and resolution into the controversy surrounding the localization of language abilities because the interval between ictus and examination was often not documented in early autopsy studies, and there was a lack of specificity with regard to the nature of the aphasic deficits.[10,21] Despite renewed interest in aphasia and localization following World War II, significant advances in our views regarding the localization of language abilities in specific cortical areas, such as Broca's area, remained somewhat stagnant until modern advances in brain imaging techniques permitted in-vivo studies of cerebral changes following brain injury. The following overview of recent computerized tomography (CT) and positron emission tomography (PET) studies outlines representative trends in this area.

Computerized Axial Tomography (CT) Studies

The advent of computerized axial tomography (CT) has led to new insights into brain-behavior relationships in aphasia and it has led to a refinement of our view of the role of Broca's area in language processing and aphasia (see refs. 4, 10, 11, 22). Naeser and Hayward,[23] for example, examined the relationship between CT findings and language profiles in nineteen stable aphasic subjects who had suffered a single left hemisphere stroke. The subjects of this study were classified by aphasia type on the Boston Diagnostic Aphasia Examination.[9] After reviewing their subjects' CT scans, the authors concluded that their results supported the classical schema for localization of Wernicke's, Broca's, conduction, and global aphasia. The three Broca's subjects examined in this study had extensive lesions involving prerolandic and inferior frontal regions including Broca's area (cortical and deep) but sparing more posterior language zones including Wernicke's area.

Although subsequent research has replicated the finding that there is a significant correlation between lesion localization and type of aphasia,[24,25] the seminal work of Mohr and his colleagues has modified our view of the role of Broca's area in language production and aphasia.[21] Mohr et al[22] published an extensive review of the literature in conjunction with the results of physical examinations, and autopsy and neuroradiodiagnostic findings from twenty subjects exhibiting Broca's area infarction. CT data were presented for fourteen of the cases, and angiograms were available for the remaining subjects. Standardized and nonstandard behavioral–language test results were also examined in this report. The results of these analyses demonstrated that subjects with small lesions confined to Broca's area exhibited a transient mutism that evolved into a mild apraxia of speech. Lasting language impairments were not found in this group of subjects. By contrast, subjects with larger lesions ". . . encompassing much of the frontal operculum, insula, and subjacent white matter in the territory of the upper division of the middle cerebral artery . . ." (p. 322) exhibited a global aphasia that evolved into persistent Broca's aphasia. Mohr et al concluded that, "Personal observation, hospital autopsy data, and autopsied cases in the literature all suggest that infarction of the Broca area or its environs does not cause what is traditionally and currently believed to be Broca aphasia. (Rather) the principal deficit in this syndrome is best described as dyspraxia of speaking aloud" (p. 321).

Ludlow, Rosenberg, Fair, et al[26] reported speech-language test results and CT findings for patients who had suffered penetrating head wounds 15 years earlier. Although all demonstrated nonfluent aphasia within 6 months of their injuries, 13 had persistent nonfluent aphasia, and the remaining 26 did not have residual signs of aphasia at the time of follow-up testing. Of interest here is the fact that Broca's area was equally involved in both the recovered and the nonrecovered patients. These results agree with the findings of Mohr and his colleagues that some individuals exhibiting lesions in Broca's area may have a near-total language recovery.

Naeser et al[5] examined the relationship between extent of lesion within specific neuroanatomical areas on CT scans and persistent limitations in spontaneous production for 27 aphasic subjects. In general, they found that severe, persistent deficits in spontaneous production were associated with a lesion affecting both the medial subcallosal fasciculus and periventricular white matter deep to the motor/sensory cortex for the mouth (i.e., the lateral angle of the frontal horn). Although the combined lesion extent in these two areas was less for subjects with Broca's aphasia than it was for those with minimal speech output or verbal stereotypes, the Broca's subjects consistently exhibited a deep subcortical white matter lesion. That is, the subjects with Broca's aphasia exhibited lesions that were not confined to Broca's area. These observations confirm speculations by early aphasiologists[18] that Broca's aphasic subjects typically have deep subcortical lesions in addition to their well-known frontal lobe involvement.

In general, Naeser et al's findings support and extend Mohr et al's[21] conclusion that an extensive lesion is typically found in subjects with Broca's aphasia. However, Naeser et al describe one subject from a previously published study[27] who "recovered to scores of seven on the BDAE in phrase length, grammatical form, articulation and melodic line . . . despite large lesions in Broca's area, surface and deep, and large lesion in the lower motor cortex area for the mouth area surface and deep" (p. 19). Thus, while large lesions in Broca's cortical area are typically found in subjects with persistent Broca's aphasia, some patients with extensive Broca's area lesion but who have sparing of other specific neuroanatomical areas recover speech fluency to a remarkable degree. Naeser et al suggest that the combined extent of lesion in the subcallosal fasciculus and its periventricular white matter and the middle one-third of periventricular white matter may play a critical role in the recovery of spontaneous speech.

While the results of CT studies demonstrate a significant correlation between lesion sites and aphasia classification, we now know that there are many exceptions to predictions based on classical localization of the aphasias. For example, several cases of Broca's aphasia without Broca's area infarction have been reported.[5,26,28–30] Moreover, individuals having lesion in Broca's area have exhibited transcortical motor aphasia rather than Broca's aphasia as traditionally expected.[23] Freedman, Alexander and Naeser[31] hypothesize that individual differences in cerebral localization may, in part, account for the unusual localization findings in these cases. They state that ". . . the cytoarchitectonic field of Broca's aphasia (may be) displaced onto the orbital aspect of the frontal operculum. Such displacement would permit entire or partial sparing of (Broca's) area" (p. 416). Recent localization studies using positron emission tomography (PET) provide additional data that bear on this issue. A review of this information is provided in the following section.

Positron Emission Tomography (PET) Studies

The traditional means of determining the pathophysiology of language disturbances in aphasia has been to correlate the results of autopsy or CT localization data with clusters of language deficits that create identifiable syndromes. Recent technical advances have permitted examination of the metabolic status of patients with brain lesions and have made significant contributions to our understanding of the pathoanatomy of the aphasias. PET scans, for example, have been used to measure the rate of glucose metabolism in the brain, thereby providing a better understanding of how structural lesions affect cerebral metabolism. PET studies have demonstrated that areas of depressed metabolic activity extend well beyond the areas of damaged cerebral tissue.[32] Areas of reduced metabolic functioning that are not structurally damaged are, in effect, functional lesions that may affect language and other abilities in brain-damaged individuals. Hanson, Metter, Riege, et al[33] demonstrated that many aphasic subjects with left hemisphere cortical lesions exhibit hypometabolism in the right cortical and subcortical regions as well. These data have led to the suggestion that both structural and functional (i.e., metabolic) lesions must be considered in any comprehensive account of the pathophysiology of the aphasias.

Metter, Kempler, Hanson, et al[34] compared structural (CT) and metabolic (PET) disturbances in Broca's, Wernicke's and conduction aphasia. Aphasia classifications were based on performance on the Western Aphasia Battery (WAB),[10] and neuroimaging data were obtained at least 1 month post onset. The PET data analyses revealed a striking similarity in regional hypometabolism in the temporal and parietal areas of all groups of aphasic subjects. In addition, the 8 Broca's subjects in this study demonstrated a left/right metabolic asymmetry in prefrontal, Broca's, and parietal areas that was more severe than the metabolic asymmetry apparent for Wernicke's and conduction patients. One can conclude from these data that the language deficits of Broca's aphasic subjects cannot be accounted for by a lesion in Broca's area or, for that matter, by structural lesions alone.[36] This conclusion was supported by data from a follow-up of 11 Broca's subjects by Metter, Kempler, Jackson, et al.[35] They reported that "(the Broca's subjects) lesions seen on computerized tomography demonstrated consistent damage to the anterior internal capsule and the lenticular nuclei with variable cortical changes, whereas glucose metabolism was found to be decreased throughout the hemisphere" (p. 134). These findings provide further evidence that changes in the brain's metabolic activity in regions outside of Broca's area also may contribute to the pattern of language impairments for at least some subjects with Broca's aphasia.

Summary

The results of studies using modern neuroradiographic techniques have led to a reexamination of the commonly held notion that Broca's aphasia results from a lesion to Broca's area. Circumscribed lesions to the posterior portion of the third frontal convolution of the dominant hemisphere generally result in minimal residual aphasia.[21] Furthermore, some individuals with Broca's aphasia have lesions that do not impinge on the third frontal convolution.[26,28,30] To complicate matters even further, there are documented cases of subjects with Broca's area lesions who have transcortical motor aphasia rather than Broca's aphasia.[23,31] Taken together, these data support the conclusion that a lesion to Broca's area is neither necessary nor sufficient to produce Broca's aphasia.

The cumulative results of recent localization studies of Broca's aphasia reinforce Kertesz'[10] caution that, "only lesions causing impairment are localizable, not the impairment itself" (p 142). Classical pathoanatomic descriptions of the aphasias, including Broca's aphasia, are gradually yielding to more sophisticated models of brain and language relationships. While far from complete, these models have attempted to account for recent findings regarding the influence of distant, especially subcortical, regions on language ability and patterns of aphasic impairments.[5,37,38]

Nature and Differentiating Features

Although the classical taxonomies of aphasia are less than adequate in terms of current models of language processing,[11,39] the technical tools and overall conceptual structure of linguistic theory are also evolving.[40] As a result, a cogent theory of normal or pathologic language that accounts for the rich variety of aphasic impairments does not exist currently, and it is unlikely that a universally agreed-upon alternative to the classical taxonomies of aphasia will be forthcoming in the near future. Moreover, the classical classification system continues to provide a valuable heuristic approach for clinicians faced with the day-to-day care of aphasic persons. As Benson[7] reminds us, aphasia syndromes such as Broca's aphasia, provide valuable localizing information, particularly when combined with other relevant history and diagnostic information. The classical descriptions of aphasic syndromes have also enhanced cross-disciplinary dialogue by providing a common vocabulary for communication and interaction, thereby encouraging multidisciplinary research and patient care efforts. Finally, the recent re-emergence of the classical taxonomies[18,41] has coincided with an increased effort by clinical researchers to develop and investigate increasingly specific language treatment approaches for subtypes of aphasic individuals (see Treatment section). It appears, therefore, that the classical taxonomies will continue to serve an important role in the clinical arena. In the remainder of this section, we will examine the nature and underlying features of Broca's aphasia, perhaps the most widely studied of all aphasia subtypes.

Nature

For ease of discussion, hypotheses relating to the nature of Broca's aphasia are described below as nonlinguistic and linguistic explanations. This dichotomy is, of course, somewhat arbitrary since nonlinguistic explanations of agrammatism are not totally void of linguistic or psycholinguistic descriptions or explanations, and varying degrees of linguistic rationale are included in most of the following nonlinguistic explanations. The nonlinguistic theories discussed herein are not, however, based on models of linguistic processing per se; their emphasis is on the nonlanguage factors that contribute to the pattern of deficits in Broca's aphasia. Only representative examples of the range of linguistic and nonlinguistic explanations of Broca's aphasia are presented below. However, comprehensive reviews of the nature of agrammatism and Broca's aphasia are available elsewhere.[11,42-45]

Nonlinguistic Hypotheses

Explanations of the nature of Broca's aphasia have stressed the importance of nonlinguistic factors, such as the disconnection of cortical areas, memory capacity, the effect of stimulus variables on verbal output, and compensatory strategies on patients' language production. For example, in his treatise "Disconnection syndromes in animals and man," Geschwind[41] examined the aphasias from the perspective of the disconnection of cortical language zones from one another. Geschwind's disconnection account of the aphasias was described most clearly for conduction aphasia, which was hypothesized to result from an interruption of deep intrahemispheric fibers, the arcuate fasciculus that connect Broca's area with Wernicke's area. A lesion to this fiber bundle would spare Broca's and Wernicke's areas and thereby leave auditory comprehension or speech fluency essentially intact. However, a lesion between Wernicke's and Broca's areas would interrupt the transfer of information between these centers and cause the verbal repetition problems that characterize conduction aphasia (see Simmons, Chapter 3 of this volume). Similar to the mid-nineteenth century localizationists,[15,16] Geschwind emphasized the localization of language processes in specific areas of the brain. He argued, for example, that specific sensory and linguistic functions that underlie naming ability are localized in the inferior parietal lobe. Geschwind[41] also provided a detailed description of important neuroanatomical pathways involved in aphasia and related disorders.

To date, a data base supporting a comprehensive disconnection model of the aphasias has not been firmly established; many authors have been content to correlate general aphasic symptoms with cortical language areas.[46] Geschwind's seminal work did, however, revitalize interest in a localizationist approach to aphasia classification, and this approach has resulted in proliferation of both clinical and research effort.[9,10,47]

In attempting to understand the nature of Broca's aphasia, aphasiologists often have scrutinized syntactic aspects of aphasic language impairments, particularly the components of agrammatism. As noted earlier, agrammatism is a frequent sequela of Broca's aphasia and is characterized by the omission from speech of low information lexical items and grammatical morphemes. The verbal output of agrammatic Broca's individuals may sound "telegraphic" because the paucity of articles, conjunctions, auxiliary verbs, and word endings results in seemingly, isolated production of short strings of nouns and verbs. Agrammatism, which is primarily viewed as a syntactic impairment, has been studied extensively as a vehicle for understanding Broca's aphasia. Many aphasiologists feel that a better understanding of the syntactic deficits in agrammatism will lead to greater appreciation of the underlying nature of Broca's aphasia.

Pick[48] provided one of the earliest nonlinguistic explanations of agrammatism when he postulated that the deletion of low-information lexical items from agrammatic speech resulted from patients' attempts to conserve effort during speech production (see ref. 49). This proposition has intuitive appeal because the nonfluent speech output of Broca's subjects is halting, hesitant, and apraxic, and an economy of effort explanation suggests that agrammatism is a compensatory strategy to circumvent these expressive problems. Several contemporary aphasiologists also have adopted explanations of the grammatical deficits of Broca's aphasia that attribute agrammatism to learned compensatory strategies. Heeschen,[50] for example, proposes an avoidance hypothesis that purports that Broca's subjects learn to speak agrammatically by monitoring their aphasic utterances and then adapting to the language problem by producing only constructions that present relatively little difficulty for them. Heeschen's position is similar to the "economy of effort" theory. He writes that, "Agrammatism is something that must be learned by the patient. . . . The advantage to the patient is obvious; his speech gains a certain systematicity for the listener and the patient spares himself enormous efforts by simply omitting all these "terrible small words," the production of which is really vexing for the patient" (p 241). The avoidance hypothesis is based, in part, on evidence that shows that agrammatic speakers who are experimentally deprived of the opportunity to avoid difficult words and syntactic constructions show marked reductions in the number of omissions of grammatical items.

Kolk, van Grunsven and Keyser[51] propose an "adaption" theory of agrammatism as a "new theory of Broca's aphasia." Three specific claims about agrammatism serve as the basis for this theory. First, the omissions of functors (articles, conjunctions, auxiliaries, etc.) and grammatical morphemes (word endings such as --ing) by agrammatic speakers is the result of an unimpaired system that is unaffected by the brain damage. In other words, the adaption theory claims that speakers with Broca's aphasia adapt to their condition by utilizing residual, unimpaired processes to adopt a "telegraphic register." Second, the adaption hypothesis assumes that agrammatism is the result of a delay in the processes that underlie sentence production as opposed to being caused by the loss of syntactic knowledge or ability. Delayed processes that underlie agrammatism may include a slowing down of the application of syntactic rules, or there may be a general slowing of lexical retrieval. The adaption theory contends that, by opting to speak agrammatically, aphasic speakers minimize the effect of delayed processing. The third assumption of this hypothesis is that individuals decide to adapt or speak agrammatically. Kolk et al[51] contend that agrammatic speakers may not be fully conscious of their decision to speak agrammatically.

Kolk et al[51] support their adaption hypothesis with a detailed case study of an expressively agrammatic subject who demonstrated minimal impairment on currently accepted tests of receptive agrammatism. One of the most popular linguistic theories of agrammatism, the central linguistic hypothesis, rests on the assumption that expressive agrammatism should be accompanied by a parallel receptive deficit (see linguistic explanations), but this was not found by Kolk and his colleagues.

Kolk et al's[51] adaption theory of agrammatism, and Broca's aphasia is similar to the avoidance theory espoused by Heeschen.[50] For example, both theories propose that agrammatism results from the patient's reaction to impairment rather than being a manifestation of impairment per se. In addition, the adaption and avoidance theories are also clearly similar to the economy of effort view of agrammatism.[48,49]

Goodglass and his colleagues argue against economy of effort explanations for agrammatism noting that the speech of Broca's subjects rarely improves to any significant degree with prompting, and even repeated attempts at self-correction are largely unsuccessful.[52,53] Goodglass[43] describes his alternative explanation of agrammatism, the stress-salience hypothesis, as follows, ". . . a basic feature of Broca's aphasia is the increased threshold for mobilizing the speech output system, . . . and the response threshold . . . requires an emphatic or salient element in the message to overcome the elevated threshold and begin the flow of informational load, affective tone, and increased amplitude and intonational stress" (p 253). The stress-salience hypothesis has been formulated on the basis of numerous research studies with Broca's aphasic subjects; this information has been reviewed extensively elsewhere (see refs. 43, 46).

Thus far we have sampled several nonlinguistic explanations of the nature of agrammatism and Broca's aphasia. It is clear that no single account can satisfactorily explain the variety and complexity of behaviors that occur in Broca's aphasia. In the following section we will examine representative linguistic theories that attempt to account for the same phenomenon.

Linguistic Hypotheses

Jakobson[54] provided the earliest linguistic description of aphasic disorders. He used the term "paradigmatic" to refer to the selection of verbal symbols, and he used the term "syntagmatic" to refer to the process of sequentially combining linguistic elements to express grammatical relationships. In applying this linguistic dichotomy to aphasia, Jakobson labeled word retrieval problems as "similarity" disorders because the paradigmatic aspect of language was seen as involving selection of words from a number of lexical choices having similar meanings. Conversely, aphasic disturbances involving impairments of sequencing (i.e., syntagmatic aspects of language) were labeled contiguity disorders because they involved disruption of a contiguous string of elements. Thus agrammatism, in which there is a deficit in the sequential combining of words into grammatical sentences, was viewed as a contiguity disorder. Jakobson's definition of a contiguity disorder was actually quite inclusive. It subsumed all disturbances involving inappropriate combinations of linguistic elements, from the phoneme level to the sentence level.[45] Jakobson's typology did however, provide one of the first principled linguistic accounts of aphasia and agrammatism (see ref. 45).

Following Jakobson's[54] writing numerous other authors applied linguistic explanations of aphasic impairments, particularly following the formulation Chomsky's[55] generative transformational grammar (see refs. 11, 45). Since that time, formal linguistic theory has played an increasing important role in aphasia research, and studies of aphasic individuals have been used with increasing frequency to examine theoretical linguistic constructs.[41,56,57] Broca's aphasia in which detailed studies of aphasic subjects have been used to formulate and explore linguistic and psycholinguistic explanations of syntactic deficits. Of particular relevance to the current discussion, researchers have extensively examined the hypothesis that agrammatism in Broca's aphasia is the result of a syntactically based, central linguistic deficit (see refs. 42, 58–61).

Although several versions of the central syntactic deficit theory exist, the primary assumption underlying each is that agrammatism is a manifestation of a ". . . central disruption of the syntactic parsing component of the language system . . ."[59] (p 225). If the syntactic impairments of Broca's individuals results from a single central deficit, then one would predict that parallel deficits would be found across language modalities. This position has been supported by research that documented a receptive component to agrammatism that parallels the expressive problems of these subjects. Thus, expressively agrammatic speakers who delete functors and grammatical markers from their speech have exhibited difficulty comprehending semantically reversible sentences that require dependence on grammatical morphology for correct interpretation.[62] Further support for the central syntactic hypothesis has been obtained from studies that demonstrate that some Broca's subjects have marked difficulties on metalinguistic tasks that require them to process syntactic relationships.[63,64]

The central syntactic deficit hypothesis has been challenged recently by data from numerous sources. For example, recent reports of patients who are expressively but not receptively agrammatic provide counter evidence to the parallelism assumption.[51,65] That is, a dissociation of impairments across modalities is problematic for theories ascribing agrammatism to a central deficit that presumably causes similar impairments in expressive and receptive modalities. Further evidence against the central syntactic deficit position comes from studies requiring Broca's subjects to make judgements of the grammaticality or well-formedness of sentences. In particular, recent studies have demonstrated that some Broca's patients retain the ability to identify syntactic and morphological violations despite the fact that they are receptively agrammatic.[66-69] It is difficult for the various forms of the central syntactic deficit hypothesis to accommodate findings of retained syntactic competence in individuals who are both expressively and receptively agrammatic (see ref. 61). Equally damaging are recent findings that demonstrate that Broca's subjects retain some sensitivity to grammatical aspects of sentences on auditory comprehension tests when task structure and demands are controlled.[70,71]

A final source of data that is incompatible with the central syntactic deficit hypothesis comes from studies that have failed to find qualitative differences in the linguistic performance of nonfluent Broca's subjects and fluent aphasic speakers. The central deficit theory carries with it the claim that levels of linguistic processing can be impaired selectively across the various types of aphasic subjects. Thus, whereas the language problems of Broca's subjects are purported to result from a central syntactic deficit, Wernicke's individuals may be viewed as manifesting a central deficit in semantic knowledge with relative preservation of syntactic abilities.[72] This claim would be considerably weakened by data that shows, for example, that despite presumed differences in the nature of their language impairments, Broca's and Wernicke's subjects perform similarly on syntactic and semantic language tasks. Although there is not total agreement, a body of data demonstrates that nonfluent Broca's and fluent aphasic subjects are not necessarily distinguishable on tests of comprehension or on analyses of speech output. For example, some comparisons of Broca's and Wernicke's subjects on tests of auditory comprehension for sentences have shown similar rather than qualitatively different patterns of impairment.[73,74] Relatedly, a recent comparison of Broca's and anomic patients on a test of auditory comprehension revealed that both groups are impaired in their ability to identify grammatical relations.[11]

If deficits in Broca's aphasia can be attributed to an impaired syntactic parser and those in Wernicke's aphasia to a disruption of semantic processes, then the verbal output of these groups should also be qualitatively different. Clinical and research observations of English speaking aphasic subjects generally demonstrate expected differences between these groups. That is, fluent Wernicke's subjects tend to make syntactic errors of substitution while non-fluent Broca's speakers frequently omit functors and grammatical morphemes. However, cross-linguistic comparisons of the verbal output of these aphasia types have found more similarities than differences (see refs. 56, 58). Bates et al[75], for example, compared English speaking aphasic subjects with aphasic subjects from two highly inflected languages, Italian and German. They found negligible differences between Wernicke's and Broca's speakers in terms of the number of article substitution errors produced by German and Italian aphasic subjects. These results are problematic for central deficit hypotheses that propose selective impairment at different levels of language (i.e., syntactic vs. semantic) for Broca's and Wernicke's subjects.

Although the central syntactic deficit theory appears to have been too extreme a position, the theory has stimulated a tremendous of amount of linguistically based research into the nature of Broca's aphasia.[58,76,77] Alternative linguistic explanations of the nature of agrammatism and Broca's aphasia have examined phonological factors,[78] retrieval difficulties for so-called closed class (e.g., functors) morphology,[79,80] difficulty mapping semantic roles onto sentence constituents,[61,68,81] and violations of phrase structure rules.[40,82] Like the central syntactic deficit hypothesis, however, none of these theories of agrammatism alone appears to explain sufficiently the nature of syntactic deficits in Broca's aphasia. As Rizzi[40] notes, syntactic theory is evolving rapidly, and a definitive theoretical linguistic account of agrammatism is neither available nor does it appear to be forthcoming. However, research in this area has contributed greatly to our understanding of the nature of Broca's aphasia from a linguistic perspective, and our understanding will continue to grow as new theoretical postulates are proposed and tested experimentally.

Summary of Nonlinguistic and Linguistic Hypotheses

Aphasiologists have examined a wide range linguistic and nonlinguistic hypotheses regarding the nature of agrammatism in Broca's aphasia. Nonlinguistic models of agrammatism have considered neuroanatomical explanations, the role of learned compensatory strategies, and the influence of stress and salience on verbal performance. Linguistic explanations of agrammatism also have proliferated since Jakobson's[54] seminal work in neurolinguistics. In particular, considerable research effort has been expended on testing various forms of the central syntactic deficit theory of agrammatism. Although this theory has not proven to be totally satisfactory, numerous alternative psycholinguistic explanations of syntactic deficits in Broca's aphasia have evolved from research in this area.

At the present time no single theory can fully account for the variety of research findings and clinical observations regarding agrammatism and Broca's aphasia. The current status of research in this area is aptly summarized by Goodglass and Menn[83] who state, "One thing is certain: No single explanation of agrammatism, whether based on syntax, phonology, or economy of speaking effort, can yield the observed intricate patterns of within-modality and cross-modality dissociation. Parsimony as a metatheoretical principle in neurolinguistics is dead . . ." (p. 19).

Although specific evaluation and treatment issues are addressed in subsequent sections of this chapter, it should be noted that clinicians can obtain valuable clinical information from research in this area despite the lack of theoretical parsimony. They can, for example, evaluate the effects of stress and salience on speech production and/or assess compensatory strategies exhibited by their individuals with Broca's aphasia[53,84] and incorporate the obtained information into treatment planning. We begin our discussion of related clinical issues by considering the distinguishing characteristics of Broca's aphasia.

Differentiating Features

As noted earlier, the hallmark of Broca's aphasia is nonfluent, effortful, and slow speech output with reduced phrase length and awkward articulation. When agrammatism is present, verbal output may include an overabundance of content words, especially nouns and verbs, and relatively few functors and grammatical word endings. Despite a tendency toward "telegraphic" speech, the verbal output of Broca's subjects usually contains sufficient informational content to communicate reasonably well. Repetition and confrontation naming are often moderately to severely impaired. In comparison with verbal skills, auditory comprehension ability is relatively preserved and often functional for everyday conversation. Reading and writing ability often parallel auditory comprehension and verbal output respectively.[7-10]

Broca's aphasia can be differentiated from other types of aphasia by examining the relative performance on spontaneous verbal output (i.e., speech fluency), auditory comprehension, confrontation naming, and repetition tasks. It should be apparent that a comparison across language modalities results in rather broad and inclusive aphasia categories. Broca's subjects, for example, vary considerably in terms of their verbal abilities, depending on the presence and/or severity of agrammatism. Some of those classified as having Broca's aphasia may be restricted to one- or two-word responses while others may display a relatively mild interruption of speech fluency. In addition to the degree of individual variability within each type of aphasia, many individuals seen clinically do not fit unequivocally into one of the classical types of aphasia[9] since many have large lesions that result in mixed behaviors. Finally, the fact that there are no invariant features common to all individuals within a given aphasia subtype further complicates attempts to classify. These cautionary remarks should be kept in mind during the following discussion of features that differentiate Broca's from other types of aphasic subgroups.

A comparison of relative aphasic performance on speech fluency, auditory comprehension, repetition, and confrontation naming results in the classification in Table 1–1.[2,9,10,45,85]

Examination of Table 1 reveals the basic dichotomy between fluent and nonfluent

Table 1-1.   Basic Classification of Aphasic Syndromes

	Fluency	Auditory	Repetition Comprehension	Naming
Nonfluent				
Broca's	−	+	=	=
Global	−	−	−	−
Transcortical Motor	−	+	+	=
Fluent				
Wernicke's	+	−	−	=
Transcortical Sensory	+	−	+	=
Conduction	+	+	−	=
Anomic	+	+	+	=

(+): relatively unimpaired; (−): impaired; (=): variable impairment across patients.

aphasias. Speech fluency is one of the most reliable features for differentiating the aphasias,[86] and it has become an important clinical criterion for classification.[9,10] Nonfluent aphasic speech is characterized by decreased speech rate, increased effort, reduced phrase length, and dysprosody. In addition, nonfluent aphasic speakers have difficulty initiating speech production, and their overall quantity of speech tends to be reduced. As shown in the table, Broca's, global, and transcortical motor aphasia are classified as nonfluent aphasias.

In contrast to nonfluent aphasic speech, the speech rate of fluent aphasic speakers is essentially normal or even somewhat increased. Speech is effortless, melodic, and flowing. These speakers substitute inappropriate words (verbal paraphasias), nonwords (jargon), and phonemes (literal paraphasias), yet, they do so smoothly and effortlessly without interruption of the flow or melody of speech. Thus, despite near normal prosody and speech rate, there is often a considerable decrease in the amount of information conveyed. Hesitations and pauses occur but they often precede and follow uninterrupted strings of fluent, sometimes meaningless speech. The fluent aphasias include Wernicke's, transcortical sensory, conduction, and anomic aphasia (Table 1).

The nonfluent speech of individuals with Broca's aphasia can be contrasted with the fluent speech of Wernicke's aphasia to demonstrate qualitative differences between fluent and nonfluent types of aphasia. In response to the request, "Tell me what you do with a cigarette," a person with chronic Broca's aphasia replied, "Uh . . . uh . . . cigarette (pause) smoke it." Obviously this response was halting and agrammatic, but it clearly conveyed an accurate response to the request. In response to the same request, a person with chronic Wernicke's aphasia replied, "This is a segment of a pegment. Soap a cigarette." This response is strikingly different from that of the speaker with Broca's aphasia in several respects. First, despite a lack of informational content, there appears to a basic syntactic integrity to the response. That is, basic word order constraints were not, apparently, violated, and the small connective words were also retained despite the fact that the response was replete with jargon. This is in marked contrast to the Broca's speaker who simply juxtaposed a correct noun, verb, and pronoun. Finally, despite a halting, disconnected style of speaking, the person with Broca's aphasia communicated successfully. On the other hand, the Wernicke example was melodic and uninterrupted, but it was essentially devoid of any meaning.

The nonfluent, agrammatic speaking style of the Broca's aphasia in the previous example can be readily differentiated from the so-called paragrammatic style of the Wernicke's aphasia. Of course, the contrast between the verbal output of Broca's and fluent speakers is not always as dramatic as the previous example. However, it is the overall pattern of impairments that determines classification rather than performance on a single variable, and standardized tests are available to assist with the sometimes challenging task of differential diagnosis.[9,10] Thus, in addition to the fluency distinction, the person with Broca's aphasia in the previous example had a mild auditory comprehension deficit on standardized testing, while the person with Wernicke's aphasia had severely impaired auditory comprehension ability. Individuals with Broca's aphasia frequently demonstrate a high level of awareness of their language problems and tend to demonstrate varying degrees of frustration when they make errors. This is in marked contrast to those with Wernicke's aphasia, who often show little frustration or awareness of error.

Within the category of nonfluent aphasias, those with Broca's aphasia can be readily differentiated from global and transcortical motor aphasia. As the comparison in Table 1 demonstrates, persons with global aphasia are severely impaired across all language modalities. Their verbal output is limited to a few nonfunctional, automatic phrases or stereotypic responses, and they have severely impaired auditory comprehension skills. By contrast, Broca's patients often communicate effectively through the use of one- and two-word responses, and their comprehension is adequate for following simple commands and understanding basic conversations.

The clinical profile of Broca's aphasia most closely resembles the clinical profile of transcortical motor aphasia (Table 1). Both Broca's and transcortical motor aphasic speakers exhibit an overall reduction in verbal output and may be agrammatic. In addition, individuals with transcortical motor aphasia have relatively good auditory comprehension skills. One important qualitative difference between these two syndromes is that those with transcortical motor aphasia demonstrate a paucity of spontaneous speech and marked initiation difficulties.[9,10] Although in Broca's aphasia spontaneous speech is effortful and halting, they spontaneously initiate communicative interactions. Another subtle difference between these nonfluent aphasias is that the transcortical speakers exhibit a greater degree of "stumbling, repetitive, even stuttering spontaneous output," in conjunction with motor prompts, such as foot stomping.[7] Echolalia also may be present in transcortical motor aphasia, but it is rarely evident in Broca's aphasia.

In addition to these rather subtle differences, one major factor, repetition ability, distinguishes these two syndromes. Whereas the ability to repeat aurally presented information is moderately to severely impaired in Broca's aphasia, repetition ability is relatively preserved in transcortical motor aphasia. A stroking preservation of repetition skills in combination with impoverished spontaneous speech and good auditory comprehension ability are characteristic of transcortical motor aphasia.

The preceding examples demonstrate the how fluency, auditory comprehension, repetition, and confrontation naming can be used to distinguish Broca's aphasia from the other classical types of aphasia. In the next section we explore associated signs and symptoms that co-occur with Broca's aphasia. Knowledge of these associated characteristics can contribute to the differential diagnosis of aphasia and related disorders.

Associated Signs and Symptoms

Aphasia-causing lesions are often rather large; therefore, it is not surprising that aphasia frequently co-occurs with other communication, motor, and sensory problems that result from brain damage. Since lesions that cause Broca's aphasia also interrupt adjacent cortical motor fibers and deep fiber tracts, it is predictable that individuals with Broca's aphasia frequently exhibit contralateral hemiparesis. Similarly, since Broca's area lesions may disrupt one's ability to plan and implement coordinated motor activity, apraxia of speech is a common and predictable concomitant impairment. Another common sequela of large Broca's area lesions is a mild dysarthria. Although severe dysarthria and dysphagia most often occur following bilateral involvement, persons with Broca's aphasia may have difficulty with intraoral transit of food, and the possibility of increased risk for aspiration should not be overlooked.

Prior to formal speech and language testing, the astute clinician will observe the client and note any associated motoric or behavioral conditions that will contribute to the differential diagnosis of the disorder. That is, the constellation of impairments associated with Broca's aphasia may lead the clinician to explore some diagnostic possibilities and eliminate others. Thus, a person with acute Broca's aphasia may be confined to a wheelchair as a result of right-sided hemiplegia (paralysis); his right arm may be in a protective sling; his right shoulder may droop; and he may show a flattening of the nasolabial folds and other signs of weakness of the muscles of the right side of the face. In time, people with Broca's aphasia frequently recover the ability to ambulate, often with the assistance of a leg brace, cane, or walker. The amount of recovery achieved for the right arm and hand is usually less than the amount of improvement apparent for the leg and foot. The amount of obvious facial weakness, drooling, and other signs of muscular involvement also tend to subside over time until there is only a mild residual involvement. In marked contrast to the pattern of involvement seen in Broca's aphasia, in fluent Wernicke's aphasia no obvious signs of physical impairment may exist, even early in the course of the illness.

As noted above, Broca's patients often have a mile dysarthria that can impair speech intelligibility. The dysarthric involvement tends not to be severely debilitating because speech muscular is bilaterally innervated and the aphasia-causing lesion only affects one side of the speech apparatus. However, the dysarthric component of speech may interest with apraxia of speech to a degree that is greater than a simple additive effect of the two impairments. That is, the cumulative effect of even mild dysarthria and apraxia of speech can significantly impair intelligibility and complicate clinical management.

Wertz, LaPointe, and Rosenbek[87] define apraxia of speech as "neurogenic phonologic disorder resulting from sensorimotor impairment to the capacity to select, program, and/or execute in coordinated and normally timed sequences, the positioning of speech musculature for the volitional production of speech sounds. . . . Prosodic alteration, that is, changes in speech stress, intonation, and/or rhythm, may be associated with the articulatory disruption either as a primary part of the condition or in compensation for it" (p 4). Unlike dysarthria, apraxia is not a result of muscular weakness, slowness, or incoordination and, although linguistic factors interact with apraxia, the disorder is most often viewed as being distinct from aphasic language impairments. Consequently, apraxia of speech requires an approach to clinical management that is quite distinct from language intervention strategies for aphasia.

Although exact figures are not available, it is clear that apraxia of speech frequently coexists with Broca's aphasia. Wertz, Rosenbek, and Deal,[88] reported that nearly two-thirds of a large sample of unclassified aphasic subjects presented with characteristics of apraxia of speech. The incidence of coexisting apraxia of speech and aphasia would be expected to be even higher in Broca's aphasia than that found in overall co-occurrence figures for clinical populations such as the one studied by Wertz and his colleagues.

The diagnosis and treatment of apraxia of speech is a complex area of study that has been thoroughly summarized elsewhere.[22,87,89] The following cursory description of the characteristics of apraxia of speech is presented as means of differentiating Broca's aphasia from other clinical populations. The effortful, dysprosodic, nonfluent speech of Broca's aphasia is frequently the result of the combined effects of language impairment and apraxia of speech. Apraxic speakers may exhibit extreme struggle to initiate and continue the flow of speech. The motoric timing difficulties experienced by these individuals affects prosody and articulatory ability as well. Speech prosody may sound "mechanical" as the apraxic speakers struggles in vain to execute and coordinate precisely timed neuromuscular sequences that are necessary for the production of normal articulation and prosody. The resultant dysprosody is characterized by a slowed speech rate, inappropriate stress patterns, pauses between syllables, a marked interruption of the inflectional contour and reduced loudness.[90-92] Apraxic speakers demonstrate a considerable degree of articulatory variability within and across speaking tasks. On the surface, their articulatory error appear to change from trial to trial, even during the same speaking task. Distinctive feature and phonological process analyses demonstrate, however, apraxic errors are usually related to target phonemes.[93] Relatedly, although phonemic (i.e., substitution) and phonetic (i.e., motoric timing) errors are produced by apraxic speakers, clinical analysis and apraxic speech reveals a preponderance of perceived articulatory substitutions. Apraxic speakers also characteristically make articulatory errors of omission.

A distinguishing characteristic of some apraxic individuals is a marked difference in performance across volitional versus nonvolitional speech tasks.[94] Apraxic speech and prosodic impairment are generally much more severe during volitional as compared with nonvolitional speaking conditions. For example, an apraxic person may perform automatic speech tasks, such as counting or reciting the days of the week, with minimum difficulty. Yet, the same person may hesitate, struggle, reapproach, and finally make several articulatory errors during the production of the same words during a repetition. It should be noted that not all apraxic speakers demonstrate clinically significant changes on volitional versus nonvolitional speech tasks.[87] Other parameters that can influence an apraxic individual's performance on speaking tasks include the length and phonetic complexity of stimulus items as well as linguistic factors, such as grammatical form class.

Whereas apraxic speakers appear to suffer from a disturbance in the sequential programming of motor movements. Those with Wernicke's aphasia erroneously select target phonemes.[95] As noted above, individuals with both Broca's aphasia and apraxia of speech and those with Wernicke's aphasia produce phonetic distortions and true phoneme substitutions. However, qualitative differences in the nature of these errors may distinguish these two groups. There is a tendency for the perceived substitution errors of apraxic speakers to approximate more closely the intended target sounds as compared to the paraphasic errors of Wernicke's and conduction aphasic individuals.[96] In addition, Broca's-apraxic speakers may appear to produce considerably more errors of articulatory distortions when compared with fluent

Wernicke or conduction speakers. This difference may be especially pronounced when the Broca's individual exhibits a coexisting dysarthria and apraxia of speech. Another subtle but clinically useful rule of thumb for distinguishing the speech of apraxic and fluent aphasic individuals is that many people with Broca's aphasia produce "transitionalization" errors that interrupt the flow of speech. These errors include, insertion of pauses within consonant clusters and insertion of neutral vowels between syllables, as well as sound and syllable prolongations.[91,92,96]

Persons with Broca's aphasia and apraxia generally have a much higher level of error awareness than that exhibited by persons with Wernicke's aphasia. As a result, apraxic speakers often reapproach and attempt to correct articulatory errors, while fluent paraphasic speakers often continue their speech flow without hesitation or interruption. Although there is not total agreement in the literature, some qualitative analyses of consecutive attempts to produce the same word have distinguished Broca's aphasia from Wernicke's and conduction aphasia. Joanette, Keller, and Lecours,[97] reported that although subjects with conduction aphasia more progressively approximated intended targets across repeated trials, subjects with Broca's aphasia did not. Those with Wernicke's aphasia reportedly produced somewhat random errors during successive attempts to produce a target word, and their successive attempts became increasingly dissimilar to intended target responses over time.

As is the case with all differential diagnostic endeavors, clinicians interested in distinguishing Broca's aphasia with apraxia of speech from other clinical populations should examine the overall pattern of involvement before affixing a diagnostic label. The presence of any single differentiating feature alone is insufficient for diagnosing apraxia of speech and distinguishing Broca's – apraxic individuals from other categories of aphasia. With this in mind, Wertz et al[87] have summarized the clinical characteristics of apraxia of speech as follows:

1. Effortful, trial and error, groping articulatory movements and attempts at self-correction.
2. Dysprosody unrelieved by extended perioss of normal rhythm, stress, and intonation.
3. Articulatory inconsistency on repeated attempts of the same utterance.
4. Obvious difficulty initiating utterances (p. 81).[87]

This cluster of behaviors provides a useful clinical guideline for diagnosing apraxia of speech in Broca's aphasia, and it should also prove useful for differentiating apraxia of speech from the speech characteristics of fluent aphasic individuals. More specific evaluation procedures for diagnosing Broca's aphasia and developing appropriate intervention strategies are considered below.

Evaluation

The clinical evaluation of aphasia is undertaken for aiding differential diagnosis, planning treatment, establishing a prognosis, monitoring change, and evaluating the maintenance of treatment gains. More often than not, evaluations serve these and other purposes simultaneously. Given the multifaceted nature of the evaluation process, it is not surprising that formal assessment measures are often supplemented with informal procedures including nonstandardized tests, behavioral observations, and clinical probes. The variety and complexity of assessment procedures underscores the need to view the evaluation process within the framework of a generalization planning approach to patient management.[98-100]

Traditional approaches to the clinical process often consider evaluation, treatment, and generalization, and maintenance as discrete, relatively independent and sequential phases of client management. This view is at variance with a generalization planning approach in which each phase of the clinical process is integrally related and overlapped with all other phases. Unlike the traditional approach, a generalization planning approach views generalization of treatment effects as the primary goal of intervention. Consequently, formal test results are supplemented with probes of performance in the clinic, in natural environments, and in simulated natural environments. The evaluation phase of a generalization plan is ongoing; it involves periodic administration of formal tests and probes so that online adjustments can be made in therapy as soon as they are needed.

The remainder of this section will focus on a description of representative tests and procedures that are commonly used for diagnosing and planning intervention for individuals with Broca's aphasia. Ideally the assessment suggestions discussed here would be administered in conjunction with clinical probes and in-vivo observations of clients and significant others so that a successful generalization plan could be developed and implemented.

Aphasia Batteries and Classification

This discussion of standardized aphasia batteries is restricted to the Boston Diagnostic Aphasia Examination (BDAE)[9,101] and the Western Aphasia Battery (WAB)[102] because these tests were designed to classify performance according to the classical taxonomy that includes Broca's aphasia. Other standardized batteries that provide valuable clinical information about aphasia are reviewed elsewhere.[85,94,103,104]

The BDAE is a comprehensive test battery that can be used to examine conversational and expository speech, auditory comprehension, oral expression, understanding written language, and writing. In addition to the test proper, supplementary language and nonlanguage tasks are provided in the test manual for use at the clinicians discretion. Although the scoring procedure used for each subtest varies, the revised edition of the BDAE[101] provides percentile rankings that permit across-task comparisons of the relative severity of performance.

The primary purpose of the BDAE is to categorize those who take the best into one of the classical types of aphasia and thereby to permit inferences about lesion localization. The authors freely admit that many clients seen in the clinic may not be categorized unambiguously and hold that the classic syndromes serve "as anchor points in our thinking about aphasia"[101] (p 74). The authors provide sample profiles of the range of speech and language characteristics of Broca's, Wernicke's, conduction, anomic, transcortical motor, and transcortical sensory aphasia.

Classification of the aphasias on the BDAE is primarily based on ratings of speech from the conversational and expository subtest. This subtest provides a means of sampling responses to everyday questions, open-ended conversation, and picture description. The clinician evaluates melodic line, phrase length, articulatory agility, grammatical form, paraphasias in running speech, and word finding difficulty by rating these parameters on a seven-point rating scale. BDAE test scores on repetition and auditory comprehension subtests are also considered in this classification system. The ratings of speech characteristics and performance on repetition and auditory comprehension subtests are displayed on a Rating Scale of Speech Characteristics. Individual profiles are compared to the range of profile ratings displayed by the various types of aphasia to determine classification.

In addition to the Rating Scale Profile of Speech Characteristics, an Aphasia Severity Rating Scale is also provided with the BDAE. The scale ranges from "0. No usable speech or auditory comprehension," to "5. Minimal discernable speech handicaps; patient may have subjective difficulties that are not apparent to listener." This severity scale covers a range of verbal abilities and is used in conjunction with the profile of speech characteristics to evaluate speech fluency and determine patient classification. Goodglass and Kaplan[101] note that individuals with Broca's aphasia are usually rated as severe (rating 1 or 2) on the severity rating scale because of the effortful, nonfluent nature of their verbal output. Those who are rated above a 4 on the overall severity rating scale are generally not classified as having Broca's aphasia.

An expected range of performance for Broca's aphasia on the Rating Scale Profile of Speech Characteristics is provided in the test book.[101] At the more severe end of the rating scale, those with Broca's aphasia may have essentially no intonational contour (i.e., melodic line), produce only single word "phrases," have minimal articulatory agility, and produce essentially no variety of grammatical constructions. Those less severely involved have appropriate intonational contour only for short phrases and stereotypes; their longest occasional uninterrupted phrase length is approximately four words; their articulatory agility is normal only in familiar words and phrases; and the variety of grammatical form is limited to simple declaratives and stereotypes.

Those with Broca's aphasia are rated as having few paraphasias in running speech. That is, they produce fewer than one paraphasia per minute of running speech, and they often do not produce any paraphasias. In addition, ratings on the word finding scale of the BDAE profile also may vary. The spontaneous speech of some of the more severe speakers with Broca's aphasia may be restricted to production of content words; the speech of less severe individuals may be rated as having informational content that is proportional to their fluency.

The two objective test scores that are displayed on the profile of speech characteristics represent performance on BDAE repetition and auditory comprehension subtests. On repetition subtests, those with Broca's aphasia range from not being able to repeat a single high probability phrase, such as "You know how," to being able to produce four to eight progressively longer phrases. The auditory comprehension score displayed on the rating of speech characteristics is actually the mean of percentiles on word discrimination, body-part identification, commands, and complex ideational materials subtests. The cumulative auditory comprehension percentile for those with Broca's syndrome is above the fiftieth percentile of aphasic patients in the standardization sample.

The comprehensive nature of the BDAE and its stated purpose of being a means of classifying aphasic syndromes makes the test a valuable tool in the clinical armamentarium. Of particular clinical utility is the qualitative analysis of spontaneous speech and fluency. However, syndrome classification on the BDAE is based largely on subjective clinical ratings, and classification relies to some extent on the knowledge base and experience of the examiner.

The other aphasia test that was designed with patient classification in mind, the Western Aphasia Battery (WAB),[102] attempts to circumvent this problem by using a numerical taxonomy to categorize aphasic syndromes.

Kertesz[10] indicates that the WAB was developed in an attempt to provide a taxonomic assessment tool that would be comprehensive enough for use as a research instrument and yet be practical enough for clinical use. The WAB contains two primary sections, an oral section and a visual language section. Optional nonverbal subtests, including the Ravens Progressive Matrices,[105] are also included. The oral portion of the WAB includes spontaneous speech (content, fluency), auditory comprehension, naming, and repetition subtests. Relatedly, the visual language portion includes reading, writing, calculation, and praxis subtests.

Two types of overall scores are derived from the WAB, an aphasia quotient (AQ) and a cortical quotient (CQ). The aphasia quotient is calculated from the oral portion of the WAB; it is purported to be a measure of the severity of language impairment. The AQ range is from 0–100, and the maximum cutoff score for aphasic language impairment is 93.8. The CQ is a summary score of the cognitive functions measured by the entire WAB. The scores from all WAB subtests are factored into the calculation of the CQ.

The scoring procedures vary across the WAB subtests that enter syndrome classification. One unique aspect of the WAB scoring system is the assignment of a numerical score for ratings of spontaneous speech samples (information content and fluency). Assigned fluency scores are associated with relatively specific descriptions of performance; they were designed to remove some of the subjectivity from the ratings of spontaneous speech.

Performance is classified on the WAB by comparing scores on fluency, comprehension, repetition, and naming subtests, and performance in each of these areas results in a score that ranges from 0 to 10. The WAB taxonomic table reveals that Broca's and other nonfluent aphasic syndromes have fluency ratings between 0 and 4. (Fluency ratings for fluent aphasic speakers range between 5 and 10.) Not surprisingly, performance by those with Broca's aphasia on comprehension tasks range from 4 to 10. This reflects the relatively well-preserved auditory comprehension abilities of these individuals. Similarly, the range of repetition (0–7.9) and naming (0–8) scores allowed for those with Broca's syndrome on the WAB reflects the considerable variability in their performance of these tasks.

Although the WAB distinguishes categories of aphasia, it does so with a forced classification system (see ref. 106). That is, nearly all test takers are placed into one or another of the WAB categories despite the fact that many have mixed symptomatology that would not be consistent with unambiguous classification. The WAB approach contrasts with Goodglass & Kaplan's[101] suggestion that nearly half of aphasic individuals seen clinically are not classifiable on the BDAE. Given apparent differences in these approaches to classification, clinical reports should reflect the basis of syndrome classification. This is particularly important because an individual who is categorized as having Broca's aphasia "according to the WAB" may not be classified as such on the BDAE.[90]

Supplemental Evaluation Procedures

The information obtained from standardized test batteries such as the WAB and BDAE is often supplemented with modality-specific and nonstandardized test results. Supplemental evaluation procedures are used to obtain additional information about known deficit areas and to probe communicative abilities that are not covered in standardized test batteries. The purpose of this section is to describe briefly selected supplemental evaluation procedures that contribute to the clinical management of individuals with Broca's aphasia. More extensive reviews of both standardized and supplemental evaluation procedures are available elsewhere.[104,107]

The verbal impairments in Broca's aphasia are often the most obvious and debilitating communication deficit, and many individuals place a high premium on obtaining as much recovery of premorbid verbal abilities as possible. Consequently, a thorough examination of verbal skills is essential to the development of a comprehensive intervention strategy. One verbal assessment procedure that is particularly relevant for the clinical management of those with Broca's aphasia is the Story Completion Test.[9,53] The test was designed to elicit grammatical constructions by having an examiner present two or three sentences of a highly predictable story and then having the client verbally complete the story. For example, the imperative intransitive (VP) is elicited as follows:

Examiner: "My cousin is at the door. I want him to come in. So I open the door and say: What?"
Target response: "Come in!"[9] (p. 197)

The Story Completion Test was originally developed for research purposes, and it has not been standardized. However, the test stimuli have been developed into an aphasia syntax training program by Helm-Estabrooks and Ramsburger.[108] The story completion format provides a means of probing specific syntactic constructions of speakers with Broca's aphasia that may not be produced in spontaneous speech samples.

In addition to probing the ability to produce specific constructions, clinicians also may be interested in examining spontaneous use of grammatical constructions, compensatory strategies used to avoid difficult constructions, ability to initiate and maintain conversational topics, and aspects of discourse. As Simmons[107] points out, the type of speech sample, elicitation procedure, stimuli, length, and conditions of sampling (eg. monologue versus dialogue) vary according to the specific goals of the evaluation. For example, a clinician could choose a picture description format to examine the content and efficiency of a language sample and also examine dyadic communication during discourse analysis. Spontaneous speech samples, however collected and analyzed, provide valuable clinical information that cannot be obtained from other more tightly controlled elicitation procedures.

Given the characteristic syntactic deficits and the interaction of semantic and syntactic aspects of language that occur in Broca's aphasia,[77] evaluation procedures that elucidate these problem areas should be explored. Crystal[110,111] has described linguistic profiling procedures that are designed to identify patterns of syntactic and semantic deficits in language-impaired patients. Crystal's Language Assessment,

Remediation and Screening Procedure (LARSP) is a procedure for examining grammatical and syntactic impairments in verbal output. This procedure involves systematically analyzing spontaneous speech samples and then tallying clause, phrase, and word elements on a summary profile. The LARSP profile allows the clinician to identify patterns of syntactic deficits within seven stages of syntactic complexity. The LARSP has been used with Broca's subjects, and the results of the analysis appear to be directly applicable to clinical intervention.[112] Crystal[111] describes a similar procedure for assessing patterns of semantic impairment deficits. Called the Profile in Semantics (PRISM), this procedure highlights the relationship between semantics and grammar and between semantics and the lexicon.

Although specialized training under a clinician who is experienced with these procedures is helpful, formal training in linguistics is not required to conduct LARSP and PRISM analyses. It appears, however, the time-consuming nature of these procedures has discouraged their adoption. Despite the apparent reluctance of clinical aphasiologists to adopt formal analyses of spontaneous speech, procedures like the LARSP are becoming a standard of practice for many clinicians working in the area of childhood language disorders. It is widely believed that the benefits derived in terms of the quality of patient care more than compensate for time invested in language sampling and analysis. Aphasiologists who avoid analyses of phonological, grammatical, and semantic aspects of spontaneous speech may miss a rich source of clinical material.

Given the frequent co-occurrence of aphasia and apraxia of speech, it is imperative that clinicians routinely screen individuals with Broca's aphasia for motor speech disorders. Wertz, Rosenbek, and LaPointe's definitive text[85] on apraxia details both evaluation and treatment procedures for apraxic individuals. At a minimum, however, the Motor Speech Evaluation[87] should be administered routinely. This battery consists of a compilation of clinical tasks that have been shown to be useful for identifying apraxia of speech and dysarthria. Furthermore, the protocol also is used to rate the severity of motor speech disorders and conduct perceptual analyses of dysarthric speech. Tasks included in the motor speech protocol range from vowel prolongation and verbal repetition, to picture description and oral reading. Of course, additional in-depth testing is necessary for individuals who exhibit signs of apraxia of speech and/or dysarthria on the motor speech protocol.

Although verbal impairments are usually the most obvious deficits in Broca's aphasia, other modalities may require additional testing beyond that provided by standardized test batteries. In particular, it is important that clinicians closely examine auditory comprehension skills because mild comprehension deficits are relatively easy to overlook in this population. The various forms of the Token Test are particularly useful for identifying subtle auditory comprehension impairments.[113,114] In addition, the Shortened Version of the Token Test is relatively quick and easy to administer (approximately 20 minutes), and severity cutoff scores and preliminary normative data are available.[115]

Other clinically useful tests of auditory comprehension ability include the Auditory Comprehension Test for Sentences (ACTS)[116] and the Functional Auditory Comprehension Test (FACT).[117] The ACTS examines comprehension of sentences that systematically vary in terms of length, vocabulary level, and syntactic difficulty. The test was standardized on Broca's and other classical types of aphasia so that clinicians can compare the performance of individuals to group normative data. The FACT was designed to overcome what the authors perceived as shortcomings of the Token Test. It consists of three levels of auditory commands that systematically increase in length and apparent complexity. The FACT appears to be more closely related to communicative skills encountered in daily living than does the Token Test.[118]

Standardized test results and initial clinical impressions provide clues to the direction of supplemental testing. The clinician's task is to interpret initial test data and follow the lead in a direction that will provide valuable differential diagnostic or treatment information. In some instances additional testing may be required for a modality that has already been carefully examined. Still other leads may take the clinician in new directions that have not been explored previously. The clinician may, for example, desire additional information about a client's reading[119] or gestural ability.[120] Whatever form and direction supplemental testing takes, however, it is imperative that the clinician does not lose sight of the need to step back from testing and observe their client's communicative abilities under more naturalistic conditions. Holland[121] spoke of this need when she suggested that we ask spouses about their partners' communication skills, observe patients with at least one other individual besides ourselves, and observe our aphasic clients in at least one naturalistic environment. These types of observations can be very enlightening with regard to realistic goal setting. More importantly, naturalistic probes also provide information needed to develop a comprehensive generalization plan that attempts to facilitate improvement of communicative abilities to people, settings, and situations where they are needed most.[98-100]

Treatment

There has been a proliferation of treatment research involving individuals with Broca's aphasia, and the vast majority of studies in this area were designed to enhance verbal abilities. For example, of 34 recent aphasia treatment studies summarized in Thompson's[122] review of the aphasia generalization literature, 19 studies (56%) included Broca's subjects, and virtually all of these studies trained verbal behaviors. Given the preponderance of studies designed to improve verbal skills, it is not surprising that reviews of treatment procedures for Broca's syndrome emphasize treatment procedures for expressive impairments. The present overview is no exception to this trend.

Although formal intervention programs for nonverbal modalities have rarely been developed specifically for Broca's patients, clinicians are routinely called upon to treat auditory and other nonverbal skills. There is a paucity of structured auditory comprehension treatment programs available, but clinicians can utilize the invaluable treatment suggestions of Schuell and her colleagues regarding auditory stimulation treatment procedures.[123,124] Stimulation and other auditory comprehension treatment strategies have been reviewed elsewhere in the clinical literature.[85,103,104,125,126]

In addition to auditory comprehension treatment procedures, various nonverbal treatment approaches are available. These include gestural training,[127,128] communicative drawing,[129] microcomputer treatment approaches,[130,131] and spouse training programs.[132] Relatedly, detailed descriptions of treatment approaches for apraxia of speech and other frequent concomitants of Broca's aphasia are available.[87,112]

The purpose of the section is to examine representative treatment approaches for the verbal impairments of Broca's clients. Our review begins with a brief discussion of a generalization planning treatment philosophy. This is followed by a brief consideration of specific treatment approaches.

A Treatment Philosophy

Language therapy for aphasia is an inexact science that is influenced by clinicians' training and their philosophy about the nature of aphasia. In addition, individual client considerations, such as the severity of language involvement, the presence of associated impairments, time postonset of aphasia, and communication environments, also influence treatment decisions. For example, a clinician who is treating an acute Broca's client with a moderately severe apraxia of speech may elect to intensely treat the apraxia prior to treating the syntactic problems. Guidelines are available to assist the clinician in making difficult treatment decisions ranging from the selection of clinical goals and choice of stimuli used in treatment, to the ordering of tasks within each treatment session.[103,104]

Another area of clinical decision-making for which clinical aphasiologists must be prepared is the development and evaluation of procedures that facilitate generalization.[99,122] Although aphasiologists have historically assumed that generalization is a natural and expected outcome of intervention (e.g., Schuell et al[123]), this has turned out to be an erroneous assumption.[122,133] Importantly, wholesale acceptance of this assumption may have inadvertently discouraged serious investigation of generalization issues in aphasia.[134] Since we now know that generalization is not an automatic byproduct of language intervention for aphasia, it is imperative that clinicians actively plan intervention in a manner that will increase the probability of obtaining generalization. Thompson[122] recently outlined the following steps for accomplishing this goal:

1. Select functional targets and plan to program response generalization, if necessary, across structurally for functionally different responses.

2. Design probes carefully for measuring generalization across response and stimulus conditions and to administer them periodically throughout treatment.

3. Establish criteria for generalization and look carefully at error responses.

4. Introduce aspects of the generalization environment into treatment or introduce aspects of the training environment into the generalization environment in early stages of treatment.

5. Use treatment methods, such as loose training [see below], that have resulted in generalization.

6. Extend treatment across settings or persons, when [generalization does not occur as planned] (p. 112).[122]

Thompson's suggestions highlight the steps involved in the development of a generalization plan and underscore the importance of clinicians becoming actively involved in programming generalization. However, as in other areas of clinical practice, we are only beginning to develop an appropriate technology for facilitating generalization. Clinicians should, therefore, incorporate measurement techniques that allow them to evaluate the success of their treatments so that they can objectively determine if, when, and where generalization occurs. Measurement techniques and design strategies associated with single-subject research designs can be adopted for this purpose.[135,136] Rosenbek, LaPointe, and Wertz[104] strongly support the notion of adapting research procedures into clinical practice as a means of improving clinical accountability. They state, "No procedure is inherently above suspicion. . . . Indeed treatments are as likely to be bad or neutral as to be good. Our nominee for the universal clinical assumption to be taught by all [training] programs is this: untested treatments are immoral, therefore clinical practice must include clinical experimentation" (p. 12). Clinicians have the responsibility to demonstrate that their treatment procedures are both effective and generalizable.

The effectiveness and generality of treatment procedures reviewed below have been examined to varying degrees. This does not, however, relieve the clinician of the responsibility of determining their success for individual clients. Published treatment procedures are rarely sufficiently detailed to permit exact duplication in the clinical arena. Furthermore, clinicians often justifiably modify published treatment programs rather than utilize them exactly as they are presented in the literature. Consequently the following approaches should be viewed as providing a beginning framework that can be changed, built upon and expanded to suit individual patient needs. However, the individual clinician is responsible for evaluating the effectiveness of the final clinical product.

General Treatment Strategies

The term "general treatment strategy" is used here to refer to intervention approaches that do not target improvement in a single modality, such as verbal production. For example, a number of authors have suggested that use of a relatively intact language or communication skill can facilitate performance of a more severely impaired ability.[47,137] This general principle can be applied regardless of the specific modality that is being treated. Skelly et al[138] provide a concrete example of how a clinician can apply treatment to one behavior and facilitate performance of a second communication skill. Specifically, Skelly et al reported that aphasic–apraxic subjects who were trained to produce iconic gestures (Amerind) also improved on verbal subtests of a standardized aphasia battery. They concluded that relatively intact gestural abilities helped facilitate improvement in more severely impaired verbal skills.

In addition to using an intact function to "deblock"[137] an impaired ability in therapy, patients can be taught a specific self-cueing strategy as a means of circumventing communicative difficulties.[139] Many clients perform well in treatment when they can rely on the clinician to provide external cues that help them successfully complete a given therapy task. Thus, for example, individuals with Broca's aphasia who are unable to produce a word spontaneously are often able to say a target word after the clinician provides a phonetic placement cue. Unfortunately, they may become "cue bound" or overreliant on external prompts. That is, they become so dependent on cues provided by the clinician that they are unable to circumvent communication difficulties without the assistance of the clinician. Since clinicians are not available to provide cues outside of the clinical setting this type of dependence sets the stage for failure when the client experiences difficulty communicating in the natural environment. A systematic program that trains clients to produce self-generated cues is one solution to this clinical dilemma. They can sometimes be taught to use a relatively intact ability consciously to facilitate communication through an impaired modality. Linebaugh and Lehner[140] taught self-generated cues to five Broca's subjects in an attempt to facilitate word retrieval with a cueing hierarchy treatment program. They organized a series of cues to facilitate confrontation naming and then worked up and down the hierarchy until sufficient progress was attained. Patients were taught to use appropriate self-generated cues to facilitate word retrieval within this program. For example, subjects were apparently taught to cue themselves to produce a target noun by trying to say the *function* of the target word. The results of this study demonstrated significant improvement in the ability to name treatment stimuli, and generalization of improved naming ability also was reported for untrained word lists. The authors speculated that the self-cueing strategies were partially responsible for improvements seen in the subjects' word retrieval abilities during group therapy.

This study demonstrates the subtle but important difference between simply using an intact skill to deblock an impaired ability during therapy and actually training a person to utilize those cues consciously. The goal of training a self-generated cueing strategy is to teach people to help themselves when they encounter communicative difficulty. Training clients to generate their own cues allows them to become less reliant on the clinician and thereby communicate more effectively in natural settings when the clinician is not available to provide assistance.

Clinicians should be familiar with the types of compensatory strategies that have been used with people with Broca's aphasia so they can incorporate them into intervention programs. Once the presence of compensatory behaviors is documented, their clinical utility can be explored by determining if the behaviors either facilitate or inhibit communicative effectiveness. Behaviors that facilitate responding or circumvent communicative difficulties can then be trained as self-generated cues that unblock an impaired ability, or they can be used as compensatory strategies that substitute for a blocked channel of communication.

Gleason, et al[53] described a number of "typical adaptive or compensatory devices" for their Broca's subjects. One of the most frequently observed compensations was the insertion of stressed words to begin an utterance. Relatedly, Meuse and Marquardt[84] described several strategies used to maintain communicative effectiveness. These included requests for clarification, verbally eliminating alternative choices, and using alternative forms of verbal communication, such as singing. In addition to the types of compensatory behaviors reported in the literature, the astute clinician will observe individualized strategies and determine their clinical usefulness.

Whitney[141] described an aphasia therapy approach in which she observed the spontaneous compensations and then systematically trained patients to use successful compensations. She described "go" strategies for Broca's subjects that were designed to help them initiate and maintain communicative interactions. For example, Whitney trained clients to use a written response to begin communicating when they were experiencing difficulty initiating a verbal response. Once a communicative attempt was begun, she subsequently employed modeling and external cues to encourage them to expand responses and continue their interactions. This treatment strategy emphasizes the importance of accepting any successful form of communication, and it rewards clients for taking communicative risks.

One final general treatment approach that may be effective with Broca's as well as other aphasia types is Davis and Wilcox's[142] PACE therapy. PACE is an acronym that stands for Promoting Aphasics' Communicative Effectiveness. As the name implies, PACE was designed to incorporate aspects of natural conversation into treatment. This interactive therapy approach adheres to four basic principles. First, clients and clinicians are equal participants as senders and receivers of messages during therapy. Stimulus materials are placed between the client and clinician, and they take turns trying to communicate information about selected items. The second principle is that there is an exchange of *new* information between the interactants. This is accomplished by having stimuli placed face down between the client and the clinician. In this way the receiver of the message does not know ahead of time what the sender is trying to communicate, and he or she must use new information provided to interact with the message sender. The third PACE principle is that the aphasic speaker is encouraged to use any available means to communicate. This may include verbal, nonverbal, or a combination of methods. The final principle is that the clinician provides naturalistic feedback with regard to the communicative success of the message. PACE therapy was perhaps the first clearly articulated and well-known treatment approach for aphasia that included principles of language pragmatics. It can be easily adapted to those of varying severity levels because it does not require high level verbal skills for participation.

Specific Treatment Tasks

The vast majority of recent treatment studies for individuals with Broca's aphasia have targeted improvements in verbal skills, and many of these studies have examined syntactic abilities. Helm-Estabrooks and her colleagues, for example, described a syntax training program called the Helm Elicited Language Program for Syntax Stimulation (HELPSS).[108,143] This program is based on the results of previous research by Gleason et al[53] that identified a relatively specific order of difficulty of grammatical structures for people with Broca's aphasia. The HELPSS program uses the previously described story completion format to elicit multiple exemplars of 11 different syntactic structures. These structures are then systematically trained at two levels of difficulty until a criterion for successful production is achieved. Helm-Estabrooks and Ramsburger[108] report that six chronic agrammatic subjects achieved significant improvement on formal language measures after completing the HELPSS. Other researchers have found that the order of difficulty of the HELPSS syntactic constructions may vary for individual Broca's subjects,[144] and that a limited amount of generalization may result from training with the HELPSS.[145] This latter finding is consistent with the results of studies of various other approaches to syntax training in aphasia.[146–149]

Melodic Intonation Therapy (MIT)

Melodic Intonation Therapy (MIT) is an aphasia treatment approach that uses intoned melodies as a means of improving verbal production.[150,151] The use of melody and intonational contours in this program is based on the notion that the intact right cerebral hemisphere, which is associated with melodic functions, can be tapped as a means of facilitating verbal response. The four levels of MIT are designed to increased a speaker's ability to independently produce high probability phrases and sentences. Programmed instruction methods are employed, and the amount of cues provided by the clinician are gradually reduced at each step of the MIT program. A variety of prompts are included ranging from intoning a melodic line and hand tapping to having the client answer questions using drilled phrases and sentences. MIT appears to be the most effective for individuals with Broca's aphasia and apraxia of speech who have very restricted verbal output and poor repetition ability, in the context of relatively preserved auditory comprehension ability.[152]

Changing Criteria

Several recent treatment approaches have been designed to increase the length and amount of informational content produced by clients with Broca's aphasia. Rosenbek et al[104] describe in detail A Program of Changing Criteria that was designed to increase the amount and quality of verbal output. This program systematically establishes the stability of increasingly longer utterances at four criterion levels. Realistic picture stimuli of everyday activities are used throughout the program, and relevant questions are used to elicit specific answers at each criterion level. Finally, a series of increasingly powerful cues are used to elicit responses when a client fails to respond accurately to the clinician's questions. Rosenbek and his colleagues provide a detailed clinical example that will benefit clinicians interested in using this approach. They note that the program is designed to teach strategies for communicating, and that it is not just intended to increase the length of responses.

Response Elaboration Training (RET)

Response Elaboration Training (RET) is a program that was developed to increase the length and information content of verbal responses of nonfluent aphasic patients.[153,154] RET is a "loose training" program[155] that was designed in reaction to treatment programs in which the clinicians treat a narrow range of predetermined responses. An important underlying assumption during the development of RET was that overly structured treatment programs may actually inhibit aphasic clients from using language creatively and flexibly by severely limiting their response options. Loose training procedures, such as RET, are designed to facilitate generalization by providing a wider variety of stimuli and responses than are encountered within overly didactic treatment approaches.

Procedurally, loose training translates into an attempt to loosen the control over stimuli and response during therapy in an effort to expose the client to numerous and varied parameters that occur in naturalistic settings. RET loosens response parameters of therapy by using client-initiated responses as the primary content of therapy rather than restricting responding to a narrow range of clinician-selected target responses. Those enrolled in RET are encouraged to elaborate on "whatever they are reminded of" when picture stimuli are presented; they are discouraged from simply describing or naming elements of the stimulus pictures. In fact, RET stimuli consist of line drawings of transitive and intransitive verbs that contain minimal contextual information so that clients can not simply describe the stimuli. Instead, they must rely on their personal history and world knowledge to respond. RET stimuli depict individuals involved in everyday activities (e.g., eating or pouring) and sports (e.g., hit ball; run); they also include a separate set of related items for probing generalization.

To date RET procedures have been applied for research purposes and a restricted set of line drawings have been used as a means of adding experimental control. However, the program can be expanded and the principles can be applied clinically in more naturalistic and interactive situations.

As noted above, the emphasis in RET is on shaping and chaining spontaneous, *client-initiated* responses. RET stimuli serve primarily as a catalyst for clinician–client interactions around an action concept. Consequently, the line drawings can be relied upon to "get started" but they must generate increasingly elaborate descriptions with minimal assistance from context and with minimal input from the clinician. Unlike clinician-directed approaches, the client directs the course of therapy in RET because his responses and subsequent elaborations provide the primary focus of treatment. In essence, the client is required to take the primary burden of communication during RET while the clinician merely ensures that the direction chosen is properly channeled to maximize therapeutic gain.

The basic RET sequence entails (1) eliciting spontaneous responses to minimally contextual picture stimuli, (2) modeling and reinforcing initial responses, (3) providing "wh" cues to prompt clients to elaborate on their initial responses, (4) reinforcing attempted elaborations and then modeling sentences that combine initial and all subsequent responses to a given stimulus picture, (5) providing a second model of sentences that combine previous responses and then requesting a repetition of the sentence, (6) reinforcing repetitions of combined sentences and providing a final model of the sentence. Throughout this sequence clients responses are not directly corrected by the clinician. Instead, naturalistic feedback is provided during the structured interactions through conversational modeling.

It should be noted that a number of backup or branching program steps are used to accommodate individual patterns of responding during RET. In addition, steps in the program are administered twice for each treatment trial during a given treatment session. A typical session consists of 20 trails, or the random presentation of 10 training items twice each. The basic RET sequence is demonstrated with the following example.

Individual training sessions begin by randomly presenting one of the line drawings and having the client describe the picture of "whatever it reminds you of." When a moderately impaired client with Broca's aphasia was presented with a picture of a figure swimming he responded, "Uh . . . swimming . . . boy." Following this response the clinician modeled a grammatically correct interpretation of the response and reinforced the effort. That is, the clinician responded by stating, "Super. . . . The boy's swimming. . . . Nice going!" During the next step in the sequence the clinician provided a "wh" cue in an attempt to elicit a more elaborate response. Thus, the cue was, *"Why . . .* is the boy swimming?" After a brief hesitation the client replied, "swimming . . . help." Again the clinician provided positive feedback, and then combined the two previous responses and modeled the combined sentence. Specifically, the clinician said, "Great! . . . The boy is swimming for help." He subsequently requested that the client repeat a model of the combined response by saying, "Try and say the whole sentence after me. Ready? Say, 'The boy is swimming for help.'" In turn, the client replied, "Boy . . . swim . . . help." Finally, the clinician modeled the combined sentence and reinforced the attempted repetition: "Super. . . . The boy is swimming for help." This sequence was repeated for the same item before beginning another trial with a different stimulus picture.

It is worth noting the evolution of responses during RET. Over subsequent treatment sessions the client in the previous example progressed from an average of approximately two content words per stimulus picture during pretreatment baseline sessions to his criterion level of five or more content words per stimulus picture. Thus, his pretreatment response in the above example of "Uh . . . swimming . . . boy" (two content words) evolved into more detailed responses, such as "Lois . . . swimming . . . water . . . uh . . . pond . . . stroke, butterfly" (six content words) during the final posttreatment probe. This final response is representative of the type of longer, albeit telegraphic, responses that he produced following RET.

It is noteworthy that the RET program was designed to reinforce informational content instead of linguistic form, so that highly informative, telegraphic responses are quite acceptable within this protocol. It is also of interest to observe that the client in the previous example elaborated on the topic of swimming by using vocabulary items and informational content that was not depicted in the stimulus picture. That is, he mentioned his wife and a specific swimming stroke in his final response. This type of creative responding is precisely what is targeted with RET. Moreover, it provides a marked contrast to structured syntactic programs that typically target clinician selected responses such as "The boy is swimming." Finally, note that the client actually produced a variety of responses to the same stimulus picture during treatment and on clinical probes. He was encouraged to and actually did produce novel and varied responses throughout the program rather than simply repeating a single rote response.

The results of Response Elaboration Training demonstrate that the procedure may facilitate an increase in the amount of information (i.e., number of content words) produced by individuals with aphasia. In addition, a moderate degree of generalization has been reported across stimuli, people, and settings following RET.[153,154] Furthermore, the RET format has been used with a moderate degree of success for facilitating communicative drawing ability with a nonverbal aphasic client.[99] These results, in combination with findings from other aphasia training studies, indicate that loose training procedures, such as Response Elaboration Training, may provide an effective and generalizable means of treating individuals with Broca's aphasia.[156,157]

In summary, verbal treatment programs for Broca's aphasia were reviewed and representative examples of specific approaches were considered. Treatment approaches have been designed to improve syntactic aspects of verbal impairments (HELPSS)[108] and to take advantage of intact right hemisphere processes governing intonation and melody (MIT).[150,151] In addition, several recent programs are attempting to improve the length and informational content produced by people with Broca's aphasia.[104] One of these programs, Response Elaboration Training (RET), was reviewed in depth and a clinical example was provided.[153,154] This approach was presented as an example of "loose training" treatment programs that have evolved from recent attempts to facilitate and program generalization in aphasia. Further clinical research is needed to evaluate the usefulness of these and other treatment approaches for individuals with Broca's aphasia.

Acknowledgments

The writing of this manuscript was supported, in part, by Veterans Administration Rehabilitation Research & Development grant No. 384. The helpful assistance of Ann Gaddie is gratefully acknowledged.

Suggested Readings

Bates E & Wulfek B: Comparative aphasiology: A cross-linguistic approach to language breakdown. *Aphasiology* 1989; 3:111–142.

Kean ML: *Agrammatism.* New York: Academic Press, 1985.

Kearns KP, Potechin G: The generalization of response elaboration training effects. In Prescott TE (ed): *Clinical Aphasiology.* Boston: College Hill Press, 1989, pp 223–246.

Lesser R: disorders of grammar and the lexicon. In LaPointe LL (ed): *Aphasia: Nature and Assessment. Seminars in Speech and Language.* New York: Thieme, 1986, pp 147–158.

Rosenbek JC, LaPointe LL, Wertz RT: *Aphasia: A Clinical Approach.* Boston: College-Hill Publication, 1989.

Signoret JL, Castaigne P, Lhermitte F, et al: Rediscovery of Leborgne's brain: Anatomical description with CT scan. *Brain Lang* 1984; 22:303–319.

Simmons NN: Beyond standardized measures: Special tests, language in context, and discourse analysis in aphasia. In LaPointe LL (ed): *Seminars in Speech and Language. Aphasia: Nature and Assessment,* vol 7. New York: Theime, 1986, pp 181–206.

Thompson CK: Generalization in the treatment of aphasia. In McReynolds LV and Spradlin J (eds): *Generalization Strategies in the Treatment of Communication Disorders.* Toronto: BC Decker, 1989, pp 82–115.

Wertz RT, LaPointe LL, Rosenbek JC: *Apraxia of Speech in Adults: The Disorder and Its Management.* New York: Grune & Stratton, 1984.

References

1. Benton AL, Joynt RJ: Early descriptions of aphasia. *Arch Neuro* 1960; 3:205–221.
2. Broca P: Portee de la parole. Ramollissement chronique et destruction partielle du lobe anterieur gauche du cerveau. *Bull Soc Anthropol Paris* 1861; 2:219.
3. Broca P: Remarques sur le siege de la faculte du langage articule, suivies d'une observation d'aphemie. *Bull Soc Anat Paris* 1861; 2:330–357.
4. Damasio A: The Nature of Aphasia: Signs and Syndromes. In Sarno MT (ed): Acquired Aphasia. New York: Academic Press, 1981, pp 51–65.
5. Naeser MA, Palumbo CL, Helm-Estabrooks N, et al: Severe Non-Fluency in Aphasia: Role of the Medical Subcallosal Fasciculus Plus Other White Matter Pathways in Recovery of Spontaneous Speech. Paper presented at the Annual Academy of Aphasia Meeting. Nashville, Tennessee October 1986.
6. Head H: *Aphasia and Kindred Disorders of Speech,* vol 1. New York: Hafner Publishing, 1963.
7. Benson DF: *Aphasia, Alexia and Agraphia.* New York: Churchill Livingstone, 1979.
8. Damasio H: Cerebral Localization of The Aphasias. In Sarno MT (ed): Acquired Aphasia. New York: Academic Press, 1981, pp 27–50.
9. Goodglass H, Kaplan E: *The Assessment of Aphasia and Related Disorders.* Philadelphia, Lea and Febiger, 1972.
10. Kertesz A: *Aphasia and Associated Disorders: Taxonomy, Localization, and Recovery.* New York: Grune & Stratton, 1979.
11. Caplan D: *Neurolinguistics and Linguistic Aphasiology: An Introduction.* New York: Cambridge University Press, 1987.

12. Brown JW, Perecman E: Neurological bases of language processing. In Chapey R (ed): *Language Intervention Strategies In adult Aphasia*, ed. 2. New York: William & Wilkins, 1986, pp 12–27.
13. Broca P: Sur le siege de la faculte du langage articule. *Bull Soc Anthropol Paris* 1865; 6:337–393.
14. Critchley M: Dax's law. *International J Neurol* 1964; 4:199–206.
15. Wernicke C: *Der aphasische Symptomenkomplex.* Breslau: Cohn and Weigert, 1874.
16. Lichtheim L: On aphasia. *Brain* 1885; 7:433–484.
17. Benton A: Aphasia: Historical Perspectives. In Sarno MT (ed): *Acquired Aphasia.* New York: Academic Press, 1981, pp 1–26.
18. Henschen SE: *Klinische und Anatomische Beitrage zur Pathologie des Gehirns,* vols. 5–7. Stockholm: Nordiska Bokhandel, 1920–1922.
19. Jackson H: Selected Writings of J Hughlings Jackson. Head H (ed): *Brain* 1915; 38:1–90.
20. Marie P: Revision de la question de l'aphasie: La troisienee circonvolution frontale gauche ne joue aucuen role special dans la fonction du langage. *Sem Med* 1906; 21:241–247.
21. Mohr J, Pessin M, Finkelstein S, et al: Broca's aphasia: Pathological and clinical. *Neurology* 1978; 28:311–324.
22. Rosenbek JC, Shimon D: Computerized axial tomography in aphasiology. In Brookshire RH (ed): *Clinical Aphasiology Conference Proceedings,* 1984. Minneapolis, BRK Publishers, pp 1–6.
23. Naeser MA, Hayward RW: Lesion localization in aphasia with cranial computed tomography and the Boston Diagnostic Aphasia Exam. *Neurology* 1978; 28:545–551.
24. Mazzocchi R, Vignolo L: Computer assisted tomography in neuropsychological research: A simple procedure for lesion mapping. *Cortex* 1978; 14:136–144.
25. Kertesz A, Harlock W, Coates R: Computer tomographic localization, lesion size, and prognosis in aphasia and nonverbal impairment. *Brain Lang* 1979; 8:34–50.
26. Ludlow CL, Rosenberg J, Fair C, et al: Brain lesions associated with nonfluent aphasia fifteen years following penetrating head injury. *Brain* 1986; 109:55–80.
27. Knopman DS, Selnes OA, Niccum ND, et al: A longitudinal study of speech fluency in aphasia: CT correlates of recovery and persistent nonfluency. *Neurology* 1983; 33:1170–1178.
28. Basso A, Lecours AR, Moraschini S, et al: Anatomoclinical correlations of the aphasias as defined through computerized tomography: Exceptions. *Brain Lang* 1985; 26:201–229.
29. Tramo MJ, Baynes K, Volpe BT: Impaired syntactic comprehension and production in Broca's aphasia: CT lesion localization and recovery patterns. *Neurology* 1988; 38:95–98.
30. Mazzocchi R, Vignolo L: Localization of lesions in aphasia: Clinical CT scan correlations in stroke patients. *Cortex* 1979; 627–654.
31. Freedman M, Alexander MP, Naeser MA: Anatomical basis of transcortical motor aphasia. *Neurology* 1984; 34:409–417.
32. Hanson WR, Metter EJ, Riege WH, et al: Positron emission tomography. In Brookshire RH (ed): *Clinical Aphasiology,* 1984. Minneapolis, BRK Publishers, pp 14–23.
33. Hanson WR, Metter EJ, Riege WH, et al: Comparison of regional cerebral metabolism (PET), structure (X-ray CT), and language in categories of chronic aphasia. In Brookshire RH (ed): *Clinical Aphasiology,* 1986. Minneapolis, BRK Publishers, pp 87–96.
34. Metter EJ, Kempler D, Hanson WR, et al: Cerebral glucose metabolism: Differences in Wernicke's Broca's, and conduction aphasia. In Brookshire RH (ed): *Clinical Aphasiology,* 1986. Minneapolis, BRK Publishers, pp 97–104.
35. Metter EJ, Kempler D, Jackson CA, et al: Broca's aphasia by 18F-flourodeoxyglucose positron emission tomography. *Ann Neurol* 1987; 22:134.
36. Illes J, Metter EJ, Dennings R, et al: Spontaneous language production in mild aphasia: Relationship to left prefrontal glucose hypometabolism. *Aphasiology.* 1989; 3:527–538.
37. Crosson B: Subcortical functions in language: A working model. *Brain Lang* 1985; 25:257–292.
38. Metter EJ, Riege WH, Hanson WR, et al: Subcortical structures in aphasia; An analysis based on (F-18) fluorodeoxyglucose, positron emission tomography, and computed tomography. *Arch Neurol* 1988; 45:1229–1234.
39. Badecker W, Caramazza A: On considerations of method and theory governing the use of clinical categories in neurolinguistics and cognitive neuropsychology: the case against agrammatism. *Cognition* 1985; 20:97–115.
40. Rizzi L: Two notes on the linguistic interpretation of Broca's aphasia. In Kean M (ed): *Agrammatism.* New York: Academic Press, 1985, pp 153–164.
41. Geschwind N: Disconnection syndromes in animals and man. *Brain* 1965; 88:237–294, 585–644.
42. Berndt RS, Caramazza A: Syntactic aspects of aphasia. In Sarno MT (ed): *Acquired Aphasia.* New York: Academic Press, 1981, pp 157–182.
43. Goodglass H: Agrammatism, in Whitaker H, Whitaker HA (eds): *Studies in Neurolinguistics,* vol 1, New York: Academic Press, 1976, pp 237–260.
44. Kean ML: *Agrammatism.* New York: Academic Press, 1985.

45. Lesser R: *Linguistic Investigations of Aphasia*. London: Edward Arnold, 1978.
46. Goodglass H, Geschwind N: Language Disorders (Aphasia). In Carterette EC, Friedman M (eds): *Handbook of Perception*, vol 7. New York: Academic Press, 1976, pp 389–428.
47. Luria A: *Traumatic Aphasia*. The Hague: Mouton, 1970.
48. Pick A: *Die Agrammatischen Sprachstorungen*. Berlin: Springer, 1913.
49. Brown J: *Aphasia by Aronold Pick*. Springfield, Illinois: Charles C Thomas, 1973.
50. Heeschen C: Agrammatism versus paragrammatism: A fictitious opposition. In Kean ML (ed): *Agrammatism*. New York: Academic Press, 1985, pp 207–248.
51. Kolk HHJ, Van Grunsven MJF, and Keyser A: On parallelism between production and comprehension in agrammatism. In Kean ML (ed): *Agrammatism*. New York: Academic Press, 1985, pp 165–206.
52. Goodglass H, Gleason JB, Bernholtz N, et al: Some linguistic structures in the speech of a Broca's aphasic. *Cortex* 1972; 8:191–212.
53. Gleason JB, Goodglass H, Green E, et al: The retrieval of syntax in Broca's aphasia. *Brain Lang* 1975; 2:451–471.
54. Jakobson R: *Aphasia As a Linguistic Topic*. Clarke University Monographs on Psychology and Related Disciplines, Worcester, 1955. Reprinted in *Roman Jakobson, Selected Writings, vol 2., Words and Language*. The Hague: Mouton, 1955.
55. Chomsky N: *Aspects of the Theory of Syntax*. Cambridge, MIT Press, 1965.
56. Grodzinsky Y: The syntactic characterization of agrammatism. *Cognition* 1984; 16:99–120.
57. Jarema G, Kadzielawa D, Waite J: On comprehension of active/passive sentences and language processing in a Polish agrammatic aphasic. *Brain Lang* 1987; 32:215–232.
58. Bates E and Wulfeck B: Comparative aphasiology: A cross-linguistic approach to language breakdown. *Aphasiology* 1989; 3:111–142.
59. Berndt RS, Caramazza A: A redefinition of the syndrome of Broca's aphasia: Implications for a neuropsychological model of language. *App Psycholinguistics* 1980; 1:225–278.
60. Caramazza A, Berndt RS: A Multicomponent deficit view of agrammatic Broca's aphasia. In Kean ML (ed): *Agrammatism*. New York: Academic Press, 1985, pp 27–62.
61. Schwartz MF, Linebarger MC, Saffran EM: The status of the syntactic deficit theory of agrammatism. In Kean ML (ed): *Agrammatism*. New York: Academic Press, 1985, pp 83–124.
62. Caramazza A, Zurif E: Dissociation of algorithmic and heuristic processes in language comprehension: Evidence from aphasia. *Brain Lang* 1976; 3:572–582.
63. Zurif EB, Caramazza A, Myerson R: Grammatical judgments of agrammatic aphasics. *Neuropsychologia* 1972; 10:405–417.
64. Zurif EB, Green E, Caramazza A, et al: Grammatical intuitions of aphasic patients: Sensitivity to functors. *Cortex* 1976; 12:183–186.
65. Nespoulous J, Dordain M, Perron C, et al: Agrammatism in sentence production without comprehension deficits: Reduced availability of syntactic structures and/or of grammatical morphemes? A case study. *Brain Lang* 1988; 33:273–295.
66. Berndt RS, Salasoo A, Mitchum CC, et al: The role of intonation cues in aphasic patients' performance on the grammaticality judgment task. *Brain Lang* 1988; 34:65–97.
67. Crain S, Shankweiler D, Tuller B: Preservation of sensitivity to closed-class items in agrammatism. Talk presented at the Annual Academy of Aphasia Meeting. Los Angeles, 1984.
68. Linebarger MC, Schwartz ME, Saffran EM: Sensitivity to grammatical structure in so-called agrammatic aphasics. *Cognition* 1983; 13:361–392.
69. Lukatela K, Crain S, Shankweiler D: Sensitivity to inflectional morphology in agrammatism: Investigation of a highly inflected language. *Brain Lang* 1988; 33:1–5.
70. Smith S, Mimica E: Agrammatism in a case-inflected language. *Brain Lang* 1984; 13:274–290.
71. Smith S, Bates E: Accessibility of case and gender contrasts for assignment of agent-object relations in Broca's aphasics and fluent anomics. *Brain Lang* 1987; 30:8–32.
72. Von Stockert TR, Bader L: Some relations of grammar and lexicon in aphasia. *Cortex* 1976; 12:49–60.
73. Parisi D, Pizzamiglio L: Syntactic comprehension in aphasia. *Cortex* 1970; 6:204–215.
74. Heeschen C: Strategies of decoding actor–object relations by aphasic patients. *Cortex* 1980; 16:5–19.
75. Bates E, Friederici A, Wulfeck B: Comprehension in aphasia: A cross-linguistic study. *Brain Lang* 1987; 32:19–67.
76. Grodzinsky Y, Marek A: Algorithmic and heuristic processes revisited. *Brain Lang* 1988; 33:216–225.
77. Lesser R: Disorders of grammar and the lexicon. In LaPointe LL (ed): *Aphasia: Nature and Assessment. Seminars in Speech and Language*. New York: Thieme, 1986, pp 147–158.
78. Kean ML: Agrammatism: A phonological deficit? *Cognition* 1979; 7:69–84.

79. Wulfeck B: Grammatical judgments and sentence comprehension in agrammatic aphasia. *J Speech Hear Res* 1988; 31:72–81.

80. Petocz A, Oliphant G: Closed-class words as first syllables do interfere with lexical decisions for nonwords: Implications for theories of agrammatism. *Brain Lang* 1988; 34:127–146.

81. Saffran E, Schwartz M, Marin O: The word order problem in agrammattism II: Production. *Brain Lang* 1980; 10:263–280.

82. Grodzinsky Y: Language deficits and the theory of syntax. *Brain Lang* 1986; 27:135–159.

83. Goodglass H and Menn L: Is Agrammatism a Unitary Phenomenon, in Kean ML (ed): *Agrammatism.* New York, Academic Press: 1985, pp 1–26.

84. Meuse S, Marquardt TP: Communicative effectiveness in Broca's aphasia. *J Commun Disord* 1985; 18:21–34.

85. Davis GA: *A Survey of Adult Aphasia.* Englewood Cliffs, New Jersey: Prentice-Hall, 1983.

86. Goodglass H, Quadfasel FA, Timberlake WH: Phrase length and the type of severity of aphasia. *Cortex* 1964; 1:133–152.

87. Wertz RT, LaPointe LL, Rosenbek JC: *Apraxia of Speech in Adults: The Disorder and its Management.* New York: Grune and Stratton, 1984.

88. Wertz RT, Rosenbek JC, Deal JL: A review of 228 cases of apraxia of speech: classification, etiology and localization. Paper presented at the American Speech and Hearing Association Convention, New York, 1970.

89. Rosenbek JC: Treating apraxia of speech. In Johns DF (ed): *Clinical Management of Neurogenic Communication Disorders,* 2nd ed. Boston: Little, Brown, 1985, pp 267–312.

90. Wertz RT, Deal JL, Robinson AJ: Classifying the aphasias: A comparison of the Boston Diagnostic Aphasia Examination and the Western Aphasia Battery. In Brookshire RH (ed): *Clinical Aphasiology Conference Proceedings,* 1984. Minneapolis: BRK Publishers, pp 40–47.

91. Kent R, Rosenbek JC: Acoustic patterns of apraxia of speech. *J Speech Hear Res* 1983; 26:231–249.

92. Kent R, Rosenbek JC: Prosodic disturbances and neurologic lesion. *Brain Lang* 1982; 15:259–291.

93. Kearns KP: The application of phonological process analyses to adult neuropathologies. In Brookshire RH (ed): *Clinical Aphasiology Conference Proceedings,* 1980. Minneapolis: BRK Publishers, pp 187–195.

94. Darley FL: *Evaluation of Appraisal Techniques in Speech and Language.* Reading, Pennsylvania: Addison-Wesley, 1979.

95. Itoh M, Sasanuma S, Tatsumi IF, et al: Voice onset time characteristics in apraxia of speech. *Brain Lang* 1982; 17:193–210.

96. Canter GJ, Trost J, Burns M: Contrasting speech patterns in apraxia of speech and phonemic paraphasia. *Brain Lang* 1985; 24:204–222.

97. Joanette Y, Keller E, Lecours AR: Sequences of phonemic approximations in aphasia. *Brain Lang* 1980; 11:30–44.

98. Baer DM: *How to Plan for Generalization.* Austin, Texas: Pro-ed, 1981.

99. Kearns KP: Methodologies for studying generalizations. In McReynolds LV, Spradlin JE (ed): *Generalization Strategies in the Treatment of Communication Disorders.* Toronto: BC Decker, 1989, pp 13–30.

100. Warren SF: Clinical strategies for the measurement of language generalization. In Warren SF, Rogers-Warren AK (eds): *Teaching Functional Language.* San Diego: College-Hill Press, 1985, pp 197–224.

101. Goodglass H, Kaplan E: *The Assessment of Aphasia and Related Disorders,* ed 2. Philadelphia: Lea and Febiger, 1983.

102. Kertesz A: *Western Aphasia Battery.* New York: Grune and Stratton, 1982.

103. Brookshire RH: *An Introduction to Aphasia,* ed. 2. Minneapolis: BRK Publishers, 1978.

104. Rosenbek JC, LaPointe LL and Wertz RT: *Aphasia: A Clinical Approach.* Boston: College-Hill Publication, 1989.

105. Raven JC: *Coloured Progressive Matrices.* London: HK Lewis, 1962.

106. Risser AH, Spreen O: Test review: The Western Aphasia Battery. *J Clin Exp Neuropsy* 1985; 7:463–470.

107. Simmons NN: Beyond standardized measures: Special tests, language in context, and discourse analysis in aphasia. In LaPointe LL (ed): *Seminars in Speech and Language. Aphasia: Nature and Assessment,* vol 7. New York: Theime-Stratton, 1986, pp 181–206.

108. Helm-Estabrooks N, Ramsberger G: Treatment of agrammatism in long-term Broca's aphasia. *British J Disord Comm* 1986; 21:39–45.

109. Yorkston K and Beukelman D: A system for quantifying verbal output of high-level aphasia patients. In Brookshire RH (ed): *Clinical Aphasiology Conference Proceedings,* 1977. Minneapolis: BRK Publishers, pp 175–180.

110. Crystal D: *Working with LARSP.* New York: Elsevier, 1979.

111. Crystal D: *Profiling Linguistic Disability.* New York: Elsevier, 1982.
112. Kearns KP and Simmons N: A practical procedure for the grammatical analysis of aphasic language impairment: The LARSP. In Brookshire RH (ed): *Clinical Aphasiology Conference Proceedings,* 1983. Minneapolis: BRK Publishers, pp 4–14.
113. DeRenzi E, Vignolo L: The Token Test: A sensitive test to detect receptive disturbances in aphasia. *Brain* 1962; 85:556–678.
114. McNeil M, Prescott T: *Revised Token Test.* Baltimore: University Park Press, 1978.
115. DeRenzi E, Paglion P: Normative data and screening power of a shortened version of the token test. *Cortex* 1978; 14:41–49.
116. Shewan CM: *Auditory Comprehension Test for Sentences.* Chicago: Biolinguistics Clinical Institutes, 1979.
117. LaPointe LL, Horner J: The functional auditory comprehension task (FACT): protocol and test format. *FLASHA Journal,* Spring Issue: 1978, 27–33.
118. LaPointe L, Holtzapple P, Graham L: The relationships among two measures of auditory comprehension and daily living communication skills. In Brookshire RH (ed): *Clinical Aphasiology Conference Proceedings,* 1985. Minneapolis: BRK Publishers, 1985, pp 38–46.
119. LaPointe L, Horner J: *Reading Comprehension Battery for Aphasia.* Austin, TX: Pro-ed, 1979.
120. Duffy R, Duffy J: *The New England Pantomine Test.* Tigard, C.C. Publications, 1984.
121. Holland A: Remarks on observing aphasic people. In Brookshire RH (ed): *Clinical Aphasiology Conference Proceedings,* 1983. Minneapolis: BRK Publishers, 1983, pp 1–3.
122. Thompson CK: Generalization in the treatment of aphasia. In McReynolds LV, Spradlin J (eds): *Generalization Strategies in the Treatment of Communication Disorders.* Toronto: BC Decker, 1989, pp 82–115.
123. Schuell H, Jenkins JJ, Jimenez-Pabon E: *Aphasia in Adults: Diagnosis, Prognosis and Treatment.* New York: Harper & Row, 1964.
124. Duffy J: Schuell's stimulation approach to rehabilitation. In Chapey R (ed): *Language Intervention Strategies in Adult Aphasia,* ed 2. Baltimore; William & Wilkins, 1981, pp 187–214.
125. Kearns, KP and Hubbard D: A Comparison of Auditory Comprehension Tasks in Aphasia, in Brookshire R (ed): *Clinical Aphasiology Conference Proceedings,* 1977. Minneapolis: BRK Publishers, pp 32–45.
126. Marshall RC: Treatment of auditory comprehension deficits. In Chapey R (ed): *Language Intervention Strategies in Adult Aphasia.* Baltimore: Williams & Wilkins, 1986, pp 370–393.
127. Kearns KP, Simmons N, Sisterhen C: Gestural sign (Amer-Ind) as a facilitator of verbalization in patients with aphasia. In Brookshire RH (ed): *Clinical Aphasiology Conference Proceedings,* 1982. Minneapolis: BRK Publishers, pp 183–191.
128. Tonkovich J, Loverso F: A training matrix approach to gestural acquisition by the agrammatic patient. In Brookshire RH (ed): *Clinical Aphasiology Conference Proceedings,* 1982. Minneapolis: BRK Publishers, pp 283–288.
129. Lyon J, Sims E: Drawing: It's use as a communicative aid with aphasic and normal adults. In Prescott TE (ed): *Clinical Aphasiology Conference Proceedings.* San Diego: College-Hill Press (in press).
130. Katz RC: *Aphasia Treatment with Microcomputers.* San Diego: College-Hill Press, 1986.
131. Loverso F, Prescott TE, Selinger M, et al: Comparison of two modes of aphasia treatment: Clinician and computer. In Prescott TE (ed): *Clinical Aphasiology Conference Proceedings.* San Diego: College-Hill Press (in press).
132. Simmons NN, Kearns KP, Potechin G: Treatment of aphasia through family member training. In Brookshire RH (ed): *Clinical Aphasiology Conference Proceedings,* 1987. Minneapolis: BRK Publishers, pp 106–116.
133. LaPointe LL: Multiple baseline designs. In Brookshire RH (ed): *Clinical Aphasiology Conference Proceedings,* 1978. Minneapolis: BRK Publishers, pp 20–29.
134. Kearns KP: Approaches to language rehabilitation in aphasia: A perspective on generalization. Paper presented at the University of Kansas Spring Symposium, Kansas City, 1980.
135. McReynolds LV, Kearns KP: *Single-Subject Experimental Designs in Communicative Disorders.* Austin, Texas: Pro-ed, 1983.
136. Kearns KP: Flexibility of Single-Subject Experimental Designs. Part II: Design Selection and Arrangement of Experimental Phases. *Journal of Speech Hearing Disorders,* 1986; 51:204–214.
137. Weigel E, Berwisch M: Neuropsychology and linguistics: Topics of common research. *Found of Language,* 1970; 6:1–18.
138. Skelly M, Schinsky L, Smith R, et al: American Indian sign (Amerind) as a facilitator of verbalization for the oral verbal apraxic. *J Speech Hear Disord* 1974; 39:445.
139. Berman M, Pelle LM: Self-generated cues: A method for aiding aphasic and apractic patients. *J Speech Hear Disord* 1967; 32:372–376.

140. Linebaugh C, Lehner L: Cueing heirarchies and word retrieval: A therapy program. In Brookshire RH (ed): *Clinical Aphasiology Conference Proceedings,* 1977. Minneapolis: BRK Publishers, pp 19–31.
141. Whitney J: Developing aphasics use of compensatory strategies. Paper presented at the American Speech/Language/Hearing Association Convention. Washington, 1975.
142. Davis GA, Wilcox MJ: Incorporating parameters of natural conversation in aphasia treatment. In Chapey R (ed): *Language Intervention Strategies in Adult Aphasia.* Baltimore: Williams & Wilkins, 1980, pp 169–190.
143. Helm-Estabrooks N, Fitzpatrick PM, Barresi B: Response of an agrammatic patient to a syntax stimulation program for aphasia. *J Speech Hear Disor* 1981; 46:422–427.
144. Salvatore AP, Trunzo MJ, Holtzapple P, et al: Investigation of the sentence hierarchy of the helm elicited language program for syntax stimulation. In Brookshire RH (ed): *Clinical Aphasiology Conference Proceedings,* 1983. Minneapolis: BRK Publishers, 1983, pp 73–84.
145. Doyle P, Goldstein H, Bourgeois MS: Experimental analysis of syntax training in Broca's aphasia: A generalization and social validation study. *J Speech Hear Disor* 1987; 52:143–155.
146. Kearns KP, Salmon SJ: An experimental analysis of auxiliary and copula verb generalization in aphasia. *J Speech Hear Disor* 1984; 49:152–163.
147. Loverso FL, Selinger M, Prescott TE: Application of verbing strategies to aphasia treatment. In Brookshire RH (ed): *Clinical Aphasiology Conference Proceedings,* 1979. Minneapolis: BRK Publishers, 1979, pp 229–238.
148. Prescott T, Selinger M, Loverso F: An analysis of learning, generalization and maintenance of verbs by an aphasic patient. In Brookshire RH (ed): *Clinical Aphasiology Conference Proceedings,* 1982. Minneapolis: BRK Publishers, pp 178–182.
149. Thompson CK, McReynolds LV: Wh interrogative production in agrammatic aphasia: An experimental analysis of auditory–visual stimulation and direct-production treatment. *J Speech Hear Res* 1986; 29:193–206.
150. Sparks RW, Deck JW: Melodic intonation therapy. In Chapey R (ed): *Language Intervention Strategies in Adult Aphasia,* 2nd ed. Baltimore: Williams & Wilkins, 1986, pp 320–332.
151. Sparks R, Helm NA, Albert M: Aphasia rehabilitation resulting from melodic intonation therapy. *Cortex* 1974; 10:303–316.
152. Helm NA: Criteria for selecting aphasic patients in melodic intonation therapy. *Science* 1978; 199:52.
153. Kearns KP: Response elaboration training for patient initiated utterances. In Brookshire RH (ed): *Clinical Aphasiology Conference Proceedings,* 1985. Minneapolis: BRK Publishers, pp 196–204.
154. Kearns KP, Potechin G: The generalization of response elaboration training effects. In Prescott TE (ed): *Clinical Aphasiology.* Boston: College Hill Press, 1988, pp 223–246.
155. Stokes T and Baer DM: An implicit technology of generalization. *J App Behav Anal* 1977; 10:349–367.
156. Doyle P, Goldstein H, Bourgeois M, et al: Programming "loose training" as a strategy to facilitate generalization of questioning in Broca's aphasic subjects. *J App Behav Anal* (in press).
157. Thompson CK, Byrne ME: Across setting generalization of social conventions in aphasia: An experimental analysis of "loose training." In Brookshire RH (ed): *Clinical Aphasiology Conference Proceedings,* 1984. Minneapolis: BRK Publishers, pp 132–144.

2

Wernicke's Aphasia

Lisa Graham

Introduction

Carl Wernicke, the man whose 1874 treatise leads us to this discussion, encountered death by "autopsychic disorientation."[1] An incorrect analysis of his own ability to ride a bicycle resulted in an untimely fall beneath a logging cart. An attempt to crystalize in one chapter the genesis and current status of thought on Wernicke's aphasia since his time would risk the same malady. Though its discovery was made more than 114 years ago, some clinicians have yet to find a Wernicke's aphasia they can believe in consistently. While many agree that the constellation of behaviors that creates the condition does occur, and often in the "classic" description, others find it less apparent.

As a case of confusion in point, Damasio[2] tells us that "Wernicke's aphasia is the most fundamental and least controversial of aphasic syndromes" (p. 59). But in the words of Benson,[3]: "Wernicke aphasia is widely recognized, although not so fully accepted as a name for a specific aphasia syndrome. Essentially identical aphasia syndromes have been called sensory aphasia, receptive aphasia, central aphasia, and many other names" (p. 71). Without question, there is controversy over the specifics of Wernicke's as of any defined aphasic syndrome; however, the constellation of behaviors associated with whatever one labels it tends to be the same. At least for a moment in time during the evolution of the aphasic condition, it may appear as an identifiable type. Often a patient's recovery and/or rehabilitation may take him on a course that starts with classic Wernicke's symptomotology and brings him into the more general "fluent type" classification. Sometimes, that trip may encompass only the space of a hallway between two aphasiologists. For a clinically useful description, we must settle on a set of behaviors associated with a generally similar lesion, regardless of our proclivity to name or not name. In the words of Wertz[4], "while we may not agree on what to call it, we seem to recognize it when we see it. This is fortunate, since we see alot of it" (p. 9).

Although controversy exists over the condition, it is firmly entrenched in many quarters as both a concept and a clinical reality, and knowledge of the suggested underlying mechanisms and possibilities for remediation are paramount to the clinician.

History/Pathophysiology

Until Carl Wernicke's paper in 1874,[5] aphasic behaviors had been localized and delineated most notably by Paul Broca. Broca had described the location and characteristics for frontal motor aphasia, or "aphemia" as he called it. He identified the source of defect as anterior to the central sulcus, whose location as division for motor and sensory functions was known at the time. It was left to Wernicke, at 26 years of age, to describe those aphasias apparent in individuals whose frontal lobes remained intact.

Wernicke's work, *The Aphasia Symptom-Complex; A Psychological Study on an Anatomical Basis,*[1] described the existence of sensory versus motor localized aphasias and provided post mortem evidence of this new localization. As a student of Meynert, Wernicke agreed with his teacher's suspicion that traces of sensory patterns would be stored in regions adjacent to the corresponding zone in the cortex. Meynert had suggested that the acoustic pathways would end near the Sylvian fissure. Following such logic, Wernicke postulated that traces of words would be stored near this zone, where interruption would result in loss of comprehension.

The landmark of sensory aphasia, later to become Wernicke's aphasia, was thus described by Wernicke as the result of a lesion in the dominant first temporal gyrus, the area first postulated by Meynert and subsequently named Wernicke's area for its descriptor. The primary deficit in sensory aphasia, according to Wernicke was an interruption of the central auditory projection area, or *klangfeld* (soundfield). Wernicke explained that, as Broca's areas must be the center for representation, of memory images of movement of the mouth and tongue, so the soundfield at the first temporal gyrus must be the center for representation of sounds.

Given the primary deficit of auditory comprehension loss, Wernicke maintained there would exist corresponding losses in the ability to understand written language, or produce it oneself. He felt these losses were a consequence of learning reading and writing in indivisible association with sounds. Obviously, without auditory comprehension, the ability to repeat also would be lost. Speech movements would be preserved as a function of the anterior system, and quality would be fluent, perhaps even rapid. However, speech content would be paraphasic due to loss of the internal correction of the motor process ordinarily overseen by the receptive speech zone. This paraphasic speech pattern would go unnoticed by the speaker because of impaired auditory monitoring. Owing to the posterior lesion and the location of motor function in the frontal lobes, the individual would demonstrate no obvious hemiplegia.

Wernicke did not believe the syndrome he described was a composite one which would require several equally devastating areas of lesion. In his refutation of such a composite, he broke purposefully with the localizationists of the time, who maintained that specific functions were assigned to discrete areas of brain.[6] In Wernicke's words, "Only the most elementary psychic functions can be assigned to refined areas of the cortex. . . . Everything which goes beyond these simplest functions, the association of different impressions into a concept, thinking, consciousness, is an achievement of the fiber tracts which connect the different regions of the cortex to each other, the so-called association system of Meynert."[7]

Wernicke asserted that because of the way language is learned and used, all the modalities associated with and arising from the auditory system would be affected by disturbance of the soundfield. His theoretical orientation regarding the associative system proved as important to the advancement of neurological studies as did his description of sensory aphasia. His theory allowed for the postulation and later confirmation of other as yet undiscovered syndromes.

As a formal definition of Wernicke's aphasia, these original findings on localization and behavioral hallmarks have stood the test of time. Currently, the behaviors associated with this syndrome are still considered a result of lesion to the posterior region of the left superior temporal gyrus. The resulting associated behaviors are:

- Fluent but paraphasic speech
- Defective auditory comprehension
- Defective repetition of words and sentences
- Both reading and writing usually disturbed
- Infrequent hemiparesis

Wernicke originally asserted that sensory aphasia resulted from lesion to the dominant superior temporal gyrus. In 1981, H. Damasio[8] published a summary of a series of computed tomography (CT) scans, delineating several cases of Wernicke's aphasia as well as other fluent aphasias. According to interpretation of the CT studies of those with Wernicke's aphasia, the core location for lesion was in the posterior portion of the superior temporal gyrus, the auditory association area, or Wernicke's area, contained in the Sylvian fissure. Although some overlap was shown between lesions in those individuals with Wernicke's aphasia and those with either conduction aphasia or transcortical sensory aphasia, "The core of each anatomical pattern is quite distinctive" (p. 34).

Benson[3] maintains that although damage to Wernicke's area may not result always in the symptoms known as Wernicke's aphasia, the opposite is not so. That is, those possessing communicative deficits consistent with Wernicke's aphasia nearly always have pathology somewhere in the dominant superior temporal gyrus. Assuming that is the case, an important consideration, in addition to what we may know about behavioral correlates to damage in a given area, is the degree to which such damage may play a part in the severity of disability and eventual recovery of function. In a paper delivered to the 1988 Clinical Aphasiology Conference, Chapman and Pool[9] presented preliminary findings that point to damage in the dominant superior temporal gyrus as a common factor among patients who are deemed most seriously impaired by their aphasia. A similar report[10] suggested that those with posterior superior temporal involvement have a poorer prognosis for auditory comprehension improvement, and have a slower recovery rate overall. Although many have long felt that Wernicke's aphasia was particularly resistant to recovery of function, perhaps we are closer to an understanding of whether we draw that conclusion from seeing particularly intransigent behaviors or just patients severely involved overall.

Nature and Differentiating Features

Wernicke's aphasia is differentiated primarily from the anterior, nonfluent aphasias. Once a diagnosis of fluent aphasia has been made, a person may be classified into one of three major posterior, fluent syndromes: Wernicke's aphasia, conduction aphasia, or transcortical sensory aphasia. The "core" lesion site for Wernicke's aphasia was described above, along with the indication that its lesion site may overlap with other sites. The behavioral patterns of the three aphasia types not only overlap, in some cases they mimic each other exactly. Table 2–1 outlines the behavioral hallmarks for each of these syndromes.

The level at which an aphasic person crosses from ability to impairment is sometimes judged unreliably among examiners, and other confounding impairments bring even more challenge to the task of deciding on an aphasia type. Familiarity with the characteristics of Wernicke's aphasia requires fuller description and knowledge of correlates well beyond the range of this table.

The comprehension deficit in Wernicke's aphasia may be called the most debilitating aspect of the disorder. Because of interconnections with other sensory modalities, a person with Wernicke's aphasia may be cut off from processing input of any kind. Schuell[11] maintained that the single most important factor in prognosis of recovery from any aphasia was the degree of residual auditory comprehension ability, specifically for individual words. She cited Hughlings Jackson's belief that the central processes underlying speech consisted of acoustical–motor arrangements. Thus, damage to the temporal lobe would not produce isolated symptoms, but rather patterns of deficit based on the dissolution of established neural interconnections. This was the premise of Wernicke as well in his postulate that higher functions were managed by the associative tracts instead of each function being handled by a discrete area of brain.

The severity of comprehension deficit varies in Wernicke's aphasia from inability to understand any spoken language to a less obvious shutter-effect type comprehension disorder, where some stimuli are processed adequately but others remain unprocessed. The exact quality of the deficit is sometimes not well understood. Contributing to the incomplete understanding is the fact that comprehension does not disintegrate predictably along defined lines, nor do we have adequate precision in our measurement tools or even an adequate understanding of the nature of comprehension in "normals" to precisely delineate the nature of the deficit. Evidence is emerging from language studies that highlights variation in comprehension ability related to the amount of naturally redundant material included in the evaluation. Most of our tests of comprehension emphasize linguistic neutrality, and only recently have clinicians begun combining accumulated information from those tests with observations of comprehension in more naturalistic environments, which may be richer in contextual and situational redundancy.

Table 2-1.   Behavioral Patterns of Types of Aphasia

	Wernicke's	Conduction	Transcortical Sensory
Auditory Comprehension	Severely Impaired	Slightly Impaired	Severely Impaired
Repetition	Impaired	Impaired	Intact
Speech	Fluent, Paraphasic	Paraphasic	Fluent, Paraphasic
Reading	Impaired	Intact	Impaired
Writing	Impaired	Impaired	Impaired

Fluent, but paraphasic speech is another hallmark of Wernicke's aphasia. Often the words of the fluent aphasic speaker are supplemented with extra syllables or are even fabricated anew (neologism). In addition to these problems is the confounding factor of press of speech. Also termed logorrhea, this behavior has been called characteristic of Wernicke's aphasia, though arguably it may exist with other syndromes, notably transcortical sensory aphasia. Press of speech manifests itself not so much in rate, though that is possible, but rather in the irrepressible intention of the speaker to continue in his monologue, often to the point where he must be forceably stopped by physical gesture or insistent interruption by the listener. Wernicke had explained this phenomenon as resulting from the lack of correction over output normally exercised by the sensory areas. This theory has been widely accepted, or at least not directly refuted, and the emphasis in treatment on having the patient "monitor" his output lends credence to our belief in Wernicke's explanation as a credible underlying cause.

Reading comprehension also is affected in Wernicke's aphasia. Wernicke's original explanation of this problem was based on the assumption that reading is learned in such a way as to be tied inexorably to auditory comprehension. He argued that each of us auditorizes what we process visually, and in the absence of an ability to do that, reading is no longer possible. Some argument has been made for a more localizationist cause, because the extension of the Wernicke's lesion may be into the angular gyrus where basic requisites for abilities to read may be located. This theory was questioned by Nielsen[12], who maintained that lesions of the temporal region alone may produce alexia.

Writing deficits also contribute to the mosaic of Wernicke's aphasia. The writing deficits consequent to posterior damage are strikingly dissimilar from those evidenced in anterior lesions. While the person with Broca's aphasia struggles valiantly over the production of a single legible word or letter, the person with Wernicke's aphasia may write easily and voluminously. Unfortunately, letter forms are appropriate and there may be occasional breaks to symbolize words, but the entire message may be devoid of meaning. Interestingly, here again is the aphasic writer's apparent lack of awareness or concern with the nonsense he has just distributed across the page. Explanations for this phenomenon parallel those offered for press of speech. Barring any monitoring ability, the patient is left with only the preserved anterior abilities to produce, but without the pivotal abilities to monitor and correct.

Above are the characteristics most cited as hallmarks of Wernicke's aphasia. Important as well are some of the ancillary behaviors that arise not from the lesion itself but from the behavioral profile it causes. Some of these fall into the area of disorders of mood or emotion.

Clinical lore depicts the Wernicke's aphasic as paranoid.[2,3] Because of his inability to appreciate his own errors, in the face of obvious and consistent confusion or neglect from his listener, it is easy to imagine such a prediliction evolving. However, the severity of damage to any one modality differs greatly from patient to patient, and some patients do have a preserved ability to appreciate their own errors. While this paranoid proclivity should not be discounted, neither should it always be anticipated. The apparent lack of concern in the person with Wernicke's aphasia is often short lived following initiation of treatment.

One note of caution, however, owing more to clinical experience than to documented reality. Reports have circulated that persons with Wernicke's aphasia are among those most likely to do themselves harm. Although such indications are vague and not particularly widespread, occasional reports of attempted suicide by persons with fluent aphasia are heard. In one study on mood disorders in aphasia, Fromm, Holland and Swindell[13] reported that while 48% of aphasic subjects were moderately depressed according to the Beck Inventory, the type of aphasia had no significant effect on likelihood of depression. The potential for alienation in severe cases of Wernicke's or any aphasia should be taken seriously by all health care providers and explained carefully to the family.

The final note on correlates of Wernicke's aphasia actually concerns a condition usually not present. As mentioned previously, obvious paralysis is a rare accompaniment of Wernicke's aphasia. Because of this, a lesion causing Wernicke's symptomotology may well go unnoticed in the standard, nonradiographic neurological examination. In the words of Carl Wernicke: ". . . thoroughly experienced and intelligent physicians regard this condition as a confusional state — as I myself have had the opportunity to experience. For the psychiatrically trained man who knows the clinical terms of confusional states, the diagnosis has not the least difficulty" (p. 290).[7] Unfortunately, the same error is possible today and is best countered by a complete language examination, especially examination of the auditory system.

Evaluation

As with any communicative disorder, evaluation of aphasia ideally begins upon first hearing of the patient. Anything shown, told, or warned to us becomes part of the appraisal information bank. From the general "if he walks he must be fluent" to the specifics of a CT scan depicting lesion in the dominant first temporal gyrus, each element becomes part of the equation. Appraisal will consist of everything from the very standardized comprehensive examinations, to the decidedly nonstandardized interviews with the clinician. All may contribute to important clinical decisions.

Numerous examinations for aphasia exist, each with the potential to be used for estimates of prognosis, treatment planning, or often in "labeling" the disorder. The evaluation with a standardized test serves as an excellent compass, providing information for the direction to take in further testing.

Among the most important tasks in diagnosing Wernicke's aphasia is thorough testing of auditory comprehension. While a number of comprehension tests exist, none can be said to provide a completely adequate indication of the person's status. There is an expanding body of literature on auditory comprehension, and it bears careful review. The clinician always must be aware that since auditory comprehension is not an openly observable ability, our estimates as to its status are only as good as our means of inference and prediction.

Perhaps the most widely used of the auditory comprehension tests is the Token Test, originally developed in 1962 by DeRenzi and Vignolo.[14] Another version was created in 1978 by McNeil and Prescott,[15] the Revised Token Test, which offers more precise administrative procedures as well as a multidimensional scoring system. These tests have been widely used for both clinical and research purposes. Both of these tests focus on auditory comprehension ability in the absence of linguistic redundancy or environmental cues. In an attempt to create a test with more everyday relevance, LaPointe and Horner[16] developed the Functional Auditory Comprehension Test (FACT), which utilizes stimulus items and directions more related to everyday living. The FACT has been shown to correlate highly with the Communicative Abilities in Daily Living evaluation of Holland,[17] and moderately with the Token Test. Token Test results were not shown to correlate strongly with the CADL.[18]

In 1978, Waller and Darley[19] suggested that in order to make reasonable estimates of comprehension of spoken language, nontraditional measures should be used. Brookshire and Nicholas[20-22] have reported many studies that suggest that information provided in paragraphs, or with content of personal interest to their subjects, improves comprehension ability. These and other authors[23,24] remind us that, to the fullest extent possible, our evaluations need to incorporate information about comprehension in real-life context. One example of the potential difference in comprehension estimates is illustrated by two patients in the Wilcox, Davis, and Leonard study[23] who scored at 58% and 49% levels in standard testing, and achieved 100% and 93% in "natural context." Although the correlates of natural language remain elusive, we can say that most communication contains heavily redundant and largely predictable information. The information provided in auditory comprehension testing should reflect both systematic prediction of linguistic deficits, and performance of the patient in a "best case" environment.

Supplementary verbal tests range in specificity from single word naming to picture descriptions. Most often we use these tests with the intention of cataloging whatever is uttered. Not so with the Wernicke's aphasic. Output is most often abundant, and before deciding on any measure of language production, one is well advised to decide what it is they want to know. The tests can certainly be adapted to account for amount of superfluous language, awareness of errors by the patient, and type of errors. Unfortunately, all methods of such evaluation have their drawbacks, with the universal disadvantage being that there is no less-efficient way to find out how someone talks than to ask them to do so. The clinician is advised to collect samples not only from structured tasks, which have the obvious advantage of duplication over time, but also to take advantage of unstructured situations for observing language output.

Supplementary tests for reading and writing are less available. The Reading Comprehension Battery for Aphasia,[25] the only test of its kind, has tasks ranging from single word sections to sentences and "functional" tasks. Some clinicians use reading tests developed for normal populations, and attempt to extrapolate scores to their patients. Bogdanoff and Katz[26] have suggested a procedure by which these tests scores might be adapted for an aphasic population. Writing tests are most often the invention of a clinician. Almost all the comprehensive inventories have some minimal writing assessment, and this is often the extent of formal testing in that modality.

A focus for testing of equal importance to the comprehensive language examination is the collection of information which leads a clinician to a judgment of the patient's functional competence. This goal is well stated in the words of instruction for the Communicative Abilities in Daily Living (CADL),[17] "We are trying to find out how you get along in everyday situations. Since I can't go along and actually watch, we'll use pictures and photographs and ask you some questions." The CADL is the only comprehensive test of its kind; it is an excellent starting point for orienting the clinician to think in terms of how a patient makes it in the outside world. In addition to the information it provides, the CADL may encourage some of us to get up and observe some "real-life" interactions of the patient. Whether that means a walk back to a room with the patient, or even to the canteen, it may be the one way to find out that when he tells us about that *?!!* kitchen crew mixing up his order, he is actually asking for french fries when he wants a chocolate shake. Unfortunately, no standardized therapy or evaluation technique exists that will replace the simple orientation of a clinician to observations of functional competence.

Treatment

> I sure wish I knew somebody who would tell me what I'm talkin' about.
>
> —H.S., a person with Wernicke's Aphasia, 1986

Often severely impaired aphasic individuals with no predictable reason for being so, are quite lucid. Ultimately, the patient with Wernicke's aphasia retains the hope that his problem will go away, or at least that somebody will help him understand and adapt. Designing effective treatment in quest of addressing that hope is what motivates many clinicians.

Treatment for any of the aphasias is not a longstanding clinical science, though strides have been made on gathering evidence on the efficacy of our efforts. In the literature on treatment of Wernicke's aphasia, there is much to create discouragement. We know from a Schuellian perspective[11] that recovery from aphasia depends mostly on the ability to comprehend language. Evidence accumul⁻ ⁻es on severity being associated with lesions to the dominant temporal region and on the relationship of recovery to the integrity of this region.[10] In addition, few treatment suggestions exist in the literature. These observations caution us with good reason, but the search continues for understanding of the system.

If it is assumed that a person has been rendered unable to process language alone in either spoken or written form, how will the clinician communicate with this person? Evaluation may reveal some modality of at least faint promise. The person's output will range from nearly on target to completely inappropriate, whether in spoken or written form. How does the patient effectively communicate with the clinician? Again, close analysis of the initial interchange with the clinician often will indicate some informational exchange. The task, then, is to replicate that exchange and expand it. The key to clinical success that may provide reasons to continue the process of treatment may not be clear in one visit. A danger is in generating a hasty conclusion based on faulty expectations. Certainly some individuals may not benefit from treatment, but before arriving at that conclusion we must be assured that we have exhausted reasonable possibilities for affecting positive change.

The clinician begins treatment development with information from interviews, chart review, and an accumulation of test results. It is not possible to make a classification of aphasia type and then turn to page Wernicke in the Book of Therapy. In their chapter, "Treating Auditory Comprehension Impairment," Rosenbek, La-Pointe, and Wertz[27] stress that stimulus manipulation has the most potential for control over an aphasic person's performance on a given task. As they point out, the ability to set up appropriate tasks is a skill born of experience but may be the most critical part of treatment. When an initial pool of information about abilities has been analyzed, specific treatment tasks can be developed.

Specific Treatment Tasks

Martin[28] admonished that the most common goals for people with Wernicke's aphasia are to "improve comprehension" and "improve self-monitoring." He emphasized that with such unspecified goals in place, it is easy to see why no obvious improvement in treatment can be reported. Without question, the comprehension and internal monitoring deficits in Wernicke's aphasia are of predominant concern. The presence of these deficits, however, affects all interactions and should be addressed within the confines of selected treatment tasks and not approached as though manageable in a task or two.

Rate and Alerting

We know that reduction in rate of speech improves comprehension for the aphasic listener when that reduction is achieved through pauses between meaningful segments.[29] These clinical research observations are buttressed by comments from our patients, "Why does everybody talk so fast?"; "You know, your words are on top of each other!" In addition to slowing rate, some clinicians alert a patient to incoming information nearly automatically, ("Hey, Mr. Green, here's the next one."), a technique confirmed to enhance attention by Loverso and Prescott in 1981.[30] Explanation and modeling of these techniques for family members is an effective first step in therapy. Press of speech is most often addressed with a stop technique, wherein the clinician quite literally stops the patient, usually by means of gesture, and then indicates that he should slow down, perhaps in order to listen to himself. Doyle and Holland[31] suggest that a pacing board similar to those used with dysarthric individuals may be another way to address the problem. They report on a patient with severe press of speech who achieved an immediate reduction of rate and extraneous speech through the use of a pacing board. They suggest transfer of this technique to a less cumbersome method for functional use. All methods for enhancing comprehension and controlling speech output should be incorporated by the clinician into strategies that can be generalized to communication outside the clinic.

Treatment Planning

Regularly scheduled treatment goals should incorporate as much emphasis on the generalization of skills as on traditional language drill. Fortunately, the two complement each other. While we rely on language to communicate, we also make use of gesture, prosody, volume, and silence. The object of effective treatment is to foster maximum success in sending and receiving information, however possible. One way to develop a preliminary treatment outline based on successes and failures in evaluation is simply to sit down with accumulated tests and notes and begin writing. These notes on possible remedial techniques and their effectiveness during treatment trials form the groundwork for a strong intervention program.

Samples of preliminary treatment development notes have been taken from a Wernicke patient's chart and are presented below:

- Counting is good when the items are ordered for him . . . he's somewhat messy; didn't organize cards logically for himself to count, but usually got them once started. Automatic language tasks are starters?

- Suprised me! He was related on naming today — table for chair, truck for car; (dismal in testing) got some outright. Slight tendency to perseverate . . . especially on error response. Some bizarre responses ("piano toast" for "butter") Semantic cues helpful?

- Asked repeatedly for nail polish for sore finger . . . even when confronted with nail polish. Never did realize error. Has tendency to go off task, perseverate on his own conversations. Self monitoring seems like it could come around. Once or twice he corrected errors and knew it. Add monitoring component to tasks at start?

- Very social. Seems to be making sense when he's NOT! Explain to family. Will he be able to manage description tasks now?

- Ugh! Unreliable for yes/no, even personal. Talk to family and NURSES. Begin yes/no personal questions.

- Big explanations, small reality. But a lot of semantic related and appropriate gesture. Watch not to close him down too much.

- Drastic change in naming without warm up and semantic cued sentence completion. Initial phoneme cues completely ineffective. "Don't show it to me, just understand it to me!"

Writing these notes at the beginning of treatment development reinforces the observation that even within major deficit parameters, each aphasic individual behaves differently and will respond to treatment based only on his or her own idiosyncracies.

Task Set-Up

After initial refinements have been made to trial treatment tasks, a series of more structured, hierarchical tasks can be set up. A tool for delineating task parameters and performance is the Base-10 Response Form.[32] At a minimum, the daily task sheets should contain information on task description (including input and output modalities requested), treatment plans, and performance results. An advantage of the Base-10 Response Forms is their room for all the above parameters plus places for listing stimulus items and charting results graphically which the patient and his family can understand. A few examples of Base-10 tasks provided for the Wernicke's patient follow:

- Task: Auditory comprehension. Choose correct picture from field of three unrelated stimuli.
  Input: Auditory   Output: Gestural
  Criterion: 90% over three sessions
  Scoring: PICA (conversion scores) 1
  Tx: Repeat target word, point to correct response, eliminate foils, provide seman-

tic cues and redundancy for stimulus, restimulate without foils, restimulate with foils (original form of request)

• Task: Auditory Comprehension. Point to picture from field of three after word is spelled.
  Input: Auditory   Output: Gestural
  Criterion, Scoring: Same as above
  Tx: Remove foils, spell and name target stimulus, write name as spelled aloud, pt points to picture alone, restimulate with two foils, then three foils. (Pt had shown that spelling aloud was a good cue and sometimes attempted to spell a word he couldn't say. He rarely spelled correctly on his own, but was undoubtedly helped when spelled to . . . a nice hint from the patient to the clinician, regardless of his inability to spell himself.)

• Task: Complete task without any verbal. Match related noun picture cards in field of three.
  Input: Visual   Output: Gestural
  Criterion: 95% over three trials
  Scoring: PICA (conversion scores)
  Tx: Eliminate foils, show related together. Put the two together in a sentence. "Eggs and bacon"; "For breakfast I have eggs and bacon." Pt. remains silent, pt places correct items together alone. Replace foils, restimulate in original form.

• Task: Object naming. Sentence completion with visual prompt of picture (familiar nouns). Accept only target noun or lead-in sentence plus target noun.
  Input: Auditory plus visual   Output: Verbal
  Criterion: 95% over three trials
  Scoring: PICA (conversion scores)
  Tx: Expands noun use to other sentences: (phone) "I talk on the phone, I'll call you on the phone. I hear the phone!" Pt points to picture after prompt: "I talk on the (point)" Clinician repeats target: "Right, you talk on the phone." Pt repeats after clinician. Restimulate in original form.

• Task: Response to personal yes/no questions.
  Input: Auditory   Output: Verbal
  Criterion: 95% over two trials
  Scoring: PICA (conversion scores)
  Tx: Write key words (You — Nebraska?) from question and present while repeating the question "Are you from Nebraska?" Model head shake and response "Yes, you are from Nebraska." Repeat question with print again; pt responds; restimulate as original.

• Task: Supplement to above task. Response to "no" questions (as result of delay and self-correction responses consistently only on "no" questions.) Series of five questions, all negative. Need to place in juxtaposition to yes/no task so that the instruction doesn't become one of simply answering "no" to everything.
  Input, Output, Criterion, Scoring, Tx: same as above

1-PICA conversion scores are described by LaPointe,[32] and allow for use of the multidimensional Porch Index of Communicative Ability (PICA) scoring system on these tasks.

There is a need for an extensive number of available tasks for treatment. The preceding are but six of about 50 such tasks used in a six-month treatment period, and the Base-10 tasks require only one-third of the session. The point is that they capitalize in a systematic way on the nature and range of the aphasic client's capabilities. Their utility lies in the efficiency and organization they impose on a treatment session, and in the time they create for more open-ended communication, which seems to be pivotal for the person with Wernicke's aphasia.

Setting a PACE

Davis and Wilcox[33] first described a method of encouraging more "real world" conversations in the clinic in 1978, with their description of "PACE: Promoting Aphasics Communicative Effectiveness." The method was further described in 1981, and has been used widely and reviewed since that time. Among the unique qualities of this program are the emphases on free choice of communicative modality, and equal opportunity to send and receive messages for the client and the clinician or other partner. Another feature of the method is that the information passing between the two participants must be novel. This aspect of the program departs radically from traditional approaches, where the clinician quite literally gets to hold all the cards. The method is highly reinforcing for the client and is usually equally reinforcing for the clinician. PACE therapy easily can incorporate techniques developed in more structured therapy, such as intentional pause before speaking, use of a pacing board, and requests for repeats.

Because the person with Wernicke's aphasia is often determined to communicate regardless of success, a PACE method can capitalize on this enthusiasm while imposing facilitating controls. The initial interaction with a person who exhibits press of speech on a PACE task can be a disheartening and frustrating experience for a beginning clinician. With experience, however, one can manipulate the amount of shared knowledge between the client and his communication partner so that success arrives before the session ends. Examples of two restricted PACE tasks are given below:

- A stack of ten picture cards is placed between the patient and the clinician. Corresponding objects are in a loosely arranged group at one end of the table, printed words of each are arranged at the other end of the table. Paper and pencil are available for writing. The partners take turns selecting items from the stimulus pile and demonstrating what they have selected by matching with print or object, writing, speaking, or gesturing. Any cue that results in the message being passed is rewarded as correct.

- A barrier is placed between partners so that they are prevented from seeing contents of identically marked blotters in front of each. Matching objects are given to both partners, to be placed by one partner where he wishes on his blotter. Information is then exchanged between the two with the goal of matching "object on blotter" configuration. Complexity is easily increased with the use of more objects, different designs on the blotters, etc. As always, exchange of information is in any modality chosen by either participant.

Family Inclusion

Derivatives of PACE therapy can be used quite successfully to incorporate family members into treatment. Participation in therapy by those who communicate most often with the client is a critical aspect of treatment with any aphasic person. With the often confusing behaviors of the person with Wernicke's aphasia, the family members benefit particularly well from understanding their part in successful communication. An excellent assessment of communication between partners can be made with Flowers and Peizer's "Strategies for Obtaining Information from Aphasic Persons." [34] The requisites of conversation for both the aphasic person and the speaking partner are well outlined and can be addressed by the clinician.

The following are factors to consider when assessing the aphasic person:

1. Are adequate clues available in the first attempted message to give information on content?
2. Are yes/no questions accurate?
3. Can the client indicate when his partner is "on the right track" in pursuit of a message?
4. Does the client expand beyond yes/no in response to questions?
5. Will the client voluntarily switch modalities when one is unsuccessful?
6. Does the client spontaneously use his best expressive modality?

The following are factors when considering the partner:

1. Does the partner make best use of the information given when seeking clarification?
2. When asking yes/no questions to clarify, is there a logical procession from general to specific?
3. Is the frequency of redundant questions appropriate for the client?
4. If the client does not spontaneously use an effective modality, does the partner request it?
5. Is the strategy of encouraging the aphasic person to continue or of asking for a repeat or elaboration likely to result in the aphasic person's giving relevant and intelligible information?

The factors that will facilitate successful communication between the aphasic person and his family differ radically from the conversational techniques of days gone by. No treatment plan can succeed unless the people who communicate with the client are taught how to adjust their own expectations and to benefit from compensatory strategies.

A Final Note

I take exception to the notion that a Wernicke's syndrome is less amenable to treatment than are other aphasias. While it may be shown eventually that more severe aphasias result from lesions in the superior temporal gyrus area, the Wernicke's behaviors themselves certainly can be managed in treatment. An effective treatment program needs to incorporate numerous styles of communication, all of which might be suggested by the aphasic person's characteristics and responses to treatment.

As a case in point, the client whose treatment program is partially described in this chapter improved from a 24th to 58th percentile overall on the Porch Index of Communicative Abilities[35] in six months of treatment, with treatment initiated two months after his stroke. More importantly, the quality of communication between himself and his family was greatly improved as judged by their reports and my observations. Perhaps because the direction of therapy follows the many paths of the client, work with a person with Wernicke's aphasia is much less predictable in its course than that with behaviors associated with more anteriorly placed lesions. This necessitates use of a much more comprehensive variety of clinical tasks and strategies.

Introspection on this issue revolves mostly around attempts to improve observation of client characteristics. Treatment of the person with Wernicke's aphasia is never easy, and sometimes may demand a greater degree of creativity and tolerance than treatment with our quieter, more plodding clients. With the extroverted, excessive, exceptionally off-task, and occasionally exhausting client, we may see ourselves more in a struggle to keep up and perhaps out of the way than in our preferred position as director of production.

For our clinical science to advance, we must continue our attempts to understand change in all our clients. For the advancement of individuals, we must continue to discover and establish the validity of whatever makes a difference — using the best of our knowledge, techniques, and creativity, regardless of the limitations of our insight as to precisely when and where we are able to influence meaningful change in this most puzzling but fascinating condition.

Suggested Readings

Darley, FL (1982). The treatment program. In FL Darley, (ed), *Aphasia* (pp. 237–278). Philadelphia: W. B. Saunders Co.

Davis, GA and Wilcox, MJ (1981). Incorporating parameters of natural conversation in aphasia treatment. In R. Chapey (ed.), *Language Intervention Strategies in Adult Aphasia* (pp. 169–193). Baltimore: Williams & Wilkins.

Rosenbek, JC, LaPointe, LL, Wertz, RT (1988). Treating auditory comprehension impairment. In JC Rosenbek, LL LaPointe and RT Wertz, *Aphasia: A Clinical Approach* (1989). Boston: College Hill Press.

Martin, D. (1981). Therapy with the jargonaphasic. In JW Brown (ed.), *Jargonaphasia* (pp. 305–326). New York: Academic Press.

References

1. Wernicke C: The aphasia symptom complex: A psychological study on an anotomic basis. In Eggert GH (trans): *Wernicke's Work on Aphasia: A Sourcebook and Review*. The Hague, Netherlands: Mouton, 1977.
2. Damasio A: The nature of aphasia: Signs and syndromes. In Sarno MT (ed.): *Acquired Aphasia*. (pp. 51–66). New York: Academic Press, 1981.
3. Benson F: *Aphasia, alexia, and agraphia*. New York: Churchill Livingstone, 1979.
4. Wertz RT: The state of the clinical art. In Holland AL (ed.): *Language Disorders in Adults*. San Diego: College Hill Press, 1984, pp. 1–78.
5. Wernicke C: Der aphasische symptomkomplex. Breslau: Kohn & Neigart, 1874.
6. Geschwind N: Carl Wernicke, the Breslau School and the history of aphasia. In Carterette EC (ed.):

Brain Function, Volume III: Speech, Language and Communication. Berkeley: University of California Press, 1963 pp. 1–16.

7. Geschwind N: (1967). Wernicke's contribution to the study of aphasia. *Cortex* 1967; 3:449–463.
8. Damasio H: (1981). Cerebral localization of the aphasias. In Sarno MT (ed.): *Acquired Aphasia.* New York: Academic Press, 1981, pp 27–50.
9. Chapman SB, Poole K: Comparison of language profiles and localized electrocortical dysfunction in aphasia. Paper presented at the Clinical Aphasiology Conference, Cape Cod, Massachusetts, 1988.
10. Selnes OA, Niccum NE, Rubens AB: CT scan correlates of recovery in auditory comprehension. In Brookshire RH (ed.): *Clinical Aphasiology: Conference Proceedings,* Minneapolis: BRK Publishers, pp 112–118, 1982.
11. Schuell H: Aphasic difficulties understanding spoken language. *Neurology* 1953; 3:176–184.
12. Nielsen JM: The unsolved problems in aphasia: II. Alexia resulting from a temporal lesion. *L. A. Neurological Soc* 1939; 5:78–84.
13. Fromm D, Holland AL, Swindell CS: Depression following left hemisphere stroke. In Brookshire RH (ed.): *Clinical Aphasiology: Conference Proceedings,* 1984. Minneapolis: BRK Publishers, pp 268–270.
14. DeRenzi E, Vignolo LA: The Token Test: A sensitive test to detect receptive disturbances in aphasics. *Brain* 1962; 85:665–678.
15. McNeil MR, Prescott TE: *Revised Token Test* Baltimore: University Park Press, 1978.
16. LaPointe LL, Horner J: The functional auditory comprehension task (FACT): Protocol and test format. *FLASHA Journal* 1978; pp. 27–33.
17. Holland AL: *Communicative Abilities in Daily Living.* Baltimore: Williams & Wilkens, 1980.
18. LaPointe LL, Holtzapple PA, Graham LF: The relationship among two measures of auditory comprehension and daily living communication skills. In Brookshire RH (ed.): *Clinical Aphasiology: Conference Proceedings,* 1985. Minneapolis: BRK Publishers, pp 38–46.
19. Waller M, Darley FL: The influence of context on the auditory comprehension of paragraphs by aphasic subjects. *J Speech Hear Res* 1978; 21:732–745.
20. Brookshire, RH, Nicholas LE: Comprehension of directly and indirectly pictured verbs by aphasic and nonaphasic listeners. In Brookshire RH (ed.): *Clinical Aphasiology: Conference Proceedings,* 1982. Minneapolis: BRK Publishers, pp 200–206.
21. Brookshire RH, Nicholas LE: Consistency of the effects of rate of speech on brain damaged subjects' comprehension of information in narrative discourse. In Brookshire RH (ed.): *Clinical Aphasiology: Conference Proceedings,* 1985. Minneapolis: BRK Publishers, pp 262–271.
22. Brookshire RH, Nicholas LE: Sentence verification and language comprehension of aphasic persons. In Brookshire RH (ed.): Clinical Aphasiology: Conference Proceedings, 1980. Minneapolis: BRK Publishers, pp 53–63.
23. Wilcox MJ, Davis GA, Leonard LL: Aphasics' comprehension of contextually conveyed meaning. *Brain and language,* 1978; 6:362–377.
24. Gardner H, Albert ML, Weintraub S: Comprehending a word: The influence of speed and redundancy on auditory comprehension in aphasia. *Cortex,* 1975; 11:155–162.
25. LaPointe LL, Horner J: *Reading Comprehension Battery for Aphasia.* Tigard, Oregon: CC Publications, 1979.
26. Bogdanoff M, Katz R: Modification of the Cloze procedure for measuring reading levels in aphasic adults. In Brookshire RH (ed.): *Clinical Aphasiology: Conference Proceedings,* 1983. Minneapolis: BRK Publishers.
27. Rosenbek JC, LaPointe LL, Wertz RT: Treating auditory comprehension impairment. In JC Rosenbek, LL LaPointe and RT Wertz: *Aphasia: A Clinical Approach.* Boston: College Hill Press (1989).
28. Martin D: Therapy with the jargonaphasic. In Brown JW (ed.): *Jargonaphasia.* New York: Academic Press, 1981, pp 305–326.
29. Brookshire RH: Auditory comprehension and aphasia. In Johns DF (ed.): *Clinical Management of Neurogenic Communicative Disorders.* Boston: Little, Brown, 1978, pp 103–128.
30. Loverso FL, Prescott TE: The effect of alerting signals on left brain damaged (aphasic) and normal subjects' accuracy and response time to visual stimuli. In Brookshire RH (ed.): *Clinical Aphasiology: Conference Proceedings,* 1981. Minneapolis: BRK Publishers, pp 55–67.
31. Doyle RJ, Holland AL: Clinical management of a patient with pure word deafness. In Brookshire RH (ed.): *Clinical Aphasiology: Conference Proceedings,* 1982. Minneapolis: BRK Publishers pp 138–146.
32. LaPointe LL: Base-10 programmed stimulation: Task specification, scoring, and plotting performance in aphasia therapy. *Journal of Speech and Hearing Disorders,* 1977; 42:90–105.
33. Davis GA, Wilcox MJ: Incorporating parameters of natural conversation in aphasia treatment. In

Chapey R. (ed.): *Language Intervention Strategies in Adult Aphasia.* Baltimore: Williams & Wilkins, 1981, pp 169–193.

34. Flowers CR, Peizer ER: Strategies for obtaining information from aphasic persons. In Brookshire RH (ed.): *Clinical Aphasiology: Conference Proceedings,* 1984. Minneapolis: BRK Publishers pp 106–113.

35. Porch BE: *Porch Index of Communicative Ability, vol. II: Administration, Scoring and Interpretation (revised ed.).* Palo Alto, California: Consulting Psychologists Press, 1971.

3

Conduction Aphasia

Nina N. Simmons

Introduction

In 1874 Carl Wernicke[1] hypothesized the existence of a distinct type of aphasia based on his neuroanatomic model of language localization in the brain. Thus, began the concept of conduction aphasia, not as a clinical entity, but as a predicted outcome of a lesion that disconnects the two primary speech centers. The first actual description of a patient with conduction aphasia was provided some years later.[2] Although numerous descriptions have appeared subsequently,[3-5] debate continues over the underlying mechanisms responsible for conduction aphasia. There does, however, appear to be agreement on the symptoms that define classic conduction aphasia. The major differentiating feature is a significant impairment of verbal repetition, which is disproportionate to the fluency of spontaneous speech, and relatively good auditory comprehension (Table 3–1). In addition, literal paraphasias and word retrieval problems appear in the context of the fluent, melodic speech. The condition has been considered rare relative to other aphasia types. Benson et al[6] estimated that between 5% and 10% of new aphasic patients admitted to their facility fit the classification of conduction aphasia.

Pathophysiology

The localization of the brain lesion associated with conduction aphasia has received substantial attention. The focus has been on identifying the neuroanatomic site of lesion through postmortem studies and brain imaging techniques, as well as developing anatomic models to explain symptoms.

Neuroanatomy

Computed tomography (CT) scan studies have reported lesions most frequently associated with the postrolandic areas of the left hemisphere.[7-10] In addition, there are reports of lesions compromising deep structures.[7,8,10] Based on a review of reported cases, Strub and Black[11] summarized two lesion sites most often associated with conduction aphasia. One involves the supramarginal gyrus and the arcuate fasciculus of the left hemisphere. The second involves damage to the insula, contigu-

Table 3-1. Comparison of General Characteristics of Broca's Aphasia and Apraxia of Speech with Conduction Aphasia

Broca's / Apraxia	Conduction
Nonfluent	Fluent
Dysprosody	Intact prosody (with self corrections; and word search)
Agrammatic	Preserved grammar
Comprehension good	Comprehension good
Repetition impaired proportionate to other verbal tasks	Repetition disproportionately impaired
Error recognition	Error recognition
Probably anomic	Probably anomic

ous auditory cortex, and underlying white matter of the left hemisphere. When Wernicke's area is involved in conduction aphasia, the lesion size appears smaller than that associated with Wernicke's aphasia.[12] In fact, Kertesz[13] concluded that the "lesions causing conduction aphasia are similar but smaller, and, at times, more anterior and inferior to those of Wernicke's aphasia" (p. 142).

The Disconnection Model

Wernicke's original hypothesis described conduction aphasia as a disconnection between the auditory "comprehension" region (Wernicke's area) and the speech "production" region (Broca's area.). According to the disconnection theory of conduction aphasia, the arcuate fasciculus is the probable site of damage.[14] This fiber tract connects Wernicke's area in the left temporal lobe with Broca's area in the left frontal lobe. Thus, an interruption in these connecting fibers might inhibit information received in an intact Wernicke's area from being transported anteriorly to an intact Broca's area for speech production. The sparing of Wernicke's and Broca's areas would account for relatively intact auditory comprehension and fluent, melodic speech production. On the other hand, the disconnection between the two speech centers would result in a disproportionate impairment in activities requiring the interaction of audition and production, such as verbal repetition. Also, phonemic paraphasias might result when the intact speech production area functions without the feedforward guidance from the auditory speech area.[15]

In support of an expansion of the disconnection model, Benson et al[6] reported conduction aphasia with lesion sites other than the arcuate fasciculus. Similar to earlier suggestions,[16,17] the authors postulated that in some cases the right temporal lobe assumes the role of auditory comprehension. Because the right temporal lobe is disconnected from the left hemisphere Broca's area, the symptoms of conduction aphasia are exhibited. Later, Mendez and Benson[18] reported three additional cases representing "atypical" lesion sites in support of the disconnection theory if the theory is expanded to include any interruption in circuits linking language comprehension and speech production.

The "Central Center" Model

Goldstein[5] disagreed with the proposal that the deficits in conduction aphasia were a result of two speech centers disconnected from each other. He attributed conduction or "central aphasia" to a disruption of a central center which was responsible for "inner speech." Inner speech would constitute a hypothetical way-station where auditory comprehension, speech production, and nonverbal mental processing meet. Green and Howes[19] reviewed the literature on site of lesion in conduction aphasia, and arrived at a conclusion similar to Goldstein's model of "central aphasia", suggesting that an area exists that integrates meaning and form of language. Thus, some have regarded the repetition deficit in conduction aphasia as one feature of a more general "central" language deficit.[5,19,20]

The Bimodal Distribution Model

Others have postulated that conduction aphasia results from damage along a continuum extending from Wernicke's area to Broca's area. Kertesz, Lesk, and McCabe[21] correlated radionucleide localization of infarcts with aphasia classification based on the Western Aphasia Battery[22] for 11 conduction patients. Consistent with earlier neuroanatomical reports, lesion location was primarily between Broca's and Wernicke's areas. However, there appeared to be variability in the degree of fluency, with the less fluent patients exhibiting more anterior lesions; those with higher fluency scores had more posterior lesions. In addition, four patients had lesions overlapping into Broca's area and four overlapping into Wernicke's area suggesting that conduction aphasia might not represent a discrete problem.

Kempler et al[23] studied ten conduction patients using positron emission tomography (PET) to measure glucose metabolism, and CT scans to assess structural lesion locus. Structural damage in the temporoparietal areas agreed with prior reports.[10] However, glucose metabolism was variable across patients. The authors proposed that variation in location of lesion along the perisylvian cortex accounted for variation in results, offering support for the "continuum" model.

Similarly, Levine and Calvanio[12] suggested that language is mediated by overlapping auditory and sensorimotor systems that comprise the perisylvian region from Wernicke's area to Broca's area. Conduction aphasia might result from damage anywhere along the continuum producing a repetition deficit as the invariable feature. "Patients with posterior lesions would have more fluent speech and poorer auditory speech comprehension . . . because of the relative predominance of neurons related more closely to auditory processing. . . . Patients with more anterior lesions would have less fluent speech . . ." (p. 105). In other words, the clinical picture in conduction aphasia might shift toward that of Broca's aphasia or that of Wernicke's aphasia depending on the locus of the lesion. This concept of a "bimodal distribution" of conduction aphasias representing a continuum of lesion locales between and overlapping the primary speech/language centers is attractive; it includes concepts of both the "central center" and disconnection models, yet allows for the variation in behavior observed among patients.

Canter, Trost, and Burns[15] combined aspects of these pathophysiological models with a linguistic model. They hypothesize that speech begins with a premotor stage where an item is retrieved in phonological form possibly as a sensory representation in Wernicke's area. The phonological pattern is then transmitted anteriorly via conduction fibers of the arcuate fasciculus to the anterior cortex. Since the arcuate fasiculus represents a complex multisynaptic and bidirectional tract, the authors suggest that it is likely that this area contributes to the actual processing as well as transmission. Broca's area then translates the received auditory pattern into a motor program or movement pattern. Conduction aphasia results from faulty transmission of the phonological form to the anterior cortex. The authors warn that "given the complex structure of the arcuate fasciculus, lesions at different loci might well be expected to produce different patterns of speech disturbance" (p. 219).

Nature and Differentiating Features

The label of conduction aphasia denotes an individual who speaks with good intonation and understands what others say, but has trouble retrieving words. He produces paraphasic errors that he recognizes and tries, though often abortively, to correct. While the hesitations and correction efforts might mimic nonfluent disorders, the combination of fluency, preserved melody, and variety and complexity of syntactic structures found in the spontaneous speech of conduction aphasia distinguish it from Broca's aphasia and apraxia of speech. Also, Benson et al[6] suggested that the use of many filler words with relatively few substantive words often discriminates these patients from Broca's aphasia. The preservation of auditory comprehension assists in distinguishing this disorder from Wernicke's aphasia, but the marked repetition deficit is a cardinal feature differentiating conduction aphasia from transcortical problems. The degree of reading and writing problems appears to vary from patient to patient. The primary criteria for diagnosis of conduction aphasia have been delineated by Benson et al[6] as follows:

1. Fluent, paraphasic conversational speech.
2. No significant difficulty in comprehension of normal conversation.
3. Significant verbal repetition disturbance.

Further Description of Salient Characteristics

FLUENCY

The term fluent aphasia has been used to describe "plentiful output (100 – 200 words per minute), easy production, good articulation, normal phrase length (averaging 5 – 8 words per phrase) and normal prosodic quality but a tendency to omit words (usually the meaningful, semantically significant words) plus an excessive number of paraphasias in some cases" (p. 22).[24] Although conduction aphasia is considered one of the fluent aphasias, hesitations and self-correction attempts necessarily interrupt the flow of otherwise fluent speech. Thus, the output is best described as fluent but not quite as fluent as that of Wernicke's aphasia.[25]

WORD FINDING

Difficulty in word retrieval is considered a prevalent aspect of the disorder[26] with problems primarily on substantive or content words.[6] Word finding failures result in paraphasic substitutions, hesitations to access words, circumlocution, or empty speech in which content words are deleted. Interestingly, Kertesz[13] has reported that some conduction aphasic subjects do quite well on naming subtests of the Western Aphasia Battery[22] suggesting variability across patients.

PARAPHASIAS

Phonemic or literal paraphasias appear to predominate in conduction aphasia[27] and are most evident on verbal repetition tasks.[28] It appears that semantic paraphasias or neologisms occur less frequently in the speech of conduction aphasia than among the other fluent aphasias.[28,29] Also, it has been reported that conduction aphasic speakers demonstrate more paraphasic errors and self-correction attempts on "target oriented" tasks (those requiring a forced choice of specific target words) than in open-ended tasks or conversation.[30]

Since the production of speech sound errors is a prevalent characteristic of conduction aphasia, Broca's aphasia, and apraxia of speech, the nature of the errors have been studied to aid in differential diagnosis and to clarify underlying mechanisms contributing to errors. It has been suggested, based on perceptual phonological analysis, that no significant differences exist among Broca's, Wernicke's, or conduction subjects in type of speech errors exhibited,[31] yet considerable evidence has accumulated to the contrary. For example, the errors in conduction aphasia have been differentiated as a product of phonological or linguistic deficit,[20,26,32,33] while the errors in apraxia of speech have been attributed to faulty programming of articulatory movement.[34-36] Table 3–2 summarizes results of several studies that analyzed speech errors of aphasic and verbally apraxic individuals. These studies appear to support the contention that the errors in conduction aphasia are attributable primarily to a linguistic or phonological processing deficit, while the Broca's aphasic patients evidence both phonological and phonetic deficits.

Relatedly, psycholinguistic models have been proposed to explain aphasic deficits.[37,38] For example, Kohn[38] analyzed phonemic errors associated with conduction aphasia during picture naming, and discussed the theoretical implications of her results. She attributed disruption in "pre-articulatory programming" (a linguistic process not to be confused with the later stage of articulatory motor programming) to a disruption between the *storage* of phonological representations in Wernicke's area

Table 3-2.   Comparison of Speech Sound Error Analysis Trends for Nonfluent Aphasia and Apraxia of Speech with Conduction or Fluent Aphasia

Nonfluent/Apraxia	Conduction/Fluent	Reference
Transitionalization or timing errors		Kent & Rosenbek, 1983; Canter, Trost and Burns, 1985
Voice onset time impaired	Voice onset time not impaired	Gandour & Dardaranada, 1984
Prevalence of substitutions	Prevalence of substitutions	Monoi et al 1983; Canter et al 1985
Substitutions differ from target by single feature	Substitutions differ by more than one feature	Monoi et al 1983; Nespoulous et al 1984
Intrusive vowels, prolongations, and artic. hiatuses	Transposition errors Sequencing errors Additions	Monoi et al 1983; Canter et al 1985; Kent and Rosenbek, 1982
Errors on word initiation	Errors toward end of word	Canter et al 1985
Primarily consonant errors	Vowel and consonant errors	Monoi et al 1983

and the coding of articulatory motor commands or programs in the frontal lobe. Thus, the paraphasic errors in conduction aphasia are distinguished from the articulatory errors of the anterior patients. Furthermore, because the errors of fluent subjects reflect disorganization at a premotor stage, errors show a trend toward more random phonemic behavior than that seen in nonfluent individuals.[15,30,39]

The phonetic nature of errors in apraxia of speech and Broca's aphasia, as distinguished from a linguistic deficit, has been further supported by acoustic and physiological studies which attribute errors to a breakdown in the timing of voicing and articulation.[40-45] For example, Kent and Rosenbek[44] attributed errors in apraxia of speech to faulty "transitionalization" or impairment in the timing of articulations for a given sound or given transition between sounds. Gandour and Dardarananda[46] found a severe impairment of voice onset time (VOT) in nonfluent aphasia (global and Broca's) yet minimal impairment in VOT for fluent aphasia including conduction and Wernicke's patients. Furthermore, the data from many of these studies suggest that many apraxic errors perceived by the "naked ear" as substitutions are actually phonetic distortions. Thus, perceptual analysis using broad transcription approaches, such as that used by Blumstein,[31] might fail to distinguish "phonetic" error types of anterior patients from "phonological" error types of posterior patients. Although the phonetic versus phonological debate might appear to be excessive, the distinction bears considerable relevance to the focus and design of treatment programs. For example, use of linguistic cues versus articulatory cues might be differentially effective depending on the nature of the errors.

ERROR RECOGNITION

Kohn[38] compared the "conduite d'approche" or sequences of self-correction attempts of individuals diagnosed with conduction, Wernicke's, and Broca's aphasia. She found that conduction patients appear to recognize their errors much more frequently but are no more successful than Broca's or Wernicke's subjects in actually correcting the errors.

While the conduction aphasic individual's attempts at self-correction result in hesitations and what might appear to be nonfluent episodes in the context of otherwise fluent speech, the behavior appears qualitatively different from the struggle and groping behavior of verbally apraxic speakers. The nonverbal posturing and timing errors of apraxia of speech are not typical of the conduction aphasic person's self-correction attempts.

REPETITION

The most discriminating feature of conduction aphasia is the significant impairment in repetition. Since several aphasia types show marked repetition difficulty, affixing the label of conduction aphasia based solely on faulty repetition would result in many mistaken diagnoses. For this reason, definitions of conduction aphasia invariably include some reference to repetition as a "disproportionate" impairment. Thus, there is a marked discrepancy between repetition and spontaneous speech production in conduction aphasia. Conversely, repetition is equivalent to performance on other verbal tasks in apraxia of speech, Broca's aphasia, and Wernicke's aphasia.

While repetition problems in conduction aphasia might occur on single words, usually the difficulty is most evident on repetition of phrases, short sentences, polysyllabic words, and unfamiliar phrases.[6] Errors tend to increase as the length and unfamiliarity of the material increases. Errors in repetition are often paraphasic or a rewording or paraphrase of the target.[6] Goodglass and Kaplan[26] suggest that number repetition might be preserved in conduction aphasia or, if impaired, take the form of word substitutions rather than literal paraphasia.

As noted previously, the classic theory of conduction aphasia attributes the repetition deficit to a disconnection between auditory and verbal systems. Others have attributed the repetition deficit to a specific impairment of memory rather than a more general language deficit. For example, selective impairment of auditory–verbal short-term memory has been designated the culprit causing the repetition deficit by some.[47-50] Heilman, Scholes, and Watson[51] disagree with the contention that faulty repetition is due to memory deficit. They found that both conduction and Broca's aphasic subjects repeat poorly on tests of immediate memory, and their "inability to repeat probably accounts for the immediate memory defect, rather than the opposite as postulated by Warrington and colleagues" (p. 205).

Other explanations for the repetition deficit include a specific impairment of memory for sequences[52] and an interruption between phonological processing and phonemic encoding, a neurolinguistic explanation consistent with the disconnection hypothesis.[53]

AUDITORY COMPREHENSION

By definition the comprehension of the individual with conduction aphasia is usually characterized as normal or near normal.[6] However, clinical experience suggests that patients frequently fail to fit into our neat definitions; thus, it is not unusual to find conduction aphasic individuals who exhibit some impairment in the auditory modality. Such is the case as a "jargon aphasia" begins to improve in the direction of conduction aphasia. Also it has been suggested that, while conduction aphasic individuals show good comprehension of lexical information,[54,55] they display difficulty understanding syntax.[54,56,57] Conversely, McCarthy and Warrington[58] found satisfactory performance by two individuals on a test of syntactic and semantic sentence comprehension.

READING

There has been controversy as to the exact nature of the reading deficit in conduction aphasia. Benson et al[6] reported good reading comprehension but paraphasic oral reading. Levine and Calviano[12] suggested that reading comprehension is relatively preserved and reading aloud less paraphasic than repetition. Green and Howe[19] reported mild to moderate oral reading impairment in conduction aphasia. Caramazza et al[50] reported a single case with no difficulty in oral reading of words and sentences. Sullivan, Fisher, and Marshall[59] also reported a case of conduction aphasia in which the "visual–verbal system" necessary for oral reading was minimally impaired. Rothi, McFarling and Heilman[60] observed in three cases that the patient could read major lexical items, but failed to comprehend when meaning depended on syntax. Possibly the degree of oral reading and comprehension deficit correlates more with the site and extent of the lesion producing conduction aphasia than with the label of conduction aphasia per se.

ASSOCIATED PROBLEMS

Frequently reported associated problems include oral and limb apraxia, parietal lobe signs, and right sensory impairment.[6,26] Mendez and Benson[18] reported facial and limb apraxia in cases involving lesions of the parietal operculum, but not in patients with involvement primarily of Wernicke's area. Poncet, Habib and Robillard[61] associated bilateral ideomotor apraxia with some cases of conduction aphasia.

PROGNOSIS

Based on a review of the literature, Davis[62] summarized that "Broca's and conduction aphasias demonstrate the largest amount of recovery" (p. 236). Similarly, Kertesz[13] reported a favorable spontaneous recovery pattern associated with conduction aphasia. Anecdotally, Benson et al[6] reported "the conditions of most of these patients improve, returning to near-normal levels" (p.339). It is probable that patients presenting with conduction aphasia immediately postonset might show significant or even complete recovery. Other conduction aphasia patients appear to "evolve" from classifications such as "jargon aphasia" or Wernicke's aphasia. The "evolved" conduction aphasias might be expected to exhibit more residual language deficit because the initial presentation tends to involve more severe aphasia symptoms, and probably more extensive brain lesions.

Barring serious complications, even the patient with residual conduction aphasia frequently becomes a functional communicator. Because of the relatively good auditory comprehension, fairly copious verbal output, and an ability to supplement speech with gestural, melodic, and facial information, these patients tend to function well in situations that do not require single-word accuracy or specific responses. In fact, information can be quite colorfully conveyed by a choice paraphasia that is perfectly inflected to transmit appropriate emotion, and is embedded in a context revealing a perfectly clear intent. What is there not to understand about "Oh no, not more MacDonald's Damburgers?". Furthermore, treatment which is appropriately designed and delivered should improve the outcome in such patients.

Evaluation

The first step toward appropriate treatment is appropriate evaluation. The major purposes of evaluation are (1) to aid the clinician in distinguishing aphasia from other neuropathologies of communication, (2) to provide information for classifying the aphasic individual according to type of aphasia, (3) to determine severity and predict outcome, (4) to provide direction in treatment planning, and (5) to measure recovery of communicative function and the patient's response to treatment. Because there is ample literature available to guide the clinician in the evaluation of aphasia[62-65] the following thoughts will serve merely as a supplement to highlight aspects relevant to conduction aphasia. Using the diagnosis of conduction aphasia to illuminate areas of concentration does not preclude assessment of individual strengths and weaknesses. Applying a label merely lights the stage whereupon one must look at, listen to, and evaluate the individual player.

Critical areas used to distinguish conduction aphasia from other aphasia syndromes include measurement of auditory comprehension, verbal repetition, confrontation naming, and spontaneous speech production. Most of the formal aphasia batteries include some aspect of these skills. In addition, supplemental measures are frequently employed to assist in classifying, planning treatment, and monitoring recovery.[66]

Formal Tests

The Boston Diagnostic Aphasia Examination (BDAE)[26] and the Western Aphasia Battery (WAB)[22] are two broadly based aphasia tests that provide approaches to traditional aphasia classification. The BDAE uses a subjective rating scale including parameters of melodic line or intonational contour, phrase length (defined as the longest uninterrupted word run), articulatory agility, grammatical form, paraphasia in running speech, and word finding. The pattern of deficits on this scale can be compared to typical profiles for each aphasia classification. The WAB employs a numerical taxonomy to classify patients with aphasia. According to Kertesz,[13] WAB test scores in the areas of fluency, auditory comprehension, verbal repetition, and naming can be used to "unequivocally" classify all aphasics. Unfortunately, experience would suggest that no aphasia test can lay claim to such a declaration. It is the clinician's judgment that ultimately must intercede in this process.

Other formal aphasia tests are useful in evaluating conduction patients as well. The highly standardized Porch Index of Communicative Ability (PICA)[67] provides useful test-retest information and predictive data, and offers excellent intermodality performance comparisons to assist in the planning of treatment. However, since the repetition subtest of the PICA is insufficient to draw attention to the problems of the conduction aphasic person, supplemental repetition testing will be required.

Supplemental Measures

AUDITORY COMPREHENSION

Since classic conduction aphasic individuals show relatively good auditory comprehension, additional testing is often required to isolate problems. For example, formal tests rarely evaluate syntactic comprehension, yet research suggests the potential for problems in this area.[54,57] Also tasks requiring retention of directions of increasing length aid in identifying short-term auditory memory deficits among these patients. Available tests such as the Token tests[68-70] or the Auditory Comprehension Test for Sentences (ACTS)[71] might prove contributory. Finally, in cases of mild to moderate aphasia, asking the client to describe problems can be remarkably helpful.

REPETITION

Repetition testing should target areas known to be affected in conduction aphasia, such as multisyllable words and low probability of occurrence phrases and words. Repetition subtests of the BDAE and the BDAE Supplementary Language Tests are particularly relevant since items were selected with conduction aphasia in mind. In addition, the influence of cues or prompts on repetition performance should be studied to aid in planning treatment.

WORD RETRIEVAL

Although confrontation naming is often considered the epitome of word retrieval testing, more comprehensive assessment of this area is generally needed for designing effective treatment. Measurement of word retrieval should focus on the severity of the deficit, types of words affected, types of errors, strategies used for repair, and potential word retrieval facilitators. The Boston Naming Test[72] has been used as an in-depth measure of confrontation naming in aphasia. It is useful for assessing the influence of word frequency and the facilitory effects of semantic and phonemic cues on naming in conduction aphasia. In addition, sampling word retrieval for word types other than nouns and in tasks other than labeling pictures is suggested.

Analysis of word retrieval error patterns and revision strategies also can assist with treatment planning. Systems have been proposed that help categorize word retrieval behavior.[73] For example, speech samples might be analyzed for the following types of problems: (1) use of a filled or unfilled pause or delay, (2) use of semantically related word(s) or semantic paraphasia, (3) phonemic or literal paraphasia, (4) circumlocution or describing something about the intended word, and (5) using a general or empty word such as "thing" in place of a target word. Furthermore, assessment of word retrieval in the context of spontaneous speech will offer information on functional communication performance.

INTERMODALITY COMPARISONS

Particularly revealing is the comparison of performance across modalities with tasks equated for difficulty and content. For example, Wener and Duffy[74] administered the Token Test, the Reporter's Test[75] (the verbal counterpart of the Token Test), and an Imitator's Test (a verbal repetition counterpart of the Token Test) to compare performance across auditory comprehension, verbal expression, and verbal repetition. Others have administered a graphic form of the Token Test to allow comparison of reading and auditory comprehension.[76] Such intermodality comparisons would appear particularly relevant to conduction aphasia due to the dissociation of performance across modes.

SPONTANEOUS SPEECH SAMPLES

Sampling spontaneous speech is critical in the evaluation of the individual with conduction aphasia. Spontaneous speech will serve as the medium for assessing fluency and serve as the standard against which to contrast repetition. Observation of language use without the constraints imposed in controlled situations allows the clinician to determine the patient's use of strategies and compare communication success to language accuracy. Moreover, sampling various types of connected speech is important in light of research which suggests that these patients perform differently in "open ended" tasks as opposed to "target oriented" or structured situations.[30] In addition, it has been shown that aphasic individuals tend to show variations in performance across different social contexts, topics, and tasks.[77] Thus, samples should include measures of social communication, possibly including several contexts, as well as more structured tasks, such as picture descriptions, question answer formats, barrier activities (i.e., describing a picture or object not visible to the listener), narratives (i.e., describing an event), or role playing.

Suitable methods of measuring the spontaneous speech of individuals with conduction aphasia are numerous. Subjective rating scales such as the Profile of Speech Characteristics from the Boston Diagnostic Aphasia Examination, or the fluency and information content scales used on the Western Aphasia Battery can be employed independent of the formal test. Judgments of the degree of success in communicating an idea can be used instead of traditional measures of response "accuracy." More objective measures might consist of actual frequency counts of specific error types, measures of response speed, or counts of content units. For example, Yorkston and Beukelman[78] provide efficiency "norms" for judging the amount of information conveyed per minute during a picture description task. Similarly Linebaugh[79] compares number of syllables per content unit used for "cookie theft" picture descriptions (BDAE[26]) to averages for normal (4.8), geriatric (5.7) and mild aphasic (6.3) speakers. Bernstein-Ellis, Wertz, and Shubitowski[80] elaborated on Yorkston and Beukelman's procedure for scoring content units in connected speech; they provide guidelines for scoring content units and an adapted PICA scoring system to be used with high-level aphasic patients. Another approach is to measure the number of occurrences of specific error types in spontaneous speech. For example, Golper et al[81] tallied the number of revised phrases and words, use of noncontent filler words, and phoneme errors used by aphasic speakers.

More comprehensive analysis of connected speech might take the form of phonological process analysis[31,82] as an approach to analyzing phonemic paraphasias, or discourse analysis as a means of identifying problems in verbal or written expression that are not apparent at the sentence level of analysis. Discourse analysis might focus on features such as organization, amount, complexity, efficiency, or cohesiveness of information conveyed.

CLINICAL PROBES

Finally, the use of clinical probes or individually designed "tests" is an essential approach for determining relative "power" of various stimuli, accumulating baseline and progress data on specific activities, and assessing the individual's personal hierarchy of task difficulty. Particularly relevant to this population are probes designed to determine the best facilitators of accurate word retrieval and the most successful self-correction strategies.

NONVERBAL TESTS

To identify disorders frequently associated with conduction aphasia, evaluation of praxis is suggested. Many clinicians use nonstandard measures of oral and limb praxis to assess this aspect. In addition, the Supplementary Nonlanguage Tests of the BDAE could prove useful in assessing limb apraxia and parietal lobe symptoms.

Treatment

Like the mating ritual of the albatross, treatment for aphasia can range from quick and productive, to protracted and disappointing. Of particular importance in achieving a productive outcome is an understanding of the purpose and rationale of treatment. The treatment of conduction aphasia shares the general goals common to the treatment of all aphasic individuals. Treatment is designed to (1) stimulate disrupted processes to promote functional reorganization, (2) teach the use of compensatory strategies to communicate in the face of residual deficits, (3) provide education and counseling to promote adjustment of the patient and family, (4) eliminate "bad habits" that interfere with successful communication, and (5) promote a suitable communication environment. Treatment is a dynamic, organized process that facilitates recovery of language function. The clinician identifies those conditions or variables which maximize language performance, then programs therapy to manipulate events which stimulate reorganization and functional recovery. Thus, the concept of treating the underlying processes as opposed to a superficial focus on a series of tasks insures more generalized improvement.[62]

It might be useful to distinguish, at least theoretically, between stimulation treatment to build language processes and direct compensation training to "teach" alternate ways of communicating. For example treatment might be directed at improving the word retrieval process of the person *and* at teaching the person how to use circumlocution effectively when he cannot "find" the word. While the distinction is frequently blurred, it points up the practicality of integrating concepts of stimulation therapy with principles of learning theory.

Finally, it is important to view treatment as a progression towards the ultimate goal of more functional communication. Thus, an overall hierarchy or plan of treatment should be designed to identify where to start in treatment, where to end (long term goals), and what steps to follow in the interim. As Rosenbek[83] observes "the consummate clinician prepares for the end of treatment simultaneously with planning its beginning (p. 319). For further discussion of philosophical foundations and general treatment principles, the reader is referred to Duffy,[84] LaPointe[85] and Brookshire.[86]

Treatment Principles

General principles of aphasia management dictate that treatment should be flexible, organized, relevant, intensive, successful, and efficient. *Organized* treatment implies that there is an overall plan that is designed to build systematically toward an end goal. It implies the need to identify a hierarchy of treatment tasks that reflects individual difficulty levels and accounts for variables known to influence the individual's responses. *Relevant* means not only choosing stimuli that bear some practical importance to the individual, but also choosing activities that show a direct relationship to the goal. *Flexible* suggests that the session should "go with the patient" not vice versa. For example, management of an aphasia therapy session has been likened to a pro tennis match.[87] The player approaches the game with a "game plan" given a thorough knowledge of the opponents strengths and weaknesses; while on the court, however, the plan is adjusted and modified to "play" to the opponent's performance at the time. Thus, the "winning" clinician approaches a session with a well-conceived, organized plan tailored to the individual, sometimes to be diverted skillfully onto other paths following the patient's lead. Sessions should provide *successful* experiences of sufficient *intensity* and frequency to promote change. Finally the *efficient* session is one that allows intensive stimulation and practice with the least reliance on clinician control, yet maximum success for the patient.

Session Organization

The treatment session follows a general framework[84,86] involving an initial period of adjustment possibly consisting of conversation to find out "what's been happenin'."

The patient's mood, energy level, and relevant news can be important determinants of the direction of the session. From here, one can move to easy warm-up activities, slowly increase the difficulty of activities, and finally ease off into relatively simple cool down activities. Sessions should conclude on a successful note.

Basic to this format is an understanding of the task hierarchy concept. This is a method of organizing therapy tasks which slowly increase in difficulty level by small steps until the clinician fades control, and the patient has increased his level of independent performance.[88] Thus, therapy activities begin where the patient can function successfully; they evolve out of an understanding of what makes a response easier or more difficult, and they evolve out of an understanding of the many variables affecting the patient's performance. There are inumerable variables that can be manipulated to help the aphasic client produce a communication response.[84,85,89] For example, Table 3–3 lists some of the more popular choices in the area of word retrieval and repetition. It is the clinician's job to determine what is

Table 3–3.   Variables that Might Influence Word Retrieval in Conduction Aphasia

Modality of stimulus (auditory, visual, gestural, graphic)
Modality of response (verbal, written, gesture, drawing)
Unimodal vs. combined modes
Frequency of occurrence of target word or phrase
Syntactic complexity
Word type (noun, verb, etc.)
Concrete vs. abstract
Semantic category (food, numbers etc.)
Open-ended vs. target specific response
Imagery
Similarity of response choices given
Number of response choices given
Length of word, phrase, sentence
Meaning of word
Temporal relationships of stimulus and response
Association "power" of stimulus
Personal relevance
Emotional content
Physical characteristics of stimulus
Length of exposure time to stimulus
Sequence of treatment tasks
Divergent vs. convergent
Functionality or realism
Type of feedback
Type of cues
    Within modality
    Through another mode
Contextual influences
    Setting
    Attitudes
    Roles of interactants
    Concurrent activity
    Intent or purpose of communication
    Pragmatic/discourse requirements
    Emotional context
    Internal context (knowledge, motivation, interest, fatigue)

more or less powerful in influencing the individual. Then the variables can be used in an organized fashion to precede a response to make the task less difficult, or follow an error response as a "correction cue." The easy tasks must build toward promoting performance of "harder" tasks to ultimately work towards functional communication. Important parameters to consider in the choice of treatment tasks and manipulating difficulty include the stimulus and response modality, the number of items in the field, the time interval between the stimulus and response, the rate and manner of stimulus presentation, the number and sequence of trials, and the type of cues or prompts to be used.

Interestingly, most of the cues or variables described in the aphasia literature are confined to those that are directly related to the specific linguistic stimulus and response. The broader realm of setting context and pragmatic variables has been recognized only recently as powerful influences.[90] For example, the framework of a session described above might imply that the setting, interactants, and sequence of activities are held constant, while only the linguistic variables are manipulated to achieve language recovery. This, in fact, is erroneous. As the client improves in the structure of the clinic room, other variables, such as unfamiliar listeners, new environments, should be introduced and incorporated into the hierarchy (while maintaining the overall format of easy–difficult–easy) to gradually work toward natural communication.

A final word on choosing tasks. It is important that the clinician avoid becoming too "task bound"; that is, viewing treatment as a sequence of tasks rather than recognizing how the activity taps the underlying deficits which are to be remediated. Davis[90] warns that tasks must be designed with some knowledge or hypothesis about the underlying process which is disrupted. For example, if one believes that a short-term memory deficit produces the repetition problem in conduction aphasia, then treatment might focus on tasks felt to improve or compensate for auditory–verbal memory rather than focus on language treatment per se.

Measurement of Progress

The clinician must determine what will constitute acceptable performance and how this will be measured. Perhaps the easiest way to identify appropriate tasks, know when to diverge, or know when to move forward, is to score each response using a system such as PICA scores and the Base-10 format.[85] Parameters identified as relevant to the individual's communication goals, such as measures of success versus accuracy, speed of response, or efficiency, might also be monitored.

Feedback

Feedback should be relevant, specific, positive, and immediate. General encouragement should foster the client's motivation and build communication confidence. Aphasic individuals deserve ongoing information on test results, daily scores, and progress. In addition, the type and manner of feedback relative to specific responses can greatly influence how a person responds in treatment. Feedback for specific errors should be directed at facilitating a correction rather than emphasizing or describing the error. In fact, numerous errors suggest a need to alter the requirements of the activity or to slip in preventative cues. Reinforcement should promote a relaxed, communicative atmosphere; a monotonous, hollow series of "good job" is boring at best. Humor and variety will not only add life to the session, but foster a more realistic environment.

In addition to feedback delivered by the clinician, patients will no doubt receive most of their consequences for communication behavior from others, such as family members and friends. It is helpful for the clinician to attempt to determine how such feedback is influencing the patient's response to treatment. For example, if the clinician has encouraged gestural self cues to facilitate word retrieval, yet the family considers this behavior annoying and weird, it is unlikely that the strategy will be as efficient as desired.

Education and Counseling

Relatedly, a major issue that must be addressed early on and continue throughout treatment is counseling and educating the client and family. This should include:

1. A general discussion of characteristics of brain damage, possibly with relevant literature and referral to outside sources such as stroke clubs or support groups.
2. Facts on the nature of the disorder with specifics about what is wrong and what is right with the patient.
3. Information on goals and expectations, which includes the aphasic person's input in goal setting and treatment planning.
4. Acquiring information on family interaction, and how their strategies promote or hinder communication.
5. Direct family training in ways to facilitate communication, such as recognizing when to allow the patient more time to elaborate or when to stop and ask for clarification.

Specific Treatment Approaches

With a broad understanding of aphasia treatment principles and procedures, those approaches that have shown particular utility for conduction aphasia can be defined.

Auditory Comprehension

Although auditory comprehension is not by definition a classic characteristic of conduction aphasia, obviously if an auditory comprehension problem exists, this modality should be considered a target of treatment. Traditional point to and direction following task continuums can be employed with sentence or word length, syntactic complexity, rate of speech, field, stimulus–response interval, redundancy, etc. systematically manipulated to build responses. High-level activities, such as comprehension of complex information or listening with a distracting background, might be appropriate also. Listening tactics, such as asking for repeats, simplifications, or pauses, can be taught as compensatory measures. More extensive descriptions of auditory comprehension treatment are available elsewhere.[91]

Verbal Repetition

Unlike the treatment of other aphasia types, therapy for conduction aphasia does not include verbal imitation as a powerful technique in deblocking access to spoken words. Because repetition is a primary deficit, it becomes a target of treatment rather than an approach to treatment. Although proficiency in repeating after other people is not a particularly useful skill, as verbal repetition improves other behaviors (such as successful self-correction and word retrieval) follow suit. One study[92] proposed that treatment of repetition and word retrieval might be interrelated in conduction aphasia suggesting that maximum improvement might be gained by targeting both areas in treatment.

Focusing therapy on verbal imitation involves (1) determining the level at which repetition begins to deteriorate, (2) determining the influences of such variables as word length, frequency of occurrence, phonemic complexity and part of speech, and (3) determining what facilitates the client's verbal repetition. For instance, in spite of problems in reading aloud, repetition is frequently facilitated when the written words are provided. Utilizing the task continuum approach, difficulty is altered by varying the length or complexity of the words or phrases, speaking the word in unison with the patient, "priming" the system by using the stimulus in other tasks prior to repetition work, enforcing delays (and even "filled" delays) between the spoken word and the patient's response, and varying syntactic complexity. In some cases, the repetition deficit seems incredibly resistent to our best efforts; obviously in these situations attention is redirected to more functional areas.

Word Retrieval

Activities that provide practice of word retrieval under facilitory conditions (e.g., using word association, high imagery pictures, written cues, gesture cues) and systematically increase the demand for "independent" word finding should improve the process of retrieving words. An infinite variety of tasks are suitable for this sort of program. For example, Table 3–4 provides several examples of tasks based on word association.

Table 3–4.   A Sample of Verbal Word Retrieval Tasks of Varying Association Strength

Task	Example
1. Paired associates	"Shoes and _____."
2. Contrastive associates	"Hot and _____."
3. Complete a spoken sentence with the written word provided.	"You drive a _____." (Show written word CAR.)
4. Complete a spoken sentence with a picture provided.	"You drive a _____." (Show picture of car.)
5. Complete a spoken sentence.	"You drive a _____."
6. Answer a structured question.	"What do you drive?"
7. Answer a question.	"You drive this. What do you call it?"
8. Answer a low-association question.	"What do you call this?" (Show picture of car.)
9. Semantic category	Name a mode of transportation.

Similarly, Helm-Estabrooks, Emery, and Albert[93] use strategies known to influence responses for individual clients to build a hierarchy of semantic categories and to promote nonperseverative responding on word retrieval tasks. They report favorable results of the approach called Treatment of Aphasic Perseveration Program (TAP) with one conduction aphasia patient.

In choosing word retrieval facilitators, one might wish to consider previous discussions related to the source of paraphasic errors. If we attribute errors to limited access to the lexion, then semantic cues might prove most powerful in eliciting target words. On the other hand phonetic, timing, and "facial" posture cues would probably prove more helpful when errors are articulatory in nature. Interestingly, research shows that phonemic cues (producing the initial sound) are usually less powerful cues for conduction patients than they are with the "anterior" aphasias[94]; however, initial phoneme cues appear to be more powerful cues for conduction aphasia than for Wernicke's patients.[27,94]

When specific cues prove successful in facilitating word recall in treatment, the patient can often learn to use or elaborate on these facilitators as self-cueing strategies. For example, if clinician-provided word associations ("drive a _____ ") or gestures (pantomime driving) promote word recall, the patient should be taught to use these in natural situations to assist with word finding. Similarly, the patient who recognizes a paraphasic error and compounds the error on repeated self-correction attempts, might redirect efforts to finding an associated word (what do I do with this?) or producing a gestural self cue. Since additional information is often communicated in the process, the self cue also serves to augment communication when word retrieval fails.

Although most word retrieval programs focus at the single word level, it is important to recognize the need to "find" words within and communicate at the sentence level. Productive circumlocution is an approach to compensating for failure to retrieve specific words in conversation. The purpose is to maintain the flow of conversation while preserving the communicative content. The patient is taught to talk around the inaccessible word purposefully though efficiently rather than dwell on trying to access it. Improvement can be measured in terms of the degree of success and the efficiency of conveying ideas.

Another approach to treatment of word finding deficits has been discussed in terms of improving "divergent" word retrieval.[95] Most traditional word-retrieval programming emphasizes "convergent" naming; that is accessing a preselected target word, such as naming a pictured object or filling in an incomplete sentence. Divergent tasks are designed to stimulate the ability to provide a variety of alternate words or concepts. For example, one might think of as many items in a given category (e.g., foods) as possible. Facilitators such as using visual imagery (e.g., imagine walking through the grocery store) can be provided to expand the behavior. Linebaugh[79,96] suggests a "lexical focus" approach, which involves divergent naming of progressively narrower categories (food, fruits, citrus fruits). Similar to Wepman's[97] thought-centered therapy, the process can be broadened to approximate the creative requirements of natural communication by providing open-ended topics or questions for the individual to elaborate on (e.g., What do you think about non-smoking policies in office buildings?).

While people with conduction aphasia show most difficulty with convergent or target-specific tasks, practice in divergent retrieval assists in effectively substituting acceptable alternative words when the target is inaccessible. This approach also seems to stimulate more creativity, flexibility, and generativity. Kearns[98] applied the concept of divergent processing in Response Elaboration Training (RET), a program designed to build more elaborate conversational content. Subsequently, Kearns and Potechin[99] demonstrated that RET was successful in improving the number of content words conveyed in a verbal picture description task with a conduction aphasic individual.

Sentence Production

Although circumlocutory or divergent strategies assist in promoting successful communication, another approach might sometimes be necessary to counter these patient's tendency to "overtalk." The patient with conduction aphasia uses a variety of grammatic and syntactic structures and an abundance of words, but often, in the barrage of fluent speech, the good gets lost in the bad. Thus, treatment might need to target production of specific responses such as verbalization of a specific sentence structure [such as, "the (noun) is (verbing)"] using whatever variables assist in production. For instance, the patient might read each word of a sentence, or form a sentence given a noun, with the goal of *controlling* fluency, reducing occurrences of nonproductive verbalizations, and avoiding unsuccessful self-corrections. Judicious use of pauses and slow rate inhibit the tendency to launch furiously into verbiage. Instead of using "stop strategies" requiring exclamations of "slow down," "think," or other equally annoying reminders, the clinician might employ pacing or use gestural accompaniment as a form of stop strategy. Pointing to each word as it is spoken or using a pacing board to slow the rate allows processing pauses and focuses attention. When the patient successfully formulates structured sentences, the stop strategies can be incorporated into more extended verbalization, such as picture description, answering questions, and other open-ended tasks. During these activities, awareness that vague responses are as noncommunicative as errors can be fostered; however, it is important that the individual is ready for this type of approach. It would be unwise to inhibit fluency and circumlocutory strategies without a foundation of retrieval potential.

In a similar format, Bernstein-Ellis, Wertz, and Shubitowski[80] reported a single case study of a mildly aphasic individual described as fluent with frequent hesitations, revisions, and paraphasias. They employed a pacing board[100] as a "delay" strategy to slow the speaking rate and eliminate "noncontent" words, such as fillers (uh, er) and incomplete revisions in connected speech. After pacing treatment their subject spoke slower and required fewer verbalizations to convery more information. The occurrence of syntax errors and paraphasias was also reduced.

Reading and Writing

Treating the person with conduction aphasia covers all areas of deficit including reading and writing. These areas are treated within the structure of language therapy; therefore, stimulus items used on reading comprehension tasks might be carried over into verbal and writing activities to "prime" the system for responses later in the session. Short words and phrases from repetition and word retrieval work can be incorporated into copying and writing tasks to minimize the need for "shifting." Reading and writing tasks are also excellent choices for homework and independent computer practice. As in the verbal realm, such activities might focus on accuracy as well as success and efficiency. For example, progress might be measured in terms of the time it takes to comprehend a paragraph or write a note, as well as the correctness of responses. Treatment of the graphic mode reflects the same orientation as that used in the treatment of the auditory verbal channel; therefore, further discussion here would be redundant.

Facilitory Channels

VERBAL CUES

As noted previously, there are numerous types of verbal prompts available to facilitate word retrieval with aphasic patients. For example, word association has been used in a variety of formats, such as sentence completions (cup of _____), opposites (hot and _____) and semantic association (giving a synonym).

Roberts and Wertz[101] reported successful application of a program called the Texas Contrastive Language Series (TACS) to improve spontaneous speech production in a case of conduction aphasia. The program is based on the use of semantic contrasts to facilitate sentence production. It consists of several phases designed hierarchically from a preparation stage in which the client is primed with auditory and graphic presentations of stimuli, followed by verbal imitation of a sentence (such as, "the door is open"), with subsequent production of a "contrasted" sentence ("the door is closed"). Their results appear to support the observation[102] that using "opposites" training is superior to using general semantic or rhyming association for persons with posteriorly-based aphasia.

VISUAL CUES

In spite of impairment in reading comprehension or oral reading, graphic cues often prove helpful in strengthening access to desired responses. Reports indicate that oral reading tasks improve word productions in some cases of conduction aphasia.[103,104] Initially providing written cues during verbal language tasks, then slowly fading the written cues, seems to help. Perhaps shifting some responsibility for accessing words to another system and practicing at this level alters response patterns somehow. Using a single-subject treatment study, Sullivan, Fisher and Marshall[59] attempted to test the hypothesis that a relatively intact "visual–verbal system should assist in reorganizing the auditory–verbal system in conduction aphasia. They reported that their subject's verbal repetition of treatment stimuli was improved by using oral reading. For one conduction patient reported by Boyle,[105] a treatment program using oral reading to "reorganize" connected speech resulted in fewer paraphasias and slower rate of speech on picture descriptions.

GESTURAL CUES

Gesture has proven to be a useful channel with some conduction aphasia patients. Although these patients often exhibit limb apraxia and may not spontaneously use symbolic or creative gestures, this modality can be strengthened and incorporated into treatment to facilitate word recall. The best approach probably involves building fast and accurate recognition and production of symbolic gestures (such as, Amerind signs[106]) by structuring tasks around pictures of sign production, written word, and sentence cues, by producing the sign in response to spoken or written words or questions, and finally by including the sign in verbal expressive tasks. Initial practice of gestures without encouraging simultaneous verbal responses often reduces useless or "empty" verbiage. When used to facilitate verbal output, gestures seem to help direct the listener's and the speaker's attention to the specific idea to be communicated. Use of gesture to augment verbal communication in conversation has also been reported in a case of chronic conduction aphasia once verbal improvement had ceased.[107]

RHYTHM AND SONG

Melodic intonation therapy[108] or prosodic cueing have not proven to be particularly useful approaches in improving the verbal expression of the patient with conduction aphasia.

Functional Communication

Because the goal of treatment is to promote communication outside of the structure and support of therapy, attention should be directed at the natural communication setting. Attention to functional communication enhancement should be integrated with language stimulation from the onset of treatment.[109] For instance, the ability to name a line drawing of a fire is certainly less useful than the ability to yell "fire" when one's car is about to explode. Obviously an effective word-retrieval program must positively influence the client's ability to access vocabulary in many situations. Thus, the clinician monitors the influence of treatment on the individual's communicative function on tasks, in settings, and with people outside of those used in treatment. Also, parameters should be incorporated into treatment to facilitate improved communication accuracy and/or success in such conditions. Carry-over is facilitated by programming realistic activities into treatment, such as discussing a TV show with a volunteer, making a phone request, writing letters to friends, or role playing problem situations. The approach called Promoting Aphasics' Communicative Effectiveness (PACE)[90] incorporates rules of natural communication into treatment; it is recommended as a means of improving functional communication in conduction aphasia. The goal of functional communication activities might be to promote carry-over, to encourage use of channels in addition to verbal ones, to point out nonproductive self-correction behavior, to reinforce successful communication strategies, as well as to desensitize the patient to unfavorable listener responses.

Summary

The previous sections have attempted to identify characteristics of conduction aphasia and assist in the difficult but rewarding job of management. However, no single chapter can possibly encapsulate every aspect of evaluation and treatment. In treating individuals with conduction aphasia, it becomes readily apparent that there are as many variations in approaches as there are conduction aphasia people and clinicians. However, there are many things that are successful with other types of aphasia, such as extensive auditory work with Wernicke's aphasia or syntax production programs with Broca's aphasia, that seem less useful with conduction aphasia. Perhaps the purpose of this chapter is simply to narrow the "field" of therapy choices a bit without providing the proverbial cookbook. Perhaps in aphasia treatment "knowledge is power"; the more we know about the disorder and how others handle it, the less time we need spend sifting through the ever-growing bag of aphasia therapy tricks. Thus, treatment that integrates a knowledge of prognostic variables, an understanding of aphasia treatment principles, a grasp of learning theory, and a familiarity with relevant research into a caring, sensitive, and creative mixture assures the person with conduction aphasia of getting the most out of treatment.

References

1. Wernicke C: The aphasia symptom complex: A psychological study on an anatomic basis, 1874. In G. Eggert (Trans.) *Wernicke's Works on Aphasia: A Sourcebook and Review.* The Hague: Mouton, 1977, pp 91–145.
2. Lichtheim L: On aphasia. *Brain* 1885; 7:433–484.
3. Potzl O: Uber parietal bedingte Aphasie und ihren einfluss auf das sporechen mehrerer sprachen. *Z Gesamte Neurologie Psychiatrie* 1924; 96:100–124.
4. Stengel E, Lodge-Patch I: "Central" aphasia associated with parietal symptoms. *Brain* 1955; 78:401–416.
5. Goldstein K: *Language and Language Disturbances.* New York: Grune and Stratton, 1948.
6. Benson F, Sheremata W, Bouchard R, et al: Conduction aphasia: A clinicopathologocial study. *Archives of Neurology* 1973; 28:339–346.
7. Murdoch B, Afford R, Ling A, et al: Acute computerized tomographic scans: Their value in the localization of lesions and as prognostic indicators in aphasia. *Journal of Commun Disorders* 1986; 19:311–345.
8. Naeser M, Hayward R: Lesion localization in aphasia with cranial computed tomography and the B.D.A.E. *Neurology* 1978; 28:545–551.
9. Mazzochi F, Vignolo L: Localization of lesions in aphasia: Clinical C.T. scan correlations in stroke patients. *Cortex* 1979; 15:627–654.
10. Damasio H, Damasio A: The anatomical basis of conduction aphasia. *Brain* 1980; 103:337–350.
11. Strub R, Black F: *The Mental Status Examination in Neurology.* Philadelphia: FA Davis, 1985.
12. Levine D, Calvanio R: Conduction Aphasia. In Kirshner H, Freemon F (eds): *The Neurology of Aphasia: Neurolinguistics.* Netherlands: Swets and Zeitlinger, 1982.
13. Kertesz A: *Aphasia and Associated Disorders.* New York: Grune and Stratton, 1979.
14. Geschwind N: Disconnexion syndromes in animals and man. *Brain* 1965; 88:585–644.
15. Canter, Trost J, Burns M: Contrasting speech patterns in apraxias of speech and phonemic paraphasia. *Brain and Language* 1985; 24:204–222.
16. Kinsbourne M: Behavioral analysis of the repetition deficit in conduction aphasia. *Neurology* 1972; 22:1126–1132.
17. Kleist K: *Sensory Aphasia and Amusia.* New York: Pergamon Press, 1962.
18. Mendez M, Benson F: Atypical conduction aphasia: A disconnection syndrome. *Archives of Neurolo* 1985; 42:886–891.
19. Green E, Howes D: The nature of conduction aphasia: A study of anatomic and clinical features and of underlying mechanisms. In Whitaker H, Whitaker H: (eds): *Studies in Neurolinguistics.* New York: Academic press, vol. 3. 1977 pp 123–156.
20. Dubois J, Hecean H, Angelergues R, et al: Neurolinguistic study of conduction aphasia. In Goodglass H, Blumstein S (eds): *Psycholinguistics and Aphasia.* Baltimore: Johns Hopkins Press, 1973.
21. Kertesz A, Lesk D, McCabe P: Isotope localization of infarcts in aphasia. *Archives of Neurology* 1977; 34:590–601.
22. Kertesz A: *The Western Aphasia Battery.* New York: Grune and Stratton, 1982.
23. Kempler D, Metter J, Jackson C, et al: Disconnection and cerebral metabolism; the case of conduction aphasia. *Archives of Neurology* 1988; 45:275–279.
24. Benson F: Aphasia. In Heilman K Valenstein E (ed): *Clinical Neurophsychology.* New York: Oxford University Press, 1985 pp 17–47.

25. Deal J: The nature of aphasia: Primary deficits and differentiating features. In LaPointe L (ed): *Aphasia: Nature and Assessment. Seminars in Speech and Language* 1986; 7:111–122.
26. Goodglass H, Kaplan E: *The Assessment of Aphasia and Related Disorders,* 2nd ed. Philadelphia: Lea and Febiger, 1983.
27. Kohn S, Goodglass H: Picture naming in aphasia. *Brain and Language* 1985; 24:266–283.
28. Boller F, Vignolo L: Latent sensory aphasia in hemisphere-damaged patients: An experimental study with the Token Test. *Brain* 1966; 89:815–830.
29. Williams S, Canter G: Action-naming performance in four syndromes of aphasia. *Brain and Language* 1987; 32:124–136, 1987.
30. Monoi H, Fukusako Y, Itoh M, et al: Speech sound errors in patients with conduction and Broca's aphasia. *Brain and Language* 1983; 20:175–194.
31. Blumstein S: *A Phonological Investigation of Aphasic Speech.* The Hague: Mouton, 1973.
32. Brown J: The problem of repetition: A study of "conduction" aphasia and the "isolation" syndrome. *Cortex* 1975; 11:37–52.
33. Lecours A, Rouillon F: Neurolinguistic an analysis of jargonaphasia and jargonapgraphia. In H Whitaker and H Whitaker (eds): *Studies in Neurolinguistics.* New York: Academic Press, vol. 2. 1976; pp 95–144.
34. Darley F, Aronson A, Brown J: *Motor Speech Disorders.* Philadelphia: Saunders, 1975.
35. Johns D, Darley F: Phonemic variability in apraxia of speech. *Journal of Speech and Hearing Research* 1970; 13:556–583.
36. LaPointe L, Johns D: Some phonemic characteristics in apraxia of speech. *Journal of Commun Disord* 1975; 8:259–269.
37. Caplan D: *Neurolinguistics and Linguistic Aphasiology.* Cambridge: Cambridge University Press, 1987.
38. Kohn S: The nature of phonological disorder in conduction aphasia. *Brain and Language* 1984; 23:97–115.
39. Nespoulous J, Joanette Y, Beland R, et al: Phonological disturbances in aphasia: Is there a "markedness" effect in aphasic phonemic errors? In Rose F (ed): *Progress in Aphasiology: Advances in Neurology,* vol 42. New York: Raven Press, 1984.
40. Blumstein S, Cooper W, Zurif E, et al: The perception and production of voice-onset time in aphasia. *Neuropsychologia* 1977; 15:371–383.
41. Blumstein S, Cooper W, Goodglass H, et al: Production deficits in aphasia: A voice-onset time analysis. *Brain and Language* 1980; 9:153–170.
42. Itoh M, Sasanuma S, Hiroe H, et al: Abnormal articulatory dynamics in a patient with apraxia of speech: X-ray microbeam observation. *Brain and Language* 1980; 11:66–75.
43. Itoh M, Sasanuma S, Tatsumi I, et al: Voice onset time characteristics in apraxia of speech. *Brain and Language* 1982; 17:193–210.
44. Kent R, Rosenbek J: Acoustic patterns of apraxia of speech, *Journal of Speech and Hearing Research* 1983; 26:231–249.
45. Duffy J, Gawle C: Apraxic speaker's vowel duration in consonant–vowel–consonant syllables. In Rosenbek J, McNeil M, Aronson A (eds): Apraxia of Speech: *Physiology, Acoustics, linguistics, Management.* San Diego: College Hill, 1984, p 167.
46. Gandour J, Dardaranada R: Voice onset time in aphasia: Thai II. Production. *Brain and Language* 1984; 23:177–205.
47. Warrington E, Shallice T: The selective impairment of auditory verbal short-term memory. *Brain* 1969; 92:885–896.
48. Shallice T, Warrington E: Auditory-verbal short-term memory impairment and conduction aphasia. *Brain and Language* 1977; 4:479–491.
49. Saffrin E, Marin O: Immediate memory for word lists and sentences in a patient with deficient auditory short-term memory. *Brain and Language* 1975; 2:420–433.
50. Caramazza A, Basili A, Koller J, et al: An investigation of repetition and language processing in a case of conduction aphasia. *Brain and Language* 1981; 14:235–271.
51. Heilman K, Scholes R, Watson R: Defects of immediate memory in Broca's and conduction aphasia. *Brain and Language* 1976; 3:201–208.
52. Tzoris C, Albert M: Impairment of memory for sequences in conduction aphasia. *Neuropsychologia* 1974; 12:355–366.
53. Strub R, Gardner H: The repetition deficit in conduction aphasia: Mnestic or linguistic. *Brain and Language* 1974; 1:241–255.
54. Heilman K, Scholes R: The nature of comprehension errors in Broca's, conduction and Wernicke's aphasics. *Cortex* 1976; 12:258–265.
55. Carramazza A, Zurif E: Dissociation of algorithmic and heuristic processes in language comprehension: Evidence from aphasia. *Brain and Language* 1976; 3:572–582.

56. Berndt R, Caramazza A: Syntactic aspects of aphasia. In Sarno M (ed): *Acquired Aphasia*. New York: Academic Press, 1981 pp 157–181.
57. Naeser M, Mazurski P, Goodglass H, et al: Auditory syntactic comprehension in nine aphasia groups (with CT scans) and children: Differences in degree but not order of difficulty observed. *Cortex* 1987; 23:359–380.
58. McCarthy R, Warrington E: The double dissociation of short-term memory for lists and sentences. *Brain* 1987; 110:1545–1563.
59. Sullivan M, Fisher B, Marshall R: Treating the repetition deficit in conduction aphasia. In Brookshire R (ed): *Clinical Aphasiology Conference Proceedings, 1986*. Minneapolis: BRK Publishers, pp 172–180.
60. Rothi L, McFarling D, Heilman K: Conduction Aphasia, syntactic alexia and the anatomy of syntactic comprehension. *Archives of Neurology*, 39:272–275, 1982.
61. Poncet M, Habib M, Robillard A: Deep left parietal lobe syndrome: Conduction aphasia and other neurobehavioural disorders due to a small subcortical lesion. *Journal of Neurology, Neurosurgery and Psychiatry*. 50:709–713, 1987.
62. Davis G: *A Survey of Adult Aphasia*. Englewood Cliffs, NJ: Prentice-Hall, 1983.
63. Wertz R: Language disorders in adults: State of the clinical art. In Holland A (ed): *Language Disorders in Adults*. San Diego: College Hill Press, 1984, pp 1–78.
64. Wertz R: Neuropathologies of speech and language: An introduction to patient management. In D Johns (ed): *Clinical Management of Neurogenic Communicative Disorders*. Boston: Little, Brown, 1985, pp 1–96.
65. LaPointe L: (ed) *Aphasia: Nature and Assessment. Seminars in Speech and Language*. New York: Thieme, 7: 1986.
66. Simmons N: Beyond standardized measures: Special tests, language in context and discourse analysis in aphasia. In LaPointe L (ed): *Aphasia: Nature and Assessment. Seminars in Speech and Language*. 7:181–206, 1986.
67. Porch B: *Porch Index of Communicative Ability*. Palo Alto, California: Consulting Psychologists Press, 1981.
68. DeRenzi E, Faglioni P: Normative and screening power of a shortened version of the Token Test. *Cortex* 1978; 14:41–49.
69. DeRenzi E, Vignolo L: The token test: A sensitive test to detect receptive disturbances in aphasia. *Brain* 1982; 85:556–678.
70. McNeil M, Prescott T: *Revised Token Test*. Baltimore: University Park Press, 1978.
71. Shewan C: *Auditory Comprehension Test for Aphasia (ACTS)* Chicago: Biolinguistics Clinical Institutes, 1979.
72. Kaplan E: Goodglass H, Weintraub S: *Boston Naming Test*. Philadelphia: Lea and Febiger, 1983.
73. Marshall R: Word Retrieval Behavior of aphasic adults. *Journal of Speech and Hearing Disord* 1976; 41:444–451.
74. Wener D, Duffy J: An investigation of the sensitivity of the Reporter's test to expressive language disturbances (Abstr). In Brookshire R (ed): *Clinical Aphasiology Conference Proceedings, 1983*. Minneapolis: BRK Publishers.
75. DeRenzi E, Ferrari C: The Reporter's test: A sensitive test to detect expressive disturbances in aphasics. *Cortex* 14:279–293, 1978.
76. Odell K, McNeil M, Collins M, Rosenbek J: Some comparisons between auditory and reading comprehension in aphasic adults. (Astr). In Brookshire R. (ed): *Clinical Aphasiology Conference Proceedings, 1984*, Minneapolis: BRK Publishers, p 276.
77. Glosser G, Wiener M, Kaplan E: Variations in aphasic language behaviors. *Journal of Speech and Hearing Disorders* 1988; 53:115–124.
78. Yorkston K, Beukelman D: An analysis of connected speech samples of aphasic and normal speakers. *Journal of Speech and Hearing Disord* 1980; 45:27–26.
79. Linebaugh C: Mild Aphasia. In Holland A (ed): *Language Disorders in Adults*, San Diego: College Hill Press 1984, pp 113–131.
80. Bernstein-Ellis E, Wertz R, Shubitowski V: More pace, less fillers: A verbal strategy for a high-level aphasic patient. In Brookshire R (ed): *Clinical Aphasiology Conference Proceedings, 1987* Minneapolis: BRK Publishers, 1987, pp 12–22.
81. Golper L, Thorpe P, Tompkins C, Marshall R, Rau M: Connected language sampling: An expanded index of aphasic language behavior. In Brookshire R (ed): *Clinical Aphasiology Conference Proceedings, 1980*. Minneapolis: BRK Publishers, pp 174–186.
82. Kearns K: The application of phonological process analysis to adult neuropathologies. In Brookshire R (ed): *Clinical Aphasiology Conference Proceedings, 1980*. Minneapolis, BRK Publishers, pp 187–195.
83. Rosenbek J: Some challenges for clinical aphasiologists. In Miller J, Yoder D, Schiefelbusch R (eds): *Contemporary Issues in Language Intervention*. Rockville, Maryland: ASHA, 1983, pp 317–325.
84. Duffy J: Schuell's stimulation approach to rehabilitation. In Chapey R (ed): *Language Intervention Strategies in Adult Aphasia*. Baltimore: Williams & Wilkins, 1986, pp 187–214.

85. LaPointe L: Aphasia therapy: Some principles and strategies for treatment. In Johns D (ed): *Clinical Management of Neurogenic Communicative Disorders.* Boston: Little, Brown, 1985, pp 179–241.
86. Brookshire R: *An Introduction to Aphasia,* 2nd ed. Minneapolis: BRK Publishers, 1978.
87. Vignolo L: Aphasia Rehabilitation: Results and perspectives. Special Session presented at the Annual Meeting of the American Speech Language and Hearing Association, Houston, Texas, 1976.
88. Bollinger R, Stout C: Response contingent small step treatment: Performance based communication intervention. *J Speech Hear Disord* 1976; 41:40–51.
89. Darley F: *Aphasia.* Philadelphia: WB Saunders, 1982.
90. Davis G, Wilcox J: *Adult Aphasia Rehabilitation: Applied Pragmatics.* San Diego: College Hill Press, 1985.
91. Marshall R: Treatment of auditory comprehension deficits. In Chapey R (ed): *Language Intervention Strategies in Adult Aphasia.* Baltimore: Williams & Wilkins, 1986, pp 370–393.
92. Sanders S, Davis G, Hubler V: A study of the interdependence of word retrieval and repetition in conduction aphasia. In Brookshire R (ed): *Clinical Aphasiology Conference Proceedings, 1979.* Minneapolis, BRK Publishers, pp 270–277.
93. Helm-Estabrooks N, Emery P, Albert M: Treatment of Aphasic Perseveration (TAP) program. *Archives of Neurology* 1987; 44:1253–1255.
94. Li E, Canter G: An investigation of Luria's hypothesis on prompting in aphasic naming disturbances. *Journal of Communication Disorders* 1987; 20:469–475.
95. Chapey R: Cognitive intervention: Stimulation of cognition, memory, convergent thinking, divergent thinking, and evaluative thinking. In Chapey R (ed): *Language Intervention Strategies in Adult Aphasia.* Baltimore: Williams & Wilkins, 1986, pp 215–238.
96. Linebaugh C: Treatment of anomic aphasia. In Perkins W (ed): *Current Therapy of Communication Disorders: Language Handicaps in Adults.* New York: Thieme-Stratton, 1983.
97. Wepman J: Aphasia: Language without thought or thought without language. *Asha.* 1976; 18:131–136.
98. Kearns K: Response elaboration training for patient initiated utterances. In Brookshire R (ed): *Clinical Aphasiology Conference Proceedings, 1985,* Minneapolis: BRK Publishers, pp 176–183.
99. Kearns K, Potechin G: The generalization of response elaboration training. Paper presented at the Clinical Aphasiology Conference. Harwich Port, Massachusetts, 1988.
100. Helm N: Management of palilalia with a pacing board. *Journal of Speech Hear Disord* 1979; 44:350–353.
101. Roberts J, Wertz R: TACS: A contrastive language treatment for aphasic adults, In Brookshire R (ed): *Clinical Aphasiology Conference Proceedings 1986.* Minneapolis: BRK Publishers, pp 207–212.
102. Logue R, Dixon M: Word association and the anomic response: Analysis and treatment. In Brookshire R (ed): *Clinical Aphasiology Conference Proceedings, 1979.* Minneapolis, BRK Publishers, pp 248–260.
103. Joanette V, Keller E, Lecours A: Sequences of phonemic approximations in aphasia. *Brain and Language* 1980; 11:30–44.
104. Nespoulas J, Joanette V, Ska B, et al: Production deficits in Broca's and conduction aphasia: Repetition versus reading. In Keller E, Gopnik M (eds): *Motor and Sensory Processes of Language.* Hillsdale, New Jersey: Erlbaum, 1987.
105. Boyle M: Reducing phonemic paraphasias in the connected speech of a conduction aphasic subject. Paper presented to the Clinical Aphasiology Conference. Harwich Port, Massachusetts, 1988.
106. Skelly M: *Amer-Ind Gestural Code Based on Universal American Indian Hand Talk.* New York: Elsevier, 1979.
107. Simmons N, Zorthian A: Use of symbolic gestures in a case of fluent aphasia. In Brookshire R, (ed): *Clinical Aphasiology Conference Proceedings, 1979,* Minneapolis: BRK Publishers, pp 278–285.
108. Sparks R, Holland A: Method: Melodic intonation therapy for aphasia. *Journal of Speech and Hearing Disorders* 1976; 41:287–297.
109. Aten J: Functional Communication Treatment. In Chapey R (ed): *Language Intervention Strategies in Adult Aphasia.* Baltimore: Williams & Wilkins, 1986, pp 266–276.

4

Transcortical Aphasias

Leslie J. Gonzalez Rothi

Whitaker[1] defines a syndrome as" . . . a set of symptoms occurring together that characterize a specific disease or condition." Heilman and Rothi[2] suggest that, in addition to avoiding the capture of extremes of random variations in behavior, a classification system must have "predictive value." The worth of syndrome identification has been questioned in the theoretical realm, especially in regard to what it can tell us about how the brain processes linguistic information.[3-5] These authors suggest that examining the "cognitive neuropsychological processes" underlying the language disorder of each patient would be more productive in helping us understand language processing in general and the mechanism of the deficit of each patient in particular. Heilman and Rothi,[2] however, state that the value of syndrome identification is never more evident than in the clinical realm where cause, lesion localization, co-occurring symptomatology, form and extent of recovery, and efficacy of treatment all can be anticipated to some extent. To the clinician it would appear that a combination of these approaches is warranted, and both versions will be attempted in this review of the transcortical aphasias.

Introduction

Kussmaul wrote:

> (These are) . . . the most essential points in the process of talking. In the first place, a thought is . . . conceived, and then (there is) an impulse of feeling urging us to express it. Next we choose and say the words which the acquired language in our memory places at our disposal. Finally, the reflex apparatuses are called into play (to) give outward utterance to the words (p. 595).

> The intellectual contents of our being slumbers unconscious in our memory until thrown into vibration by some vigorous shock from without or within. (p. 624) . . . If conceptions . . . be called upon, the extent to which they were set in motion will reflect back with such force of feeling upon the being as to awaken its interest and produce a readiness to follow up the thoughts; and to clothe them in words. . . . (These are called) the inner

preparatory processes of speech which present themselves . . . to our consciousness, and are also only partially subject to our will (p. 625).

After destruction of voluntary speech, the power of repeating words spoken aloud by others often remains . . . although unable of their own free will to utter these words. They are incapable of bringing word pictures to the recollection by conceptions. . . . By the utterance aloud of others, the acoustic picture of words which can no longer be produced from within are presented to them from without, and so the reflex start to the corresponding movements of sound is rendered possible. (p. 641)[6]

Wernicke[7] proposed that thought and language are distinct functions represented in separate anatomical brain locations. In addition, Wernicke[7] delineated two separable language functions that he also suggested were supported by separate anatomic regions in the left hemisphere. Specifically, he identified an "auditivo–verbal" center located in the first temporal convolution of the left hemisphere that contained the "stored memory images of auditory sensations corresponding to the audition of spoken language."[8] Secondly, he identified a "verbo–motor" center in the third frontal convolution of the left hemisphere that contained the "stored memory images of the sensations of movement corresponding to the production of articulated language."[8] In addition, Wernicke[7] suggested a connection between these two centers and predicted three aphasia syndromes reflecting damage to each of the centers and the connection between. Lichtheim[9] was the first to comment that Wernicke's[7] model of language processing in the brain did not account for aphasia in which repetition was spared. He postulated that these aphasias with spared repetition resulted not from a destruction of Wernicke's language centers ("central aphasias") but instead resulted from a disconnection of the language centers and the nonlanguage associations of "motivation" and/or "concepts" ("peripheral commissural aphasias"). Wernicke[10] coined the term "transcortical" aphasia to refer to aphasia with spared repetition, with transcortical motor aphasia referring to a dissociation of language and "motivation" and transcortical sensory aphasia referring to a dissociation of language and "concepts." Goldstein[11] referred to mixed transcortical aphasia as "isolation of speech."

Transcortical motor aphasia is characterized by nonfluent verbal output in the context of relatively spared comprehension (visual and auditory) and spared repetition. In contrast, transcortical sensory aphasia is characterized as a fluent aphasia where comprehension is poor in the context of relatively spared repetition. Mixed transcortical aphasia is characterized as a nonfluent aphasia where comprehension is impaired while repetition is relatively spared. Study of the syndromes of transcortical aphasia reveals anatomically and possibly psychologically distinct clinical syndromes. Therefore, each of the transcortical syndromes will be discussed separately.

Pathophysiology

Transcortical Motor Aphasia

Wernicke[10] himself questioned the transcortical explanation of transcortical motor aphasia, though continuing to endorse the use of the term in application to this form of aphasia. Bastian[12] also contradicted the transcortical explanation of transcortical motor aphasia, saying that the mechanism of this disorder actually reflected damage to the cortical speech center directly. He suggested that the two linguistic activities of spontaneous speech and repetition require differing levels of cortical excitability and that less-than-complete destruction of critical areas yields differential performance on these tasks. Therefore, transcortical motor aphasia reflects a degree of cortical speech center destruction that is enough to impair spontaneous speech but not enough to impair repetition. A different explanation was proposed by Niessel von Mayendorf[13] who suggested that spared repetition in the context of aphasia represents the contribution of the right hemisphere in these left hemisphere damaged cases (as reported by Rubens and Kertesz[14]).

More recently Goldstein[11] referred to two syndromes that could be included under the label of transcortical motor aphasia. One he considered to result from "partial damage to the motor speech area" itself, much like that proposed by Bastian[12] resulting in "a heightening of the threshold of the motor speech performances." In contrast, Goldstein[11] describes a second form of transcortical motor aphasia, which he describes as "an impairment of the impulse to speak at all" resulting from damage to the "frontal lobe itself." The second form is distinguished by a "lack of any other speech disturbance or mental defect . . . " whereas the first is distinguished by "more or less defects in the motor act of speaking." Goldstein[11] also recognized that both motor speech performance and impulse to speak also could be compromised in combination in a single case.

Botez[15-18] refers to this "impulse to speak" as "incitation to action," which can be functionally selective to speech and language. Botez and his colleagues suggest that the supplementary motor area (SMA) of the left hemisphere, a portion of premotor cortex, provides this "starting mechanism" for speech, and destruction of SMA yields a lack of "incitation to speak." Luria[19-23] calls this Dynamic Aphasia and attributes it to "a pathologic inertia" or a "disturbance of the predicative function of speech." It should be noted that there are those who question whether "aphasia" is a term appropriately applied to a syndrome such as this where the mechanism is not hypothesized to represent a deficit in the structural processing of language per se.[24-27] Others support use of the term aphasia.[28,29]

Roland and co-workers[30] present a somewhat different viewpoint on what SMA contributes to human behavior. Specifically, they hypothesize that SMA is involved in programming motor subroutines prior to execution, and the implication would be that damage to SMA precludes this preprogramming. For speech this would mean that lack of speaking in left SMA-lesioned patients did not result from a lack of impulse or intention, but instead from a lack of a plan or program to carry forth. This is similar to the explanation for limb apraxia from SMA lesions put forth by Watson and co-workers.[31]

Goldberg,[32] in reviewing what he proposes are two separable premotor systems, includes the SMA in the medial premotor system. In contrast to the lateral premotor system in which action generation is related to "external context" (as provided by the sensory systems), Goldberg suggests the function of SMA and the medial premotor system is in the "intentional process" "whereby internal context influences the elaboration of action." Goldberg[32] continues that, in addition to the role of SMA in the "intention-to-act", is the "specification and elaboration of action", which influences "the 'programming' and fluent execution of extended action sequences." Therefore, the role of SMA can be summarized as mediating limbic influence on primary motor cortex, specifically in regard to intention to act and in preprogramming action prior to its execution. In speech and language, this can be translated so that lesions of SMA would be anticipated to produce deficits of the intention to speak combined with deficits of preprogramming and planning verbal utterances prior to the act of speaking.

Possibly tying together these seemingly disparate perspectives on the mechanism of transcortical motor aphasia specifically, Stuss and Benson[33] discuss a continuum of syndrome manifestations that might be related to lesion localization within the left frontal lobe. Specifically, the frontal lobe is noted to be quite large in comparison with remaining portions of the human brain, and lesions of the frontal lobe may vary greatly in regard to the relative involvement of specific anatomic structures of interest. In regard to transcortical motor aphasia, these structures of interest include mid- and upper-premotor cortex around or including SMA.[34,35] The potential for variations in the anatomy of frontal lobe involvement and, thus, the behavioral variations of transcortical motor aphasia[36] become apparent when looking at the vascular system supplying the frontal lobes. Two vessels supplied by the internal carotid artery supply the frontal lobe exclusively. These are the anterior cerebral artery, which supplies the medial portions of the frontal lobe, and the anterior branches of the middle cerebral artery, which supplies the dorsal–lateral convexity of the frontal lobe. Thus, pathology that might impede blood flow through these vessels selectively would involve SMA and lateral convexity premotor cortex selectively producing behavioral variations such as those discussed by Stuss and Benson.[33] Stuss and Benson[33] suggest that the closer a lesion of the left frontal lobe comes to Broca's area (i.e., middle cerebral artery), the more motor speech deficits will be evident. In contrast, the closer a lesion comes to SMA (i.e., anterior cerebral artery), the more aspontaneous the patient's speech will be. Most typically, when lesions are produced by vascular pathology, individuals with transcortical motor aphasia have lesions representing the watershed region between the middle cerebral and anterior cerebral arteries.[37] In addition, significant frontal pathology resulting in transcortical motor aphasia is reported to be seen commonly in trauma.[38]

Transcortical Sensory Aphasia

That transcortical sensory aphasia simply represented a less severe form of Wernicke's aphasia (especially because it can occur as a stage in evolution from acute Wernicke's aphasia) was refuted by Bonhoeffer,[39] Heilbronner,[40] and Pick.[41] Lichtheim[9] suggested that verbal information processed by the "auditivo–verbal" center was subsequently processed via a direct link to a "verbo–motor" center and also processed by all of the association cortices linked to these two centers. Lichtheim[9] described this syndrome as resulting from a disruption of the link between association cortices and the "auditivo–verbal" center. Sparing of the link between the two "centers" allows the patient with transcortical sensory aphasia to repeat what is said to him. Lichtheim[9] named this the sensory version of "peripheral commissural aphasia"; subsequently it was renamed transcortical sensory aphasia by Wernicke.[7]

Unlike the single route of repetition described by Lichtheim,[9] McCarthy and Warrington[42] propose a two-route functional model for the repetition of sentences or word lists. The first system is a "relatively passive phonological store subserving list repetition" and second is a semantically based, "dynamic, anticipatory, and integrative memory system which underpins sentence repetition." McCarthy and Warrington[42] suggest that the transcortical sensory aphasic patient they tested displayed reliance on the phonological system during repetition.

A third, lexically mediated functional system of repetition is discussed by Kremin,[43] Coslett and co-workers[44] and Martin and Saffran.[45] In this third system, a direct association between phonology of input and output lexicons is achieved without semantic mediation.

This three-route functional model of repetition is compatible with the three-route model of oral reading proposed by Morton and Patterson[46] and expanded by many other authors to include recognition, comprehension, and production of spoken words and nonwords.[47] Patterson and Shewell[47] present a model of this expanded version, and the portion referring to spoken language, and thus relevant to the repetition skill of transcortical sensory aphasia, is reviewed in Figure 4 – 1 (p. 91). The sublexical, acoustical-to-phonological conversion system of Patterson and Shewell's model compares to the first, phonological system suggested by McCarthy and Warrington[42] where input is processed into segmental phonological representations and then converted to the corresponding output representations. Repeating words via this system allows the repetition of nonwords as well as words, is influenced by stimulus length, and is insensitive to part of speech, word frequency or imagibility. Repetition errors emanating from reliance on this system include phonological aberrations of the target. Caramazza and co-workers[48] report a case who showed a selective deficit of this system who could not repeat nonwords but who could read, write, and repeat words.

Next, the repetition system proposed by Coslett and co-workers[44] is compatible with the direct link between the auditory input lexicon and phonological output lexicon proposed in Patterson and Shewell's[47] model. In this lexical system of repetition, access to the phonological addresses of words in the input and output lexicons are linked directly without semantic mediation. This system is sensitive to word frequency but not to word length or concreteness. Repetition errors emanating from reliance on this system include such things as lexicalization of nonwords (for which there is, by definition, no lexical address). Caramazza and co-workers[49] describe a Wernicke's aphasic whose performance indicated impairment of this lexical system and sparing of semantic processing.

Finally, the second system proposed by McCarthy and Warrington[42] is compatible with the semantic system represented as the auditory input lexicon to cognitive to phonological output lexicon of Patterson and Shewell's[47] model. In this semantic system of repetition the access to output phonology is achieved via semantic mediation. As with the lexical system, this semantic system cannot process nonwords. This system is sensitive to concreteness and part of speech[49] but not to stimulus length. Repetition errors emanating from reliance on this system include semantic paraphasias. Only the semantic route, by accessing the "cognitive" system, allows us to apply meaning to what we hear as well as to produce words meaningfully and this is the system that appears to be impaired in transcortical sensory aphasia (involving deficits a or B in Figure 4 – 1). Compatible with this interpretation, it is interesting to note that Davis and co-workers[50] found that during repetition tasks patients with transcortical sensory aphasia were less able to recognize and correct semantic errors in the stimuli than were patients with transcortical motor aphasia.

Subtypes of transcortical sensory aphasia are predicted by this model. Specifically, Coslett and co-workers[44] and Berndt and co-workers[51] describe cases of transcortical sensory aphasia in which the patients are unable to comprehend what is said via the semantic system but who repeat lexically. In addition, Coslett and co-workers[44] describe transcortical sensory aphasia in which repetition is accomplished via nonlexical phonological analysis.

Regarding the anatomical substrate of transcortical sensory aphasia, Henschen[52] described two associated etiologies: one involved with "general cerebral atrophy" and the other with focal lesions. Kertesz and co-workers,[53] Rubens and Kertesz,[14] and Hiltbrunner and co-workers[54] report that transcortical sensory aphasia is associated with lesions of the left inferior parietotemporooccipital area. This area is supplied by portions of the posterior cerebral artery or represents a watershed between the posterior cerebral and middle cerebral arteries. This localization remains controversial, however,[55,56] and further research that accounts for syndrome subtyping is needed.

Mixed Transcortical Aphasia

Geschwind and co-workers,[57] studying a case of mixed transcortical aphasia resulting from carbon monoxide poisoning, anatomically confirm Goldstein's[11] hypothesis that this syndrome resulted from lesions of association cortex that isolate but spare the left hemisphere perisylvian region including Wernicke's area, Broca's area, and the connections between. Rubens and Kertesz[14] report that mixed transcortical aphasia is typically associated with multifocal or diffuse brain damage of the above-mentioned structures. Etiologies include hypoxia from such things as carbon monoxide poisoning, dementing processes (e.g., Pick's disease), and multiple infarctions involving vascular watershed zones. Others have reported the rare occurrence of mixed transcortical aphasia in association with CVAs involving the left internal carotid artery[58] and, more rarely, the left anterior cerebral artery[59,60] and left middle cerebral artery.[61] Interestingly, Bando and co-workers[62] discuss a case they labeled transcortical sensory aphasia but which they described as also disinclined to speak, a feature more compatible with mixed transcortical aphasia. Given a left-sided WADA test, the patient continued to repeat; given a right sided test, the patient could not repeat, suggesting to these authors that the repetition skill in their patient was being mediated by the right hemisphere.

Nature and Differentiating Features

Transcortical Motor Aphasia

Transcortical motor aphasia is characterized by nonfluent verbal and written output in the context of spared repetition and comprehension (auditory and orthographic). Nonfluency of verbal output is characterized by several features including a reduction in the quantity, variety, and elaboration of output, a reduction in syntactic complexity, and a lack of motor precision in the execution of verbalizations. Any or all of these features of nonfluency may be present. With intense testing methods, some deficits of auditory comprehension of syntactically complex information may be noted;[63] however, most typically, auditory comprehension is noted to be spared.

Transcortical motor aphasia is most likely to be confused with Broca's aphasia, aphemia, or the other transcortical aphasias. However, it should be noted that in cases of transcortical motor aphasia, verbal productions during repetition tasks are far better than what would be predicted from production skills during nonrepetition tasks, whereas in Broca's aphasia this discrepancy is not typically noted. Unlike in transcortical sensory or mixed transcortical aphasia, comprehension skills in transcortical motor aphasia are relatively spared.

Many times in behavioral neurology differential diagnoses are made based upon associated symptomatology. Therefore, it is important to know what behaviors are typically associated with transcortical motor aphasia. For patients with superior premotor involvement, associated signs may include transient urinary incontinence, contralateral grasp reflex, rigidity of the upper extremity, and a hemiparesis that involves the leg more than the arm. Initially, patients with SMA lesions may display mutism that quickly evolves into transcortical motor aphasia. Additionally, they may display bilateral ideomotor apraxia.[31] Akinesia (paucity of movement) and bradykinesia (slowness of movement) are also common.

Transcortical Sensory Aphasia

Lecours and Lhermitte,[64] calling this Wernicke's aphasia type II, describe transcortical sensory aphasia as including a normal flow of spoken output that is prosodically, phonetically and phonemically relatively undisturbed but contains numerous verbal and syntagmic paraphasias. Discourse appears incoherent, circumlocutory, and typically contains a limited number of contentives and a significant number of "ready-made expressions." Naming is severely impaired, and numerous word-finding pauses are noted during conversations. During naming failures, these patients are noted to repeat the correct label offered by the clinician without apparent recognition that it is the target. Written productions are qualitatively similar to verbal productions. It should be noted, however, that this deficit of verbal output is not necessarily absolute in that Heilman and co-workers[65] describe a case of transcortical sensory aphasia who displayed relative sparing of verbal output in comparison with impaired auditory comprehension. Comprehension of spoken as well as written information is, of course, impaired in transcortical sensory aphasia. Albert and co-workers[66] report that auditory comprehension in transcortical sensory aphasic patients is "fragile and context-dependent" meaning that shifts in the context of verbal interactions make previously meaningful information difficult for the patient to comprehend. Reading aloud and repetition are, of course, significantly better than all other language skills with these patients able to read aloud or repeat long, complex information that they are unable to understand.

Albert and co-workers[66] report that neurological symptoms commonly associated with transcortical sensory aphasia include elements of the Gerstmann syndrome, alexia, constructional apraxia, and ideational apraxia. Albert and co-workers[66] report that hemiparesis or hemisensory loss are rarely noted with transcortical sensory aphasia, whereas Mesulam[67] reports that they are, in conjunction with a visual field defect, "not uncommon."

Albert and co-workers[66] note that transcortical sensory aphasia is not uncommonly seen as the initial language disturbance of dementia of the Alzheimer's type. This language disturbance evolves with the disease, however, to a more severe language and cognitive disorder. In contrast, recovery from transcortical sensory aphasia from other etiologies is reported to be quite good. Rubens and Kertesz[14] report that transcortical sensory aphasia can occur as the result of trauma, but this posttraumatic syndrome is fleeting. Regarding focal ischemic lesions, several possible outcomes are described.[14] Lesions involving temporal cortex may initially result in Wernicke's aphasia that eventually evolves into chronic transcortical sensory aphasia.[68] However, persistent difficulties with repetition in aphasic patients have been noted to be associated with lesions involving damage to Wernicke's area.[69] What allows some but not all Wernicke's aphasic patients with temporal lesions to evolve to transcortical sensory aphasia remains unclear, although the size of the lesion may be related. Another version begins with transcortical sensory aphasia with some patients evolving to anomia and possibly ultimately to full recovery, whereas others remain persistently aphasic. Kertesz and co-workers[68] report that cases with this persistent form of transcortical sensory aphasia have parietal involvement.

Mixed Transcortical Aphasia

Goldstein,[11] calling this "isolation of speech," described the syndrome of mixed transcortical aphasia as characterized by severely diminished quantity of spontaneously generated verbal output, very poor auditory comprehension, and relative sparing of repetition. Echolalia is not infrequently associated with this syndrome, with automatic completion of unfinished sentences (produced by the examiner) noted.[61] Goldstein[11] described two forms of this syndrome where one has an almost "compulsive" drive to repeat that which they hear if "understanding" or "intention to repeat" (considered to be "nonspeech mental processes") are "not present." If these two factors are partially present, the mixed transcortical aphasia is characterized by "intentional repetition." Goldstein[11] thought the "compulsive" form was probably related to more extensive brain damage than the "intentional repetition" form. Although patients with mixed transcortical aphasia are noted to correct syntactically incorrect sentences during repetition tasks,[70] they are not noted to correct semantically incorrect sentences during repetition.[53,71] Although typically able to produce only a limited amount of verbal output and especially unable to name, Heilman and co-workers[72] report a remarkable case of mixed transcortical aphasia who was able to name objects. Although very unusual and not typical of this syndrome, this case made the point that it is possible to not gain meaning from object names while at the same time being able to produce those same object names.

Neurological signs possibly associated with mixed transcortical aphasia include echopraxia and grasp and suck reflexes.[73,74]

Evaluation

Transcortical Motor Aphasia

The task of differential diagnosis requires the identification of transcortical motor aphasia in contrast to other forms of aphasia, as stated above. An excellent review of assessment procedures is offered by Albert and co-workers.[66] The first task is to establish that there is a difference in performance between that obtained from spontaneous speech samples versus that obtained from repetition tasks. This differential should be such that speech obtained by repetition is better than that of spontaneous samples. Repetition tasks should compare repetition of stimulus sentences that increase in length from single words to sentences of up to ten words. The words and sentences used for these repetition tasks also should compare words of common usage versus words of infrequent usage and open- versus closed-class words. Patients with transcortical motor aphasia have greater difficulty repeating longer stimuli, sentences loaded with closed-class words, and infrequent words. To maximize the difficulty with repetition, these linguistic features should be emphasized in the stimuli. (Further information regarding the construction of repetition tasks is reviewed in the section on transcortical sensory aphasia). Spontaneous speech samples should involve response to questions as well as picture/event description or procedural discourse (e.g., "Tell me how you make your favorite sandwich"). Self-generation of sentences is recommended where the clinician provides word pair stimuli that control the number of possible sentences available to the patient. The patient is to generate a sentence using these words. For example, word pairs such as "bed and sleep" require less from the patient to construct a complete sentence than "apple and rhythm." Patients with transcortical motor aphasia who are able to produce any sentences at all will have greater difficulty with stimuli such as "apple and rhythm" than with "bed and sleep." Compatible with this, questions that do not provide information to the patient, such as "What did you have to eat today?" may be answered less completely than questions that provide information to the patient, such as "what kind of sandwich did you have for lunch?" These procedures should be repeated, having the patient write his/her response. Errors in verbal productions relevant to the clinician would include whether the patient displays any distortion of the speech signal (reflecting a motor speech disturbance), echolalia (or incorporation of the clinician's questions into the response to those questions), perseveration, reduction of syntactic complexity of those few patients able to produce such responses, and, finally, a lack of verbal elaboration in responses calling for elaboration.

When this differential in performance on repetition versus self generation of verbalization is identified, transcortical aphasia can be suspected, with the next task being to differentiate transcortical motor from sensory or mixed aphasias. This is typically accomplished by testing auditory or orthographic comprehension using any of the many tests available or procedures reviewed in the section on transcortical sensory aphasia.

Finally, verbal generativity[75] or word fluency where the patient is asked to name words beginning with a certain letter in 60 seconds, has been reported to be deficient in patients with left frontal damage.[76] Newcombe[77] suggests that tasks utilizing the generation of words belonging to semantic categories do not show a similar deficit in these patients. Therefore, it would be important to test the verbal generativity of words beginning with specific letters (see Benton[78]) of each patient suspected of transcortical motor aphasia.

Transcortical Sensory Aphasia

Transcortical sensory aphasia can be confused with Wernicke's aphasia or multimodal agnosia. Like those with Wernicke's aphasia, patients with transcortical sensory aphasia have deficient auditory comprehension and produce fluent verbal output containing numerous verbal paraphasias. However, Wernicke's aphasics do not improve with repetition tasks, whereas transcortical sensory aphasics do. Like patients with transcortical sensory aphasia, patients with a syndrome combining multimodal associative agnosia (tactile and visual modalities) and anomia (resulting from the same lesion noted above for transcortical sensory aphasia) can repeat but cannot name objects when seen/felt or point to objects when named. Unlike those with transcortical sensory aphasia, patients with multimodal agnosia utilize auditorily presented information significantly better than information presented via the visual or tactile modality.

As with transcortical motor or mixed aphasia, testing for the presence of transcortical sensory aphasia requires use of a standard language exam that allows comparisons of auditory comprehension, verbal output and repetition, such as the Boston Diagnostic Aphasia Exam[79] or the Western Aphasia Battery.[80] Auditory comprehension testing using these measures allows us to examine the differential between comprehension of words versus sentences. Further evaluation of lexical and semantic information about single words is necessary with transcortical sensory aphasia. Using word comprehension testing that is especially sensitive to semantic distinctions is discussed by Martin and Saffran.[45] They describe a Lexical Comprehension Test developed by Saffran and Schwartz in which the examiner says a word and the patient is asked to point to one of four pictures that matches the word. The four pictures are either all unrelated or are all semantically related. Patients with deficient semantic processing will confuse semantically related alternatives. In addition, Martin and Saffran[45] describe a second test of the patient's sensitivity to semantic information about words, called the Synonymy Test developed by Saffran and Schwartz. In this test the examiner says two words that may or may not be synonymous and the patient is asked to judge whether the two words mean the same thing. A comparison is made between errors on related pairs versus unrelated pairs with poorer performance on related pairs indicating semantic difficulties.

It is important that we carefully select the stimuli we use on repetition tests to evaluate the integrity of each of the systems reviewed in the Patterson and Schewell model.[47] The mechanism of the patient's spared repetition is especially important to evaluate in transcortical sensory aphasia because performance on this task also allows us to assess the integrity of the lexical system in patients believed to have deficient semantic processing or at least deficient access to semantic information (as tested above). For example, repetition testing should begin with single CVC (Consonant Vowel Consonant) words and increase to longer words and word strings to look at the influence of stimulus length. Pronounceable nonwords compatible in length with other word stimuli should be included on repetition tasks. These factors, as mentioned previously, influence the phonological conversion system, and sensitivity to these factors may imply reliance on that system. Comparisons should be made between repetition performance using high- versus low-frequency words (sensitivity to which implies reliance on the lexical system) and concrete versus abstract words (sensitivity to which implies reliance on the semantic system). The nature of the errors on all repetition tasks should be noted, the relevance of which has been discussed in the preceding section.

Mixed Transcortical Aphasia

The differential diagnosis of mixed transcortical aphasia requires distinguishing this syndrome from other forms of transcortical aphasia and also from global aphasia. Using either of the standard tests listed previously (WAB; BDAE) the diagnosis of any transcortical aphasia requires establishing that repetition is relatively selectively spared. If this is confirmed, then global aphasia can be ruled out. Depressed verbal fluency ratings will indicate that transcortical sensory aphasia can be excluded, whereas poor auditory comprehension performance excludes transcortical motor aphasia.

The same assessment procedures described for lexical comprehension and repetition in transcortical sensory aphasia would provide interesting information about those same skills in mixed transcortical aphasia. In addition, the fluency and verbal self-generativity measures described for transcortical motor aphasia would also be applicable.

Treatment

Transcortical Motor Aphasia

The prognosis for recovery from transcortical motor aphasia is considered to be good[34,81–83]; however, much of the literature represents conclusions drawn on single case studies or from groups of limited number. In contrast, one study (that did not distinguish right- from left-sided anterior watershed lesions (ACA/MCA) suggested that 82% of their 22 patients remained "moderately to severely" disabled at discharge.[37] The mean discharge date of the group was noted to be 22 days postonset, and this may have been too early to experience the significant recovery seen by other authors. However, most authors noting significant recovery also reported that this recovery occurred early in the postonset course. The prognosis for recovery from transcortical motor aphasia therefore remains unclear.

Despite limited information regarding treatment efficacy, several authors have suggested treatment methodologies for transcortical motor aphasia. Restitutive rehabilitative strategies attempt to restore impaired functions in contrast to substitutive rehabilitation strategies, which attempt to circumvent impaired functions (see Rothi and Horner[84] for a review). Several authors have suggested restitutive strategies with transcortical motor aphasia. For example, Johnson's[85] treatment program emphasized remediation of motor function deficits in general and verbo–motor skill in particular, which he felt needed to precede "traditional language retraining" methods. Specifically, he targeted those processes that "affected the volitional initiation of motoric responses, maintenance of a required motor act, and/or voluntary inhibition or termination of motor acts." "Conventional speech therapy" procedures were reportedly used by Kools[86] with self-cueing strategies for naming specifically emphasized. Lentz and co-workers[87] report their attempts to emphasize expansion of the restricted sentence structure of a case with transcortical motor aphasia by capitalizing upon the patient's spared naming skills. Huntley and Rothi[88] report their attempts to treat verbal generativity of semantic category membership and self generation of complete sentences in a case with transcortical motor aphasia of long standing. Although the behaviors specifically targeted by each of these treatment studies reported above have all responded to these intervention strategies at least temporarily, the pervasive communication deficit of verbal aspontaneity in these patients remained relatively uninfluenced. Alexander and Schmitt[83] suggest that "traditional methods" of treatment such as those using "repetition or verbal cueing" are "of limited value."

Less has been attempted using substitutive strategies. Luria and Tsvetkova[23] and Luria[21] suggest using a reorganizing technique that allows externally mediated sequencing to assist in the initiation and maintenance of speaking. For example, these authors note that a transcortical motor aphasic patient may be completely unable to generate a desired sentence on command. However, when objects (unrelated to the words in the target sentence) are placed in front of the patient equivalent in number to the number of words in the target sentence and the person is asked to touch each object while saying target words of the sentence, the patient is able to produce more words of the sentence than without the objects to touch. Alexander and Schmitt[83] note that this method was unsuccessful in their two subjects, but no further information is provided about their methodology. They conclude that "external rhythmic stimulation," which appears to be a slightly different conception of the strategy described by Luria,[21] "remains a plausible approach" for treating transcortical motor aphasia.

Recently, pharmacotherapy has been reported by Albert and co-workers[89] who treated a patient who had a two-and-a-half-year history of transcortical motor aphasia from a left frontal intracerebral hemorrhage. They gave the patient the drug bromocryptine, a dopamine agonist, and noted improvement in aphasia characterized by decreases in response latency, improved naming, and fewer paraphasias. These improvements were noted to abate when the drug was discontinued. Unfortunately, the limits of a single case study do not allow conclusions on this drug's applicability to other cases yet, but further research activity in this area is certain to be forthcoming.

Transcortical Sensory Aphasia

Treatment for the communication handicap posed by transcortical sensory aphasia has received no attention in the rehabilitation literature. One problem that may contribute to this lack comes from the fact that anosognosia is common in this syndrome, and a basic appreciation of the deficit by the patient is a necessary prerequisite to any successful treatment program. In cases in which denial of deficit impedes progress, the focus of treatment might initially be better directed at the denial rather than the aphasia.

Good treatment planning begins with an appreciation and accommodation for the etiology inducing the syndrome. In the case of progressive dementing processes, case management is very different than for transcortical sensory aphasia resulting from ischemic infarct, and treatment of dementia is not within the purview of this chapter. Regarding vascular etiologies, chronicity and syndrome evolution should be very influential in treatment planning.[84] For the person who presents initially with transcortical sensory aphasia, treatment planning should be designed to anticipate a probable evolution where verbal output and auditory comprehension of major lexical items improves. This evolution should not be anticipated for those who evolved to chronic transcortical sensory aphasia from Wernicke's aphasia. This patient likely will be left with persistent deficits in the above areas, and treatment should provide strategies designed to compensate for these deficits.

Mixed Transcortical Aphasia

Kertesz and McCabe[82] suggest that although the prognosis for recovery from mixed transcortical aphasia in general is good, mixed transcortical aphasia has a poorer prognosis than the motor or sensory forms. The patients of Geschwind and co-workers[57] and Heilman and co-workers[72] remained chronically, severely impaired. Whitaker's[70] case, due to the nature of her disease ("presenile dementia"), did not recover either. Therefore, the etiologies responsible for mixed transcortical aphasia may contribute to the lack of syndrome evolution to milder forms of language impairment. Unfortunately, mixed transcortical aphasia is another syndrome that has received little attention in the treatment literature.

Specific Treatment Tasks

Transcortical Motor Aphasia

Although a tested pathway is not yet available, it seems clear that behavioral treatments for transcortical motor aphasia need to emphasize further substitutive strategies, such as those suggested by Luria.[21,23] These strategies need to address the mechanisms proposed to account for this disorder and are described under the preceding subheading (Pathophysiology). Regarding impairments in the intention to verbalize and in verbal preprogramming, treatment methods, such as the externally mediated sequencing or external rhythmic stimulation techniques described above, seem justified. Other external mediation strategies for verbal interaction might be considered, such as listing questions to be answered by the person during discourse. Further, if the disruption of verbal intention does result from disconnection of limbic influence on the verbo–motor system as previously suggested, utilization of right hemisphere mediation of emotionally intoned verbal stimuli for treatment tasks may be considered.

Transcortical Sensory Aphasia

At the present time, there has been no study of the efficacy of specific treatment tasks for transcortical sensory aphasia and, therefore, only speculation about treatment programming is possible. The overwhelming contribution to impaired communication in transcortical sensory aphasia is the inability to apply meaning to what is heard or what is said. Rothi and Feinberg[56] suggest that if lesions a and/or B of Figure 4-1 truly represent the deficit that accounts for the patient's inability to link meaning to words in transcortical sensory aphasia, treatment programs should address the mechanisms of this deficit. For example, if a particular patient presents a disconnection between the cognitive system and the input plus output lexicons (a in Figure 4-1), treatment should emphasize pairing auditory input with another input modality or verbal output with another output mode. Although reading and writing are typically noted to be impaired in patients with transcortical sensory aphasia, even slight assistance from these and other modalities/modes would be helpful. In contrast, if the patient has a dysfunction of the cognitive system itself (B in Figure 4 – 1), emphasis should be placed on reconstruction of semantic relationships. The third possibility exists that a patient with transcortical sensory aphasia is able to repeat via the sublexical phonological conversion system but unable to utilize lexical or semantic information. These patients may represent the chronic form resulting from evolution from Wernicke's aphasia. Treatment's applicable to Wernicke's aphasia, as reviewed in Chapter 2, might be more applicable in these cases.

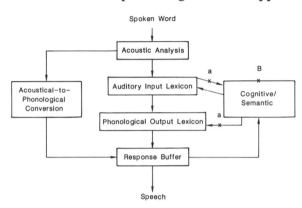

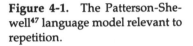

Figure 4-1. The Patterson-She-well[47] language model relevant to repetition.

Mixed Transcortical Aphasia

In this author's experience, the occurrence of the syndrome of mixed transcortical aphasia in its most complete and severe form is rare indeed, but milder versions are not completely uncommon. In those milder cases, the treatment for the verbal deficits described above under transcortical motor aphasia and the treatments for the receptive deficits described above for transcortical sensory aphasia might be relevant. Finally, we pass along a word of caution originally suggested by Alexander and Schmitt[83] regarding treatment of any person with transcortical aphasia. Treatment programs relying heavily on repetition skill will not produce significant therapeutic result because, as stated by Alexander and Schmitt,[83] "they address a function that is preserved and performed almost automatically in these patients." However, those treatment programs that possibly begin with repetition but in which the focus is to move slowly away from the automatic to the less automatic or intentional may be more likely to address the deficit of transcortical aphasia.

Conclusion

The topic of transcortical aphasias resulting from thalamic/subcortical infarction has not been discussed in this chapter. However, recognition of the occurrence of these syndromes underscores the point of Goldberg[32] (made specifically with transcortical motor aphasia but applicable to all) that subcortical and cortical structures are not only structurally but also functionally interconnected, forming systems which are dependent upon all the component parts for the functional integrity of the whole. Therefore, lesions of subcortical structures may induce syndromes that in many ways resemble, though not necessarily exactly mimic, the cortically induced syndromes. However, it is not just the subcortical/cortical connections that explain the relationship between these syndrome variants. Cortical-to-cortical connections can possibly explain the relationship within and among syndromes as well, and in this particular instance the relationships among the major categories of transcortical aphasia.

Pandya,[90] in his review of the cellular architectonic and connectional organization of the human frontal cortex, reviews the notion that " . . . in the course of evolution, the adaptation of organisms to increasingly complex conditions is reflected in concomitant morphological features of the brain . . . ". From evidence across species and within primates specifically, Pandya[90] reviews the hypothesis that all cortical regions have evolved from two sources, which he calls moieties. Therefore, cortical regions that are widely distributed anatomically may have evolved from a common source or moiety. Pandya[90] asks the important question: "Is there some organizational principle that accounts for, and interrelates, different cytoarchitectonic regions in the frontal lobe?" And we might continue, "Is there some organizational principle that accounts for and interrelates anatomically distributed portions within cytoarchitectonic regions?" Pandya[91] suggests that from one of these moieties (paleocortical) those cortical systems evolved that process sensory information, while from the other moiety (archicortical) those cortical systems evolved that process spatial information "crucial for effecting behavior in space." It is the archicortical moiety that is most relevant to the transcortical aphasias as the frontal structures evolving from this moiety include dorsolateral prefrontal cortex, implicated in transcortical motor aphasia. Pandya[90] points out that this system of connectivity projects back to (among other structures) the medial and ventral occipito–temporal region. This is the same region related to transcortical sensory aphasia and provides a structural suggestion that transcortical sensory and motor aphasias are related by more than symptom similarity. Heilman (personal communication) suggests that both syndromes, by virtue of the connectivity of the neural structures involved, possibly may represent differing levels of deficit in the same functional system; i.e., activation of the semantic field. Transcortical motor aphasics might be those in whom activation of the semantic field is possible only by externally generated stimulation. In contrast, for transcortical sensory aphasia, activation of the semantic field is possible only by internally or self-generated stimulation. The result would yield symptoms characteristic of each of these syndromes. This remains an interesting hypothesis awaiting further study.

Suggested Readings

Transcortical Motor Aphasia

Albert ML, Goodglass H, Helm, et al: *Clinical Aspects of Dysphasia.* New York: Springer-Verlag Wien, pp 94–98.

Luria AR: *Neuropsychological Studies in Aphasia.* Amsterdam: Swets and Zeitlinger BV, 1977.

Stuss DT, Benson DF: *The Frontal Lobes.* New York: Raven Press, 1986.

Transcortical Sensory Aphasia

Coslett HB, Roeltgen DP, Gonzalez-Rothi LJ et al: Transcortical sensory aphasia: Evidence for subtypes. *Brain and Language,* 1987; 32:362–378.

Kremin H: Is there more than ah-oh-oh? Alternative strategies for writing and repeating lexically. In Coltheart M, Job R, and Sartori G (eds): *The Cognitive Neuropsychology of Language.* London: Lawrence Erlbaum Assoc, 1987.

McCarthy RA, Warrington EK: The double dissociation of short-term memory for lists and sentences. *Brain* 1987; 110:1545–1563.

Mixed Transcortical Aphasia

Geschwind N, Quadfasel F, Segarra J: Isolation of speech area. *Neuropsychologia,* 6:327–340, 1968.
Goldstein, K. *Language and Language Disturbances.* New York: Grune and Stratton, 1948.
Whitaker HA: A case of isolation of the language function. In Whitaker H, Whitaker HA (eds): *Studies in Neurolinguistics,* vol 1, New York: Academic Press, 1976.

References

1. Whitaker HA: Two views on aphasia classification. *Brain and Language* 1984; 21:1–2.
2. Heilman KM, Rothi LJG: Aphasia: Syndrome subtypes. *Curr Neurol* 1987; 7:277–294.
3. Schwartz MF: What the classical aphasia categories can't do for us and why. *Brain and Language* 1984; 21:3–8.
4. Caramazza A: The logic of neuropsychological research and the problem of patient classification in aphasia. *Brain and Language* 1984; 21:9–20.
5. Caramazza A: When is enough, enough? A comment on Grodzinsky and Marek's algorithmic and heuristic processes revisited. *Brain and Language* 1988; 33:390–399.
6. Kussmaul A: Disturbances of speech: An attempt in the pathology of speech, vol. 14. In Ziemssen HV (ed): *Cyclopedia of the Practice of Medicine.* New York: Wood, 1887, pp 581–875.
7. Wernicke C: *Der Aphasische Symptomenkomplex.* Breslau: Cohn and Weigart, 1874.
8. Lecours AR, Poncet M, Ponzio J, et al: Classification of the aphasias. In Lecours F, Lhermitte F, Bryans B (eds): *Aphasiology.* London: Bailliere Tindall, 1983.
9. Lichtheim L: On aphasia. *Brain* 1885; 7:433–484.
10. Wernicke C: The Symptom-complex of aphasia. In Church A (ed): *Modern Clinical Medical Diseases of the Nervous System.* New York: Appleton, 1908.
11. Goldstein K: *Language and Language Disturbances.* New York: Grune and Stratton, 1948.
12. Bastian H: Some problems in connexion with aphasia and other speech defects. *Lancet* 1897; 1:933–942, 1005–1017, 1131–1137, 1187–1194.
13. Niessl von Mayendorf E: *Die Aphasischen Symptome und ihre kortikale Lokalization.* Leipzig: Barth, 1911.
14. Rubens A, Kertesz A: The localization of lesions in transcortical aphasias. In Kertesz A (ed): *Localization in Neuropsychology.* New York: Academic Press, 1983.
15. Botez MI: Clinical contributions of the tumoral frontal syndrome. *Psychiatria et Neurologia* 1960; 140:351.
16. Botez MI: The starting mechanism of speech. *Ldegyogyaszati* 1964; 1:13.
17. Botez MI, Barbeau A: Role of subcortical structures and particularly of the thalamus, in the mechanisms of speech and language. *International Journal of Neurology* 1971; 8:300–320.
18. Botez MI, Lecours AR, Berube L: Speech and language in the frontal syndrome. In Lecours AR, Lhermitte F, Bryan B (eds): *Aphasiology.* London: Bailliere Tindall, 1983, pp 124–140.
19. Luria A: *Human Brain and Psychological Processes.* New York: Harper and Row, 1966.
20. Luria A: *Traumatic Aphasia.* The Hague: Mouton, 1970.
21. Luria AR: *Neuropsychological Studies in Aphasia.* Amsterdam: Swets and Zeitlinger BV, 1977.
22. Luria AR, Hutton JT: A modern assessment of the basic forms of aphasia. *Brain and Language* 1977; 4:129–151.
23. Luria AR, Tsvetkova LS: The Mechanisms of Dynamic Aphasia, *Foundations of Language,* vol. 4, Amsterdam, 1968.
24. Brown JW: *Mind, Brain and Consciousness: The Neuropsychology of Cognition.* New York: Academic Press, 1977.
25. LaPlane D, Talairach J, Meininger V, et al: Clinical consequences of corticetomies involving the supplementary motor area in man. *J Neurol Sci* 1977; 34:301–314.
26. Damasio AR: Understanding the mind's will. *Behav Brain Sci* 1985; 8:567–616.
27. Damasio A, Van Hoesen G: Structure and function of the SMA. *Neurology* 1980; 30:359.
28. Masdeu JC, Schoene WE, Funkenstein H: Aphasia following infarction of the left supplementary motor area. *Neurology* 1978; 28:1220–1223.
29. Jonas S: The supplementary motor region and speech emission. *Journal of Communicative Disorders* 1981; 14:349–373.
30. Roland PE, Larsen B, Lassen NA, et al: Supplementary motor area and other cortical areas in organization of voluntary movements in man. *J Neurophysiol* 1980; 43:118–136.
31. Watson RT, Fleet S, Gonzalez-Rothi L, et al: Apraxia and the supplementary motor area. *Arch Neurol* 1986; 43:787–792.
32. Goldberg G: Supplementary motor area structure and function: Review and hypotheses. *Behav Brain Sci* 1985; 8:567–616.

33. Stuss DT, Benson DF: *The Frontal Lobes*. New York: Raven Press, 1986.
34. Rubens AB: Aphasia with infarction in the territory of the anterior cerebral artery. *Cortex* 1975; 11:239–250.
35. Naeser MA, Hayward RW: Lesion localization in aphasia with cranial computed tomography and the Boston Diagnostic Aphasia Exam. *Neurology* 1978; 28:545–551.
36. Freedman M, Alexander MP, Naeser MA: Anatomical basis of transcortical motor aphasia. *Neurology* 1984; 34:409–417.
37. Bogousslavsky J, Regli F: Unilateral watershed cerebral infarcts. *Neurology* 1986; 36:373–377.
38. Kertesz A: *Aphasia and Associated Disorders. Taxonomy, Localization and Recovery*. New York: Grune and Stratton, 1979.
39. Bonhoeffer C: Uber subkortikale sensorische aphasie. *Jahrbucher fur Psychiatrie un Neurologie* 1905; 26:126.
40. Heilbronner K: Zur Ruckbildung der sensorischen aphasie. *Archiv fur Psychiatrie und Nervenkrankheiten* 1909; 46.
41. Pick A: Ein Fall von transkortikaler sensorischer Aphasie. *Neurologisches Zentralblatt* 1890.
42. McCarthy RA, Warrington EK: The double dissociation of short-term memory for lists and sentences. *Brain* 1987; 110:1545–1563.
43. Kremin H: Is there more than ah-oh-oh? Alternative strategies for writing and repeating lexically. In Coltheart M, Job R, Sartori G (eds): *The Cognitive Neuropsychology of Language*. London: Lawrence Erlbaum, 1987, pp 295–335.
44. Coslett HB, Roeltgen DP, Rothi LJG, et al: Transcortical sensory aphasia: Evidence for subtypes. *Brain and Language* 1987; 32:362–378.
45. Martin N, Saffran EM: Factors underlying the repetition performance in transcortical sensory aphasia. (Submitted for publication.)
46. Morton J, Patterson K: A new attempt at an interpretation, or an attempt at a new interpretation! In Coltheart M, Patterson K, Marshall JC (eds): *Deep Dyslexia*. London: Routledge and Kegan-Paul, 1980, pp 91–118.
47. Patterson K, Shewell C: Speak and spell: Dissociations and word-class effects. In Coltheart M, Sartori G, Job R (eds): *The Cognitive Neuropsychology of Language*. London: Lawrence Erlbaum Associates, 1987, pp 273–294.
48. Caramazza A, Miceli G, Villa G: The role of the (output) phonological buffer in reading, writing and repetition. *Cognitive Neuropsychology* 1986; 3:37–76.
49. Caramazza A, Berndt RS, Basili A: The selective impairment of phonological processing: A case study. *Brain and Language* 1983; 18:128–174.
50. Davis L, Foldi NS, Gardner H, et al: Repetition in the transcortical aphasias. *Brain and Language* 1978; 6:226–238.
51. Berndt RS, Basili A, Caramazza A: Dissociation of functions in a case of transcortical sensory aphasia. *Cognitive Neuropsychology* 1987; 4:79–107.
52. Henschen SE: *Klinische und Anatomische Beitrage zur Pathologie des Gehirns*, vol. 5–7, Stockholm: Nordiska Bokhandel'n, 1920–1922.
53. Kertesz A, Sheppard A, MacKenzie R: Localization in transcortical sensory aphasia. *Arch Neurol* 1982; 39:475–478.
54. Hiltbrunner B, Alexander MP, Fischer RS: *Transcortical Sensory Aphasia: CT Anatomy and Neuropsychology*. A paper presented at the annual meeting of the Academy of Aphasia, Phoenix, 1987.
55. Feinberg TE, Rothi LJG, Heilman KM: Multimodal agnosia after unilateral left hemisphere lesion. *Neurology* 1986; 36:864–867.
56. Rothi LJG, Feinberg TE: Patient with left posterior circulation CVA, now with anomic dysphasia, Can you help? In Helm-Estabrooks N, Aten J (eds): *Difficult Diagnoses in Neurogenic Communication Disorders*. San Diego: College-Hill Press, 1989, 93–100.
57. Geschwind N, Quadfasel F, Segarra J: Isolation of the speech area. *Neuropsychologia* 1968; 6:327–340.
58. Bogausslavsky J, Regli F, Assal G: Acute transcortical mixed aphasia: A carotid occlusion syndrome with pial and watershed infarcts. *Brain* 1988; 111:631–641.
59. Kornyey E: Aphasie transcorticale et echolalie: Le probleme de l'initiative de la parole. *Revue Neurologique* 1975; 131:347–363.
60. Ross ED: Left medial parietal lobe and receptive language functions: Mixed transcortical aphasia after left anterior cerebral artery infarction. *Neurology* 1980; 30:144–151.
61. Stengel E: A clinical and psychological study of echoreactions. *J Ment Sci* 1947; 93:598–612.
62. Bando M, Ugawa Y, Sugishita M: Mechanism of repetition in transcortical sensory aphasia. *J Neurol Neurosurg Psychiatry* 1986; 49:200–202.
63. Rothi LJ, Heilman KM: Transcortical motor aphasia and syntactic comprehension. *A Presentation at the Academy of Aphasia*, Bass River: Massachusetts, 1980.

64. Lecours AR, Lhermitte F: Clinical forms of aphasia. In Lecours AR, Lhermitte F, Bryans B (eds): *Aphasiology*. London: Bailliere Tindall, 1983, pp 76–108.
65. Heilman KM, Rothi L, McFarling D, et al: Transcortical sensory aphasia with relatively spared spontaneous speech and naming. *Arch Neurol* 1981; 38:236–239.
66. Albert ML, Goodglass H, Helm NA, et al: *Clinical Aspects of Dysphasia*, New York: Springer-Verlag/ Wien, 1981.
67. Mesulam M-M: *Principles of Behavioral Neurology*, Philadelphia: FA Davis, 1985.
68. Kertesz A, Harlock W, Coates R: Computer tomographic localization, lesion size, and prognosis in aphasia and nonverbal impairment. *Brain Lang* 1979; 8:34–50.
69. Selnes OA, Knopman DS, Niccum N, et al: The critical role of Wernicke's area in sentence repetition. *Ann Neurol* 1985; 17:549–557.
70. Whitaker H: A case of isolation of the language function, vol. 1. In Whitaker H, Whitaker HA (eds): *Studies of Neurolinguistics*. New York: Academic Press, 1976.
71. Pirozzolo FJ, Kerr KL, Obrzut JE et al: Neurolinguistic analysis of the language abilities of a patient with a "double disconnection syndrome": A case of subangular alexia in the presence of mixed transcortical aphasia. *J Neurol Neurosurg Psychiatry* 1981; 44:152–155.
72. Heilman KM, Tucker DM, Valenstein E: A case of mixed transcortical aphasia with intact naming. *Brain* 1976; 99:415–426.
73. Schneider DE: The clinical syndromes of echolalia, echopraxia, grasping and sucking. *J Nerv Ment Dis* 1938; 88:18–35, 200–216.
74. Stengel E, Vienna MD, Edin LRCP: A clinical and psychological study of echo-reactions. *J Ment Sci* 1947; 93:598–612.
75. Thurstone LL, Thurstone T: *The Chicago Tests of Primary Mental Abilities*. Chicago: Science Research Associates, 1943.
76. Milner B: Some effects of frontal lobectomy in man. In Warren JM, Akert K (eds): *Frontal Granular Cortex and Behavior*. New York: McGraw-Hill, 1964, pp 313–334.
77. Newcombe F: *Missile Wounds of the Brain: A Study of Psychological Deficits*. New York: Oxford University Press, 1969.
78. Benton AL, Hamsher K de S, Varney NR, et al: *Contributions to Neuropsychological Assessment: A Clinical Manual*. New York: Oxford University Press, 1983.
79. Goodglass H, Kaplan E: *The Assessment of Aphasia and Related Disorders*. Philadelphia: Lea and Febiger, 1976.
80. Kertesz A: *The Western Aphasia Battery*. New York: Grune and Stratton, 1982.
81. Geschwind N, Kaplan E: A human cerebral disconnection syndrome. *Arch Neurol* 1962; 12:675–685.
82. Kertesz A, McCabe P: Recovery patterns and prognosis in stroke. *Brain* 1977; 100:1–18.
83. Alexander MP, Schmitt MA: The aphasia syndrome of stroke in the left anterior cerebral artery territory. *Arch Neurol* 1980; 37:97–100.
84. Rothi LJG, Horner J: Restitution and substitution: Two theories of recovery with application to neurobehavioral treatment. *The Journal of Clinical Neuropsychology*. 1983; 5:73–81.
85. Johnson M: Treatment of transcortical motor aphasia. In Perkins W (ed): *Current Therapy of Communication Disorders*. New York: Thieme-Stratton, Inc., 1983.
86. Kools J: Congenital transcortical motor aphasia. In Talbott R, Larson V (eds): *Communicative Disorders* 1983; 12:171–172.
87. Lentz S, Shubitowski Y, Rosenbek J, et al: *Treating Sponaneous Speech Production in Transcortical Motor Aphasia*. Paper presented at the American Speech and Hearing Association Convention, Cincinnati, Ohio, 1983.
88. Huntley RA, Rothi LJG: Treatment of verbal akinesia in a case of transcortical motor aphasia. *Aphasiology*, 1988; 2:55–66.
89. Albert ML, Bachman D, Morgan A, et al: Pharmacotherapy for aphasia. *Neurology* 1987; 37:175.
90. Pandya DN: Frontal lobe architecture and connections. A presentation to the Annual Meeting of the International Neuropsychological Society, New Orleans, LA, 1988.

5

Lexical Retrieval Problems: Anomia

CRAIG W. LINEBAUGH

In the vernacular of clinical aphasiology, *anomia* refers both to a specific clinical sign and to a specific clinical syndrome. In this chapter, the discussions of differentiating features, evaluation, and treatment will focus on the sign rather than the syndrome. The rationale for this is twofold. First, anomia is virtually universal among patients presenting a neurogenic language disorder and, for most, is a significant contributor to their reduced communicative success and efficiency. Second, the cardinal feature of anomic aphasia, the syndrome, is anomia, the clinical sign. A diagnosis of anomic aphasia requires that the patient present an impairment of lexical access (word retrieval) which is of significantly greater severity than his/her impairments of other language functions, though patients with anomic aphasia have been reported to experience particular difficulty in comprehending isolated nouns and verbs.[1]

Anomia as a clinical sign refers to an impairment of the process of retrieving words from one's lexicon. It is important to distinguish between lexical retrieval and naming. Naming is a task that involves several processes in addition to lexical retrieval. These include visual perception and recognition, phonological encoding and speech motor programming, and execution. In addition, performance on virtually any language task involves those executive cognitive functions by which one attends to specific stimuli and mediates appropriate responses. Impairments of these processes may significantly affect a patient's performances on verbal expressive tasks either independently of or coincidentally with a specific impairment of lexical retrieval. This chapter focuses specifically on the process of lexical retrieval.

It appears that lexical retrieval problems may arise from both disruption of lexical structure and interference in lexical access. Several investigators[2-5] have presented results suggesting some alteration of lexical structure in patients with focal brain lesions. It would be expected that if the representation of lexical entries is degraded they would be less readily available to the language-impaired individual. The existence of lexical retrieval problems arising from interference with the process of lexical retrieval is supported by the variable performance of aphasic individuals (Sometimes they can find the word, and sometimes they cannot.), the successful elicitation of words using a variety of prompts and the results of lexical priming studies.[6,7] In this chapter, evaluation and treatment approaches applicable to both mechanisms will be discussed.

It also should be noted that access to the lexicon can be achieved from both "below" and "above." External and internal physical stimuli evoke from us comments, requests, protests, etc. in what can be viewed as bottom-up access. Sometimes these utterances are volitional (May I see that?), and sometimes they are highly automatic (Ouch!). Access to the lexicon in the course of expressing internally generated opinions, feelings, and desires may be viewed as top-down. Here the "stimulus" exists in the speaker's mind, rather than in the internal or external physical environment. Figure 5–1 presents a model depicting various "access routes" to the lexicon. These routes should be considered in the evaluation and treatment of anomia.

Pathophysiology

Specific lexical entries, along with their semantic, syntactic, phonologic, and orthographic representations, may be viewed as being stored in the brain by means of neuronal networks. Various aspects (e.g., semantic features, grammatical form class, syllabic structure) of lexical entries may be represented within networks that are common to all lexical entries sharing specific features, but no two lexical entries are represented by identical networks. In this way, synonyms, homonyms, and homographs retain unique, albeit extensively shared, neuronal representations. Retrieval of a specific lexical entry requires activation of its neuronal representation to a level which makes the entry available for further linguistic processing. Selection of a specific lexical entry also may involve inhibition of other entries that share common features.

Three mechanisms may be hypothesized which account for anomia. The first involves "damage" to the neuronal representations of lexical entries. Lesions to

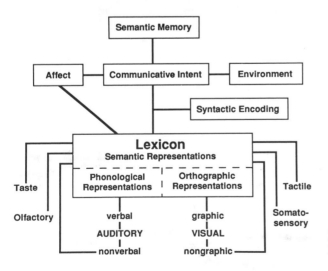

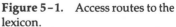

Figure 5–1.   Access routes to the lexicon.

these networks of neurons might render certain lexical entries inaccessible or at least require a higher level of activation of the residual elements of the network. This mechanism could account for several manifestations of impaired lexical retrieval, including word omissions, partial responses, semantic paraphasias, and neologisms. The second mechanism involves a delay or failure in substantially intact neuronal networks reaching an adequate level of activation. This mechanism may manifest itself in a number of ways including increased response latencies, partially accurate responses, circumlocutions, word omissions, and perhaps production of unrelated words. The third involves a failure to inhibit lexical entries which share a substantial number of common features.[8] Occurrences of this phenomenon could result in semantic paraphasias.

Anomia has been associated with a wide range of lesion patterns, both focal and diffuse, and as a result has frequently been regarded as a nonlocalizing clinical sign.[9] Persistent anomia has, however, generally been linked to large left hemisphere lesions or focal lesions of the left temporal-parietal cortex. For example, Knopman et al.[10] have reported that of 19 patients with lesions greater than 60 cm in volume, 13 named fewer than 25% of pictured items at six months post onset, while the remaining 6 patients named fewer than 75% of the items. These investigators also reported that among patients with lesions less than 60 cm in volume, semantic errors suggesting impaired lexical retrieval were most commonly associated with lesions of the posterior superior temporal-inferior parietal regions.

Differentiating Features

Differentiating anomia from impairments of other neurolinguistic processes involved in verbal expression may be complicated by a number of factors. Impairments of perceptual, cognitive, and/or linguistic processes required for the performance of tasks being used to assess lexical retrieval may interfere with performance of the task prior to lexical retrieval. For example, misperception of an object may lead to what might be interpreted as a "naming error," when in fact the patient retrieved the appropriate name for what he perceived the object to be. In an auditory responsive naming task, a breakdown in comprehension of the stimulus might result in what could be interpreted as an error in lexical retrieval. Similarly, impairments of processes lying "downstream" from lexical retrieval (e.g., phonological encoding, speech motor programming) may mask impaired lexical retrieval in much the same way lower motor neuron damage may mask involvement of other components of the motor system. Also, it may be difficult to attribute an error response to a single, specific error mechanism. For example, can *rat* produced in response to a picture of a *cat* be classified as a semantic paraphasia with any greater confidence than can *hat*? Or might both be phonemic paraphasias? Moreover, some errors may not be the result of breakdown in a single process at all, but rather a result of a concatenation of errors in two or more successive processes. It is neccesary, therefore, to determine, as best one can, the contributions of breakdowns in processes other than lexical retrieval to task performance.

In spite of these difficulties, certain features in the verbal output of aphasic people may be interpreted as signs of impaired lexical retrieval. Delayed accurate responses in naming tasks and extended interword pauses in contextual speech may be indicative of a slowing of the retrieval process. During such episodes of increased response latency, patients may be searching their lexicons actively or selecting from a group of response alternatives which are available. These covert activities may reflect failure of the target word to reach a threshold of activation and faulty inhibition of related lexical entries, respectively. Aphasic individuals also may have partial information available to them regarding a lexical entry.[3] These occurrences are similar to the "tip of the tongue" phenomenon experienced by normal speakers in which they may recall the first letter or number of syllables of a word, but are unable to retrieve the word itself.

Many aphasic speakers also engage in overt self-cueing behaviors.[11] Observation of these behaviors generally allows an examiner to verify that the person is attempting to produce a semantically appropriate response. They do not, however, permit ready discernment as to whether the breakdown is occurring in the retrieval of a specific lexical semantic representation or in the retrieval of that semantic representation's phonological form. Likewise, production of real words that are phonologically similar to target words (e.g., cap/cat, house/mouse) does not permit differentiation between retrieval of an incorrect phonological representation or a breakdown in phonological encoding. The dilemma is heightened when the word that is produced bears both semantic and phonological similarities to the target word (e.g., cat/rat; bake/cake).

Production of semantically related words and circumlocutions may be interpreted as indicating breakdown in the retrieval of lexical semantic representations. In the former, a word sharing semantic features with the target word is retrieved and produced. In the latter, either no specific word reaches a level of activation sufficient for retrieval, or the patient recognizes the inaccuracy of those words which are available and chooses to "talk around" a concept rather than produce a word that does not convey the concept accurately.

In differentiating anomia from impairments in other processes which may influence verbal expressive performance, therefore, it is essential either to (1) establish the integrity of those other processes or (2) obtain a corpus of lexical retrieval errors that permits determination of the relative contributions of breakdowns in various processes to the patient's verbal output. Although this cannot always be done with certainty, it can frequently be done with sufficient confidence to permit focusing of treatment specifically on lexical retrieval and/or certain other processes. The means by which this differentiation can be accomplished will be discussed next.

Evaluation

Evaluation of lexical retrieval requires the use of a variety of tasks in which several variables are systematically manipulated. These include: (1) the direction from which the lexicon is to be accessed (top-down vs. bottom-up), (2) the stimulus modality, (3) the nature of the stimulus, (4) the characteristics of the lexical entries to be retrieved, (5) the context in which lexical retrieval is to occur, (6) the response modality, and (7) the nature of the response. Each of these variables warrants some brief discussion.

Lexicon Access. As discussed above, the lexicon may be accessed either from "above" (top-down) or from "below" (bottom-up). Patient-initiated utterances provide the most valid sample of top-down lexical access. Here lexical retrieval is driven by communicative intent and the specific concepts to be expressed. Utterances produced in response to open-ended questions also provide a fairly good view of top-down lexical access in that patients need to formulate responses based on general knowledge. Retelling stories that have been heard or read and describing pictures represent a sort of midground between top-down and bottom-up access. These two tasks are similar because the information to be conveyed has been provided, but they are also different in some important ways. In story retelling, the patient needs to recall and organize the information and generate appropriate syntactic forms prior to lexical retrieval. Here, the burden is on information recall, and the patient has the benefit of the vocabulary that was used in the stimulus story. In describing a picture, the stimulus generally remains before the patient, alleviating recall burdens, but the patient needs to select appropriate lexical entries independent of any previous model. Responsive naming tasks also include both top-down and bottom-up elements in that the stimulus first needs to be comprehended, and then an appropriate lexical entry retrieved. Confrontation naming tasks involve mainly bottom-up access to the lexicon.

Verbal fluency measures,[12,13] which are included in many standardized tests of aphasia, bear special mention as a means of assessing top-down access to the lexicon. These tasks are essentially metalinguistic in nature; they require patients to make a controlled search of the lexicon. As such, they may provide useful information regarding lexical structure and retrieval strategies.[14-17]

Two major forms of verbal fluency measures have been used. One requires patients to produce words beginning with particular letters of the alphabet. In this form, lexical entries are retrieved based on orthographic representations, though many patients are observed to employ a phonologically based retrieval strategy (e.g., For *s*: see, soup, sew, shop, ship, shape, stop, stare, staple. For *c*: cents, cereal, ceiling, car, cart, carrot.). The other form requires patients to retrieve words from specific semantic superordinate categories. On these tasks, patients' ability to organize a lexical search can be observed through their retrieval of words from various semantic subcategories (e.g., for *animals*: farm animals, zoo animals, pets; for *clothing*: men's clothing, women's clothing). In evaluating lexical retrieval, particularly in mildly aphasic patients, it is recommended that both letter and semantic category verbal fluency tasks be employed. Normative data are available for the letter task included in the Neurosensory Center Comprehensive Examination for Aphasia[18] and for the Animal Naming subtest of the Boston Diagnostic Aphasia Examination.[19]

Stimulus Modality.   Though rare, modality specific anomias have been reported.[20] Most commonly these impairments have been attributed to disconnections between sensory and associative cortical regions.[21] When a patient presents markedly better lexical retrieval in conversation than in visual confrontation naming, it is important to determine the cause of this dissociation. First, performance on other tasks using visually presented stimuli should be compared with the performances in conversation and on tasks using auditory stimuli (e.g., responsive naming, naming environmental sounds). Should performance be consistently depressed on tasks using visual stimuli, the patient should be examined for visual agnosia. Tactile naming also may be assessed as a means of differentiating generalized from modality specific anomia.

Nature of the Stimuli.   Most studies that have examined naming of objects versus pictures have reported little or no difference between the two types of stimuli.[22,23] One advantage of using objects, however, is that they can be manipulated by the client; this seems to facilitate naming for some individuals. Picturability[24] and operativity[25] have also been shown to influence naming performance. For auditorily presented stimuli, retrieving a specific lexical entry in response to a description has generally proven to be more difficult than retrieving the entry in response to a sentence-completion stimulus.[26,27]

Characteristics of the Lexical Entries.   A number of characteristics of lexical entries themselves have proven to influence aphasic client's lexical retrieval. Frequency of occurrence has been demonstrated to influence the availability of lexical entries both on naming tasks[28,29] and in spontaneous speech.[30,31] Likewise, word length,[32] grammatical form class[33,34] and personal relevance[35] influence lexical retrieval. In evaluating lexical retrieval, it is advisable to sample performance for different grammatical form classes (e.g., nouns, verbs, adjectives) and a variety of semantic categories.

Context.   Williams and Canter[36] reported different retrieval performances for specific nouns by Broca and Wernicke aphasic patients when the nouns were depicted as isolated pictures in a confrontation-naming task as opposed to being depicted in context as part of a picture-description task. These authors suggest that lexical retrieval should be assessed both in confrontation-naming and picture-description tasks.

Response Modality.   Lexical retrieval is most commonly assessed via speech. For some individuals, however, especially those with severe motor speech impairments, speech may not be the best modality in which to assess lexical retrieval. Therefore, evaluation of lexical retrieval should include responses made by writing and/or selecting from a set of printed words, as well as through spoken responses.

Nature of the Response.   Many aphasic clients' lexical retrieval varies across communicative tasks. As Williams and Canter[36] noted, performance on tasks requiring single word responses is not necessarily predictive of performance on tasks requiring description. Some aphasic persons converse better than they can describe pictures. Some may be able to retrieve the lexical entries necessary to adequately describe a picture before them, but encounter significant anomia when faced with the additional cognitive burden of projecting what events might have preceded or could follow the pictured actions. The variable of "nature of the response" encompasses two main aspects of the task. One is the length and complexity of the response (e.g., single words, phrases, sentences, narrative). The other is the amount of responsiveness and cognitive organization (confrontation naming versus picture description versus referential communication versus conversation) required for the performance of the task.

As is apparent from the review of these seven variables affecting lexical retrieval, obtaining an accurate appraisal of a speaker's lexical retrieval abilities requires sampling performances on a number of different tasks. Selection of these tasks needs to consider the various routes to the lexicon and the other cognitive–linguistic processes involved in performance of the tasks. In this manner, the specific locus or loci of neurolinguistic impairment might be determined. Specific tasks which should be included in the evaluation of lexical retrieval are listed in Table 5–1. Of course, not all of the tasks listed in Table 1 will be appropriate for all clients, and in some cases additional tasks (e.g., tactile naming, naming environmental sounds) will be needed to delineate more precisely the nature of a patient's lexical retrieval impairment.

Examination of a patient's verbal output is also an important part of the evaluation of lexical retrieval. Identification of the conditions under which lexical retrieval is successful and analysis of the errors produced on various tasks contribute to determining the locus or loci of impairments within the verbal output system. Several different types of error responses have been identified, many of which have been attributed to breakdowns in specific neurolinguistic processes.[36–38] Table 5–2 lists these error types and the mechanisms by which they might be produced.

Tasks assessing performance in other modalities also may provide information about the nature of a speaker's lexical retrieval impairments. Gainotti et al.[5] compared the naming performance of aphasic subjects with and without a lexical comprehension impairment. Although the two groups of subjects produced similar numbers of errors, those with a lexical comprehension impairment produced more semantic paraphasic errors than did those without a lexical comprehension impairment. The authors interpreted these results as indicating an alteration of the semantic representations of the group with lexical comprehension impairments. Other tasks which may provide information regarding the integrity of the lexical semantic and/or phonological representations (e.g., categorization, identifying pictures whose labels rhyme) also may help in discerning the nature of lexical retrieval impairments.

Treatment

Treatment of anomia involves three main components which are common to the treatment of most language-impaired patients. These are (1) facilitation of the impaired process(es), (2) fostering generalization to untrained linguistic units and natural communicative situations and (3) developing effective compensatory strategies for coping with residual deficits. This section will focus on the first of these components with some attention to be given to the other two.

Table 5–1. Tasks for the Evaluation of Lexical Retrieval

Visual confrontation naming
Word naming
Responsive naming
Picture-to-word matching
Written confrontation naming
Verbal fluency
Picture description
Story retelling
Story completion
Referential communication
Conversational speech sample

Table 5-2. Error Types and Error Mechanisms

Error Type	Error Mechanism
Delayed	"Slowed" activation/selection of target lexical entry
Self-corrected	Recognition of error response; retrieval of target lexical entry
Circumlocution (sticker bush/cactus; definition)	Failure to retrieve specific lexical entry; conveys semantic information
Phonemic paraphasia	Error in phoneme selection and sequencing
Semantic paraphasia Coordinate (cat/dog) Associate (mouse/cheese; fly/bird) Super-/sub-ordinate (animal/cat; oak/tree) Part-whole (hand/finger; toe/foot)	Retrieval of a lexical entry semantically related to the target
Unrelated word	Failure to access appropriate semantic category
Neologism Lexical blend [chofa (chair + sofa)/couch]	Combination of two lexical entries
"Nonword" (grimpton/beaver)	Extreme phoneme selection and sequencing error
Perseveration	Failure to inhibit a previous response
Gesture	Compensation for failure to retrieve target lexical entry
No response	

Facilitating Impaired Lexical Retrieval

A number of procedures have been developed to facilitate impaired lexical retrieval, nearly all of which are based on the provision of some prompt or cue which is expected to enable the patient to produce a target word. In one approach, a facilitating cue is made a part of the stimulus intended to elicit a particular response. Podraza and Darley[39] demonstrated the effectiveness of "prestimulation" using the initial phoneme of a target word, an open-ended sentence, and presentation of the target word along with two unrelated foils. These and other cues (e.g., descriptive statement, printed word) can be incorporated in a task continuum in which the client progresses through a series of tasks of increasing difficulty contingent upon reaching a criterion level of performance on each preceding task.

An alternative approach calls for providing the facilitating cues contingent upon failure to produce a target word. This "cueing hierarchy" approach[40,41] is based on the rationale that long-term improvement of lexical retrieval is best accomplished by the patient's retrieving the target word with as little external facilitation as possible. It also incorporates the notion of "stimulus power." Stimulus power refers to the probability of a given stimulus eliciting a target response. In the cueing hierarchy approach, successively presented cues should be hierarchically organized according to stimulus power. Studies of cueing techniques have indicated that for aphasic subjects as a group initial phoneme cues are more powerful than sentence completion cues, which in turn are more powerful than descriptions.[26,27,42,43] Rhymes[43] and printed words[42] also have been shown to be effective cues. Of course, no cue is effective one hundred percent of the time, and cues vary in effectiveness according to the type and severity of aphasia. For example, phonemic cues are generally more effective for anomic and Broca aphasic patients than for Wernicke aphasic subjects.[38,44] Function cues are more effective for mild and moderate than severely aphasic subjects and for anomic than Broca or Wernicke aphasic subjects.[43] Combinations of cues have been shown to be more effective in some instances than single cues.[45] In addition, aphasic individuals vary idiosyncratically in their responsiveness to different cues. Therefore, cueing hierarchies should be established for each based on his or her individual responsiveness to different types of cues.

Recently, some evidence has been reported which suggests that the long-term effects of different cues may vary. In a series of studies,[46-48] the relative stability of the effects of phonologically based versus semantically based facilitators have been examined. Phonologically based facilitators which were examined included repetition of a target word prior to presentation of a picture for naming, phonemic cueing, and making rhyme judgments about a target word and another word. These cues were shown to facilitate naming performance, but their effects dissipated in as little as 15 minutes. Semantically based facilitators studied were pointing to a picture of a target word when spoken prior to naming, matching a printed target word to a picture prior to naming, and making semantic judgments about a target word (Is a *cat* an animal?). The facilitatory effects of these cues were shown to persist longer than those of the phonologically based cues. The authors of these studies suggest that cues that activate the semantic representation of a lexical entry are more effective than cues that may activate only a phonological representation. These conclusions should be regarded as preliminary, however, in that at most the patients in these studies underwent only eight treatment sessions. Nevertheless, this is an important line of investigation, and much research remains to be done to determine the efficacy of various types of cues for various types of patients.

Fostering Generalization

Generalization of improved lexical retrieval is to be sought at a number of levels. First, improved retrieval of untrained, as well as trained, lexical entries is a goal of treatment. If the process of lexical retrieval is indeed facilitated, then improved retrieval of untrained words is a logical expectation. Unfortunately, such generalization is not always achieved.[49] In these cases, improved lexical retrieval appears to be limited to those lexical entries that have been specifically facilitated during the course of therapy. Why some patients exhibit generalized facilitation and others do not remains an area of investigation. Nevertheless, it is important to assess performance on both trained and untrained items during therapy to determine the efficacy of the treatment procedures being employed. Also, it is recommended that in selecting the specific lexical entries to be used in therapy, one selects words which are functionally relevant to the client. Not only is this likely to enhance generalization to natural communicative situations, but should improved lexical retrieval be limited to trained words, far better that those words be useful to the client.

Generalization of improved lexical retrieval beyond the production of single words should also be sought. Generally, speakers are asked to produce successively longer utterances beginning with two-word combinations and gradually increasing the length of their utterances depending on their success at previous levels. Two treatment approaches whose effectiveness in eliciting longer utterances from aphasic individuals has been demonstrated are Loverso, Selinger and Prescott's[50] "verb-as-core" approach and Kearns'[51] "response elaboration training."

When developing specific tasks intended to extend improved lexical retrieval to longer utterances, it is important to weigh the demands the tasks place on other cognitive and linguistic processes. For example, picture description requires the client to organize the content to be conveyed and to hold in working memory what has been expressed and what is yet to come. "Projecting" what might have preceded the pictured events and what might follow adds additional cognitive demands. Viewed from a resource allocation perspective, such cognitive demands, along with greater phonological encoding and motor programming demands, may limit the degree to which patients can "focus" their efforts on lexical retrieval. Progressing through a continuum of tasks that place successively greater demands on patients' cognitive–linguistic resources is an important means of fostering generalization of improved lexical retrieval to more realistic communicative tasks.

Generalization of improved lexical retrieval to natural communicative situations is also of concern. A number of techniques are available by which this type of generalization can be fostered. PACE therapy[52] provides clients an opportunity to "exercise" their lexical retrieval abilities in a situation that incorporates several aspects of natural conversation. An adaptation of PACE developed at The George Washington University focuses on patients' expression of specific semantic notions (agent, number, gender, action, location) and seeks to enhance the efficiency with which they express those notions by either direct lexical or compensatory means. Role-playing,[53] simulations of natural communicative situations,[54,55] and forays into the "real world" also have been used to foster generalization.

Developing Compensatory Strategies

When lexical retrieval fails, it is essential that aphasic persons have a means of conveying information, their needs and desires, their feelings. Treatment should, therefore, prepare patients to deal with their residual lexical retrieval impairments. One means of doing so is to develop patients' use of self-generated cues.[56] Not only do self-generated cues frequently lead to successful retrieval of the intended word,[11] but they often enable listeners to discern the intended word, even when the patient is unable to produce it.[57] The use of gestures and drawing[58,59] has proven to be an effective compensatory strategy.

Specific Treatment Tasks

The tasks to be presented in this section fall into two categories, those designed to facilitate the process of lexical retrieval and those designed to foster generalization of improved lexical retrieval skills.

Facilitating Lexical Retrieval

CONFRONTATION NAMING

Confrontation-naming tasks involve presentation of a stimulus that the client is to name. Access to the lexicon is essentially bottom-up with relatively little demand on higher cognitive–linguistic processes. Goldstein,[60] however, has postulated that some patients experience difficulty with confrontation-naming because of the "abstract attitude" the task requires. Usually, confrontation-naming tasks involve visual presentation of an object or picture, but they can be accomplished also through the auditory, tactile, olfactory, and gustatory modalities. Responses in confrontation-naming tasks are usually spoken or written, but they also may be made by pointing to one of several words presented or through use of an alphabet board.

CONFRONTATION NAMING WITH PRESTIMULATION

Several variations on basic confrontation-naming tasks using some form of prestimulation also can be used to facilitate lexical retrieval. Prestimulations that might be used include (1) repetition of the target word, (2) initial phoneme, (3) sentence completion, (4) description, and (5) functional gesture. In these tasks, the prestimulation is presented first, followed either immediately or after some predetermined delay by the picture or object to be named.

SENTENCE COMPLETION

Sentence completion tasks require the patient to produce the last word of a sentence. Sentence completions are most powerful when the content of a stimulus directs the client to a specific lexical entry ("You write with a ballpoint _____ " versus "You write with a _____ "). Care should be taken when using sentence completions, however, to ensure that the client comprehends the completion stimulus. Some clients may be able to complete the stimuli in such an automatic manner as to raise questions about their use as a treatment procedure.[61]

The above tasks may be incorporated into a task continuum. Table 5–3 lists these tasks in their generally accepted order of difficulty, but it should be kept in mind that as many aphasic individuals may deviate from this order as adhere to it. In addition, the difficulty of any of these tasks can be modified by manipulating those variables discussed above that influence lexical retrieval.

CUEING HIERARCHIES

Cueing hierarchies can be used for a wide variety of tasks in all language modalities. They involve presentation of a cue selected to facilitate patient performance contingent upon the patient's production of an error response. Cues are arranged hierarchically based on their relative stimulus power and presented sequentially until the patient produces an accurate response. Table 5–4 presents two representative cue-

Table 5–3.   A Task Continuum for Facilitating Lexical Retrieval

Picture + Spoken target word
Picture + Spoken target word and two semanticaly related foils
Picture + Sentence completion with initial phoneme
Picture + Sentence completion
Picture + Descriptive statement
Picture + Functional gesture
Picture only
Descriptive statement only

Table 5–4. Two Representative Cueing Hierarchies for Visual
Confrontation Naming

Picture
Picture + "Tell me what you do with it."
Picture + "Show me what you do with it."
Picture + Descriptive statement
Picture + Sentence completion
Picture + Sentence completion + Initial phoneme
Picture + "Say ———————."

Picture + "Show me what you do with it."
Picture + Functional gesture
Picture + Sentence completion
Picture + Sentence completion + Printed target word and two foils
Picture + Sentence completion + Printed target word
Picture + Sentence completion + Printed target word + Initial phoneme
Picture + "Say ———————."

ing hierarchies. When an accurate response has been elicited, the cues are presented in order of decreasing stimulus power until the client produces an accurate response to the original stimulus. Should the person fail to produce an accurate response during this "descending" presentation of the cues, the direction of cue presentation is reversed, and the cues are again presented in order of increasing stimulus power until an accurate response is produced. This ensures that the last response for a given item is successful.

Because the relative stimulus power of cues varies among aphasic persons, it is necessary to evaluate the relative power of cues and to develop individualized cueing hierarchies when appropriate. When developing hierarchies, one should first examine the self-cueing strategies being used by a patient and incorporate those which are successful into the hierarchy. This will foster the use of self-cues, thereby potentially facilitating lexical retrieval and providing listeners with additional information.[62] The power of additional cues whose potency has been demonstrated for aphasic individuals can then be assessed, and those which are effective for the specific client added to the hierarchy.

LEXICAL FOCUS

Many aphasic clients' anomia manifests itself primarily as semantic paraphasias. These errors may be interpreted as indicating that the speaker has achieved access to the appropriate "semantic field" but has failed to retrieve the specific lexical entry to convey a particular concept. Lexical focus therapy requires clients to retrieve lexical entries from progressively narrower semantic categories. First-order categories are broad superordinate categories containing entries from several subcategories. Second-order categories are smaller subsets of first-order categories, and third-order categories are, in turn, smaller subsets of second-order categories. Table 5–5 lists examples of first-, second- and third-order categories for use in lexical focus.

During therapy, a client is presented a category and asked to name as many items contained in that category as quickly as possible. Criterion performance levels are 10 items in 60 seconds for first-order categories, 7 items in 60 seconds for second-order

Table 5–5.   Example Categories for Lexical Focus

First-order	Second-order	Third-order
Fruits and Vegetables	Fruits	Citrus fruits
		Berries
	Vegetables	Green vegetables
		Yellow vegetables
Musical instruments	Horns	Brass
		Woodwinds
	String	Played with a bow
		Plucked
	Keyboard	
Sports	Played with a ball	Played with a racket
		Not played with a racket
	Not played with a ball	

categories and 4 items in 60 seconds for third-order categories. Categories falling within the same superordinate category should not be presented consecutively. When patients experience difficulty retrieving items in a particular category, "search strategies" may be employed. These are not cues for specific lexical entries. Rather, they are devices to aid patients in organizing their search for appropriate items. For example, for the category of fruits and vegetables, a patient may be instructed to think about the produce section in a supermarket. Patients frequently develop their own search strategies. These should be identified and refined to make them as effective as possible.

The evidence cited above regarding "damage" to the lexical semantic structure itself suggests that tasks which require access to semantic representations, without necessarily requiring retrieval of lexical entries, may facilitate lexical retrieval. Indeed, Howard et al.[48] have reported that such tasks do have a facilitatory effect on lexical retrieval. Tasks of this nature which might be employed include (1) auditory word-to-picture matching, (2) printed word-to-picture matching, (3) sorting pictures and printed words by semantic category, (4) identifying semantic features shared by two or more objects and (5) making semantic judgments about individual words. In addition, Chapey[63] has described a number of cognitively based tasks that may prove beneficial in improving semantic organization and lexical retrieval.

Fostering Generalization

As discussed above, generalization of improved lexical retrieval to longer, more complex utterances and to naturalistic communicative situations can be achieved under conditions that place increasingly greater demands on cognitive–linguistic processing. The following is a series of tasks by which such generalization can be fostered.

PICTURE DESCRIPTION

This task can be used to elicit utterances ranging from a two-word phrase (e.g., man drinking, drinking coffee) to an extended narrative. Advantages of this task are that it places little demand on patients' working memory and content of patients' utterances can be controlled by that of the picture. Lexical retrieval occurs on-line. This task also can be used between sessions by having patients select their own pictures and rehearse their descriptions. They then describe them to the clinician in a PACE-like format.

PREPARED MONOLOGUE

In this task, patients have an opportunity to prepare a set of utterances about a particular topic. Topics should be chosen for patient interest and relevance. Unlike picture description, lexical retrieval is initially accomplished off-line, and strategies to facilitate retrieval of specific words can be rehearsed. This is a very useful "between sessions" task for many patients and also can be effective in group therapy.

STORY RETELLING

This task can be quite difficult for some patients. It places considerable demands on auditory comprehension and memory and requires retrieval of specific vocabulary. Visual cues can be used to reduce the memory load for details and temporal ordering of events.

STORY ELABORATION

This task requires patients to provide those events that preceded and/or will follow those depicted in a picture or in an auditorily or graphically presented story. It adds the cognitive demands of formulating a plausible sequence of events, while still maintaining relatively predictable content. A group variation on this task has group members successively adding events.

REFERENTIAL COMMUNICATION

This task employs a barrier game format in which the client must convey specific information to an uninformed listener. It adds an interactive component in that the speaker must respond to listener contingent queries intended to resolve ambiguities in the client's utterances. This task can also be useful in groups and is especially effective for training frequent communication partners in communication-enhancing strategies.

ROLE-PLAYING

This task requires a client to respond to a partner's utterances other than contingent queries. A progression from rehearsed to impromptu, from predictable to unpredictable dialogues can help prepare a client for the dynamic nature of natural communication.

In spite of the best efforts of both clients and clinicians, however, most aphasic persons will continue to experience at least some degree of residual anomia. To this end, it is important that patients learn compensatory strategies in order to deal with episodes of anomia. In addition, they need to understand those conditions that may exacerbate their communication difficulties (e.g., stress, fatigue) and learn means by which the effects of these factors can be minimized. Finally, frequent communication partners of aphasic persons may benefit from counseling regarding appropriate courses of action and perhaps training in specific strategies to enhance communicative success and efficiency.[64]

Suggested Readings

Berman M, Peelle LM: Self-generated cues: A method for aiding aphasic and apractic patients. *Journal of Speech and Hearing Disorders* 1967; 32:372–376.

Golper LA, Rau MT: Systematic analysis of cueing strategies in aphasia: Taking your "cue" from the patient. In R.H. Brookshire (ed), *Clinical Aphasiology,* 1983. Minneapolis: BRK Publishers.

Howard D, Patterson K, Franklin S, et al: Treatment of word retrieval deficits in aphasia: A comparison of two therapy methods. *Brain* 1985; 108:817–829.

Kohn SE, Goodglass H: Picture-naming in aphasia. *Brain and Language,* 1985; 24:266–283.

Linebaugh CW: Treatment of anomic aphasia. In W.H. Perkins (ed), *Current Therapy of Communication Disorders, Language Handicaps in Adults.* New York: Thieme-Stratton, 1983.

Marshall RC: Word retrieval behavior of aphasic adults. *Journal of Speech and Hearing Disorders,* 1976; 41:444–451.

References

1. Goodglass H, Gleason J, Hyde M: Some dimensions of auditory language comprehension in aphasia. *Journal of Speech and Hearing Research* 1970; 13:595–606.
2. Zurif E, Caramazza A, Myerson R, Galvin J: Semantic feature representations for normal and aphasic language. *Brain and Language* 1974; 1:167–187.
3. Goodglass H, Baker E: Semantic field, naming and auditory comprehension in aphasia. *Brain and Language* 1976; 3:359–374.
4. Whitehouse P, Caramazza A, Zurif EB: Naming in aphasia: Interacting effects of form and function. *Brain and Language* 1978; 6:63–74.
5. Gainotti G, Silveri CM, Villa G, et al: Anomia with and without lexical comprehension disorders. *Brain and Language* 1986; 29:18–33.
6. Milberg W, Blumstein SE: Lexical decision and aphasia: Evidence for semantic processing. *Brain and Language* 1981; 14:371–385.
7. Blumstein SE, Milberg W, Shrier R: Semantic processing in aphasia: Evidence from an auditory lexical decision task. *Brain and Lang.* 1982; 17:301–315.
8. Luria AR: Factors and forms of aphasia. In de Reuck AVS, O'Conner M (eds): *Disorders of Language.* London: Churchill, 1964.
9. Benson DF: (1979). Neurologic correlates of anomia. In Whitaker H, Whitaker HA (eds): *Studies in Neurolinguistics,* vol 4. New York: Academic Press, 1979, pp 293–328.
10. Knopman DS, Selnes, OA, Niccum N, et al: Recovery of naming in aphasia: Relationship to fluency, comprehension and CT findings. *Neurology,* 1984; 34:1461–1470.
11. Marshall RC: Word retrieval behavior of aphasic adults. *Journal of Speech and Hearing Disorders* 1976; 41:444–451.
12. Borkowski JG, Benton AL, Spreen O: Word fluency and brain damage. *Neuropsychologia* 1967; 5:135–140.
13. Wertz RT: Word fluency measure. In Darley FL (ed): *Evaluation and Appraisal Techniques in Speech and Language Pathology.* Reading, Massachusetts: Addison-Wesley, 1979.
14. Grossman M: The game of the name: An examination of linguistic reference after brain damage. *Brain and Language,* 1978; 6:112–119.
15. Grossman M: A bird is a bird is a bird: Making reference within and without superordinate categories. *Brain and Language,* 1981; 12:313–331.
16. Collins M, McNeil MR, Rosenbek JC: Word fluency and aphasia: Some linguistic and not-so-linguistic considerations. In Brookshire RH (ed): *Clinical aphasiology: Conference proceedings, 1984.* Minneapolis: BRK Publishers.
17. Adamovich BLB, Henderson JA: Can we learn more from word fluency measures with aphasic, right brain injured and closed head trauma patients? In RH Brookshire (ed): *Clinical aphasiology: Conference proceedings,* 1984. Minneapolis: BRK Publishers.
18. Spreen O, Benton AL: *Neurosensory Center Comprehensive Examination for Aphasia.* Victoria, BC: University of Victoria Press, 1969.
19. Goodglass H, Kaplan E: *The Assessment of Aphasia and Related Disorders,* 2nd ed. Philadelphia: Lea and Febiger, 1983.
20. Geschwind N, Kaplan E: A human cerebral deconnection syndrome. *Neurology,* 1962; 12:675–685.
21. Geschwind N: Disconnexion syndromes in animals and man. *Brain* 1965; 88:237–294, 585–644.
22. Benton AL, Smith KC, Lang M: Stimulus characteristics and object naming in aphasic patients. *Journal of Communication Disorders* 1972; 5:19–24.

23. Corlew MM, Nation JE: Characteristics of visual stimuli and naming performance in aphasic adults. *Cortex* 1975; 11:186–191.
24. Goodglass H, Hyde MR, Blumstein S: Frequency, picturability and availability of nouns in aphasia. *Cortex*, 1969; 5:104–119.
25. Gardner H: The contribution of operativity to naming capacity in aphasic patients. *Neuropsychologia* 1973; 11:213–220.
26. Barton MI, Maruszewski M, Urrea D: Variation of stimulus context and its effect on word-finding ability in aphasics. *Cortex* 1969; 5:351–365.
27. Goodglass H, Stuss DT: Naming to picture versus description in three aphasic subgroups. *Cortex* 1979; 15:199–211.
28. Rochford G, Williams M: Studies in the development and breakdown of the use of names, Part IV. *Journal of Neurology, Neurosurgery and Psychiatry* 1965; 28:407–413.
29. Newcombe F, Oldfield R, Ratcliffe G, et al: Recognition and naming of object drawings by men with focal brain wounds. *Journal of Neurology, Neurosurgery and Psychiatry* 1971; 34:329–430.
30. Wepman J, Bock R, Jones L, et al: Psycholinguistic study of aphasia: A revision of the concept of anomia. *Journal of Speech and Hearing Disorders* 1956; 21:468–477.
31. Howes D: Application of the word-frequency concept to aphasia. In DeReuck AVS, O'Conner M (eds): *Disorders of Language*. Boston: Little, Brown, 1964.
32. Goodglass H, Kaplan E, Weintraub S, et al: The "tip-of-the-tongue" phenomenon in aphasia. *Cortex* 1976; 12:145–153.
33. Miceli G, Silveri D, Villa G, et al: On the basis for the agrammatic's difficulty in producing main verbs. *Cortex* 1984; 20:207–220.
34. Williams SE, Canter GJ: Action-naming performance in four syndromes of aphasia. *Brain and Language* 1987; 32:124–136.
35. Wallace GL, Canter GJ: Effects of personally relevant language materials on the performance of severely aphasic individuals. *Journal of Speech and Hearing Disorders*, 1985; 50:385–390.
36. Williams SE, Canter GJ: The influence of situational context on naming performance in aphasic syndromes. *Brain and Language* 1982; 17:92–106.
37. Moerman C, Corluy R, Meersman W: Exploring the aphasic's naming disturbances: A new approach using the neighbourhood limited classification method. *Cortex*, 1983; 19:529–543.
38. Kohn SE, Goodglass H: Picture-naming in aphasia. *Brain and Language*, 1985; 24:266–283.
39. Podraza BL, Darley FL: Effect of auditory prestimulation on naming in aphasia. *Journal of Speech and Hearing Research*, 1977; 20:669–683.
40. Linebaugh CW, Lehner L: Cueing hierarchies and word retrieval: A therapy program. In Brookshire RH (ed): *Clinical Aphasiology: Conference Proceedings*, 1977. Minneapolis: BRK Publishers.
41. Linebaugh CW: Treatment of anomic aphasia. In Perkins WH (ed): *Current Therapy of Communication Disorders, Language Handicaps in Adults*. New York: Thieme-Stratton, 1983.
42. Love R, Webb W: The efficacy of cueing techniques in Broca's aphasia. *Journal of Speech and Hearing Disorders*, 1977; 42:170–178.
43. Pease DM, Goodglass H: The effects of cueing on picture naming in aphasia. *Cortex*, 1978; 14:178–189.
44. Li EC, Canter GJ: Phonemic cueing: An investigation of subject variables. In Brookshire RH (ed): *Clinical Aphasiology*, 1983. Minneapolis: BRK Publishers.
45. Weidner WE, Jinks AFG: The effects of single versus combined cue presentations on picture naming by aphasic adults. *J Communication Disorders*, 1983; 16:111–121.
46. Patterson K, Purell C, Morton J: Facilitation of word retrieval in aphasia. In Code C, Muller DJ, (eds): *Aphasia Therapy*. London: Edward Arnold, 1983.
47. Howard D, Patterson K, Franklin S, et al: The facilitation of picture naming in aphasia. *Cognitive Neuropsychology*, 1985; 2:49–80.
48. Howard D, Patterson K, Franklin S, et al: Treatment of word retrieval deficits in aphasia: A comparison of two therapy methods. *Brain* 1985; 108:817–829.
49. Thompson CK, Kearns KP: (1981). An experimental analysis of acquisition, generalization and maintenance of naming behavior in a patient with anomia. In Brookshire RH (ed): *Clinical Aphasiology: Conference Proceedings*, 1981. Minneapolis: BRK Publishers.
50. Loverso FL, Selinger M, Prescott TE: Application of verbing strategies to aphasia treatment. In Brookshire RH (ed): *Clinical Aphasiology: Conference Proceedings*, 1979. Minneapolis: BRK Publishers.
51. Kearns KP: Response elaboration training for patient initiated utterances. In Brookshire RH (ed): *Clinical Aphasiology*, 1985. Minneapolis: BRK Publishers.
52. Davis GA, Wilcox MJ: *Adult Aphasia Rehabilitation: Applied Pragmatics*. San Diego: College-Hill Press, 1985.
53. Schlanger P, Schlanger B: Adapting role playing activities with aphasic patients. *Journal of Speech and Hearing Disorders*, 1970; 35:229–235.

54. Ritter E: Modular therapy: A practical approach to life situations. In Brookshire RH (ed): *Clinical aphasiology: Conference Proceedings*, 1976. Minneapolis: BRK Publishers.
55. Simmons NN: A trip down easy street. A paper presented at the Clinical Aphasiology Conference, Harwich Port, Massachusetts, 1988.
56. Berman M, Peelle LM: Self-generated cues: A method for aiding aphasic and apractic patients. *Journal of Speech and Hearing Disorders*, 1967; 32:372–376.
57. Tompkins CA, Marshall RC: Communicative value of self-cues in aphasia. In Brookshire RH (ed): *Clinical Aphasiology: Conference Proceedings*, 1982. Minneapolis: BRK Publishers.
58. Morgan ALR, Helm-Estabrooks N: Back to the drawing board: A treatment program for nonverbal aphasic patients. In Brookshire RH (ed): *Clinical Aphasiology*, 1987. Minneapolis: BRK Publishers.
59. Lyon JG, Sims E: Drawing: Its use as a communicative aid with aphasic and normal adults. A paper presented at the Clinical Aphasiology Conference, Harwich Port, Massachusetts, 1988.
60. Goldstein K: *Language and Language Disturbances*. New York: Grune and Stratton, 1948.
61. Linebaugh, CW: A dissociation between auditory comprehension and sentence completion: Theoretical and clinical implications. In Brookshire RH (ed): *Clinical Aphasiology*, 1987. Minneapolis: BRK Publishers.
62. Golper LA, Rau MT: Systematic analysis of cueing strategies in aphasia: Taking you "cue" from the patient. In Brookshire RH (ed): *Clinical Aphasiology*, 1983. Minneapolis: BRK Publishers.
63. Chapey, R: Cognitive intervention: Stimulation of cognition, memory, convergent thinking, divergent thinking and evaluative thinking. In Chapey R (ed): *Language Intervention Strategies in Adult Aphasia*. Baltimore: Williams & Wilkins, 1986.
64. Linebaugh CW, Person Margulies CL, Mackisack EL: Contingent queries and revisions used by aphasic individuals and their most frequent communication partners. In Brookshire RH (ed): *Clinical Aphasiology*, 1985. Minneapolis: BRK Publishers.

6

Global Aphasia

Michael James Collins

Introduction

As in most introductions it enhances clarity to begin by "specifying your criteria" as an old professor of mine insisted. Operational definitions are one way of doing that. Global aphasia, for example, might be defined operationally as "A severe, acquired impairment of communicative ability, which crosses all language modalities, usually with no single communicative modality substantially better than any other. In addition visual, nonverbal problem-solving abilities, as well as other cognitive skills, are often severely depressed and are usually compatible with language performance." That definition will serve to characterize most globally aphasic individuals. There seems to be an additional need, however, to differentiate among what appear to be several subtypes of global aphasia. These subtypes are acute, evolutional, and chronic.

Most aphasias are severe initially, and one might ask why it is necessary to differentiate among them at all. The initial shock to the central nervous system, regardless of the size of the lesion, apparently has a profound impact on speech and language function. It may be, too, that the production of language is relatively more impaired than comprehension, but because of the initial shock that relatively well-preserved comprehension cannot be demonstrated.

The most prudent course in the early stages of recovery is to describe behaviors and label them cautiously. The process of labeling, however, has not endeared itself to many of our colleagues. Nevertheless, labeling the disorder can be useful. First, the label may be only provisional. Acute global aphasia in a patient's chart, for example, alerts hospital staff and knowledgeable family members that the aphasia is severe, and that functional comprehension, particularly in important matters, should not be assumed. Also, since the term *acute* implies that the patient is very ill, more of the communicative burden can be assumed by the patient's listeners, particularly the staff, without stigma and with the realization that this is not a permanent state of affairs.

Evolutional aphasia is a term that may be applied relatively early or relatively late in a patient's recovery. The beginning of the evolution may be seen within days and is frequently obvious because the patient demonstrates his recovering language system. Documentation of recovery is reinforcing to all those concerned. The collection of standardized data need not be dehumanizing, childish, or humiliating, but it also cannot be disguised as chit-chat.

The chronic global aphasic cannot be described as such until he is no longer acutely ill, is no longer clinically depressed, and is what neurologists call "neurologically stable." Generally, that occurs from one week to one month post onset.

Pathophysiology

The general statement that the more severe the aphasia the more extensive the lesion is an aphorism that is rarely contradicted. It suggests that the most severe lesions produce global aphasia. It may be that the single most critical factor in failure to recover is lesion size.

Generally, the lesion in global aphasia involves the frontal, temporal, and parietal lobes, areas served by the distribution of the middle cerebral artery. The middle cerebral artery nourishes a major area of the cortical hemispheres. Occlusion inferior to even one of the minor branches usually results in an area of extensive damage, not only in superficial, cortical areas but deep to the surface as well. Selnes, Niccum, and Rubens,[1] for example, found that patients whose auditory comprehension recovered least had lesions that extended into the supramarginal gyrus, and average volumes were 116 cm^3. Small, strategically placed lesions can produce severe, persisting aphasia. With few exceptions, however, lesions of greater than 60cm^3, which include frontal, parietal, and temporal lobes, and particularly the posterior temporal gyrus, result in the most serious deficits.

Nature and Differentiating Features

Some evidence exists to suggest that global aphasia is qualitatively and quantitatively different from other aphasias, but it is unclear why this is so. Diaschisis, the decreased responsiveness and dysfunction of intact neurons remote from the damaged area, is one possibility, and may play a role in preventing or inhibiting early recovery and suppressing other functions. Several authors, using regional cerebral blood flow (rCBF) seem to have substantiated this. More severe aphasias, in general, seem to have greater reduction of flow of longer duration. It also may be that "remote effects" result from damage that disrupts communication brain regions that are functionally related.

One remote effect is the lowering of metabolic rate in an area distant from a structural lesion. Hanson et al[2] found substantial hypometabolism in many of their 44 aphasic subjects. Their globally aphasic patients showed substantial impairment of metabolism in all but four of 16 areas measured, and, for these patients, hypometabolism was most severe in Wernicke's area. There is no fully adequate explanation for this, but several are plausible:

1. Focal lesions interact with other brain regions, and the combination can result in behavioral dysfunction.

2. Focal lesions damage white matter, resulting in a disconnection with interacting regions, and the distal and proximal changes cause behavioral dysfunction.

The behavioral symptoms often seen in severe, persisting global aphasia lend superficial support to the notion that diaschisis is important. Sarno and Levita[3] found that many of their globally aphasic patients made more gains in the second six months of recovery than in the first, which is contrary to the normal course of recovery. There are significant implications in that finding, which affect not only prognosis but treatment decisions.

Evaluation

A daily assessment of some critical communicative behaviors is often helpful to staff and family, for example a Rating of Communicative Ability form from the Porch Index of Communicative Ability (PICA)[4] or perhaps a graph based on a more subjective, briefer evaluation, such as portions of the Mayo Language Evaluation.[5]

Very severe aphasic individuals will fail most tests, even the simplest of standardized tests. They display a special kind of failure, rejection of the items, the tester, and the family. Sometimes, covert observation of these patients is the clinician's only recourse. Another approach, equally eclectic, is to determine whether yes–no responses are stable, to determine if the patient can follow whole body commands or gesture spontaneously, and to determine how he interacts in his present environment with family and staff.

Clinicians know that conditions evolve, and that the focus of treatment should shift in response to that evolution. Early test results are not immutable. The purpose of early testing should be to contribute to the medical management of the aphasic patient, establish baseline, measure progress, illuminate both strengths and weaknesses, and reveal those modalities most likely to be improved on. While a complete battery is probably not possible early in recovery, the tests that follow have been validated clinically.

Comprehensive Measures

The Porch Index of Communicative Ability (PICA)[4] samples performance across five communicative modalities (gesturing, speaking, writing, reading, and listening) to 10 objects, relatively homogeneous in difficulty. Responses are scored with a 16-point, multidimensional scoring system. Scores for each subtest are averaged, and modality scores are derived from them. The overall score is a mean score derived from all 180 scores. A percentile then can be determined that is based on Porch's normative sample of 357 aphasic adults. Useful information, particularly for prognosis, also can be derived from a measure of variability. Porch determines variability by subtracting each mean subtest score from the highest score in the subtest. If a patient's mean subtest score was 10.0, for example, and the highest score was 15, mean variability would be 5, times a factor of 10, or 50. Total variability scores are determined by adding up all 18 variability scores. Higher variability scores suggest a better prognosis.

The notion that variability can be related to prognosis may be analogous to the frequently noted dichotomy between competence and performance. To some authorities, McNeil[6] for example, the ability to perform at an accurate level, even if only once in numerous trials, suggests that competence is intact but cannot be demonstrated consistently.

One of the most frequent criticisms leveled at the PICA is that it is too long. For many patients in the acute stage, it is too long to endure. One alternative to sacrificing objective data from standardized tests, however, while imposing minimally on the patient, is to administer a shorter version of the PICA. Dubbed the SPICA by its early advocates,[7] the test can be administered in a fraction of the time it takes to administer the entire test, usually 15 minutes or less. There are several variations of abbreviated versions of the PICA. One that seems to be the most reliable and valid is the two-item version. In this version, only two objects, knife and pencil, are used, although six items—knife, pencil, fork, pen, key, and comb—are displayed. The test is administered in standard fashion, but subtest III, the second of the two gestural subtests, is not given. The scores for each object (knife and pencil) are added, and the sum for each divided by 17. For knife, this sum is multiplied by 0.41, and for pencil, by 0.54. These sums are then added to a constant value of 0.56, yielding an overall mean score. Percentiles can then be derived from this mean score. Recently, however, some cautions have been expressed regarding clinical use of abbreviated versions of the PICA.[8]

One of the more useful features of the PICA, mentioned above, is its usefulness in evaluating variability. Much of this ability is lost in the short version, but its loss may be compensated for by its brevity and consideration of the patient.

Two other tests that deserve consideration are the Boston Diagnostic Aphasia Examination (BDAE)[9] and the Western Aphasia Battery (WAB).[10] The WAB may be particularly appropriate because it is comprehensive, is relatively easy to learn, score, and administer, provides an adequate data base, and includes in its battery two sections particularly appropriate to the globally aphasic person: the Coloured Progressive Matrices[11] and a series of yes/no questions.

Other tests for more specific functions may be added as appropriate, including tests for speech and limb apraxia, reading comprehension, and writing. Auditory comprehension is particularly crucial, and an adequate assessment should include responses to yes/no questions, whole body commands, family names, and more salient stimuli. A series of questions for eliciting yes/no responses to personal, immediate environment, and informational questions is found in Table 6–1.

Functional Communication Assessment

Functional communication is a term that is sometimes misused, but in general it can be defined as communication, through any modality, that one uses to communicate in daily activities, that is, outside the four walls of the clinic and the confines of traditional aphasia testing. Theoretically, functional testing tells us not why a person communicates as he does, but how he communicates. The two formal tests of functional communication are the Functional Communication Profile (FCP)[12] and Communicative Activities in Daily Living (CADL).[13] Both are useful adjuncts to more traditional testing, although they are frequently administered and interpreted in lieu of other testing.

Table 6-1.   Questions for Yes/No Responses

Personal

1. Is your name (underline)correct name(underline)?
2. Is your name (underline)incorrect name(underline)?
3. Do you live in (underline)incorrect name(underline)?
4. Do you live in (underline)correct name(underline)?
5. Are you a phlebotomist?
6. Are you a (underline)correct occupation, or retired(underline)?
7. Are you wearing a _____? (underline)no(underline)
8. Are you wearing a _____? (underline)yes(underline)
9. Do you have _____ eyes? (underline)yes(underline)
10. Do you have _____ eyes? (underline)no(underline)

Immediate Environment

1. Are you in the hospital?
2. Are you in the theatre?
3. Is the light on?
4. Is the light off?
5. Do you live in _____? (underline)yes(underline)
6. Do you live in _____? (underline)no(underline)
7. Is there a 1957 Thunderbird in this room?
8. Is there a _____ in this room?
9. Is the door closed/open? (underline)yes(underline)
10. Is the door closed/open? (underline)no(underline)

Informational

1. Was George Washington our first president?
2. Is Canada part of the United States?
3. Is a window made of glass?
4. Do you light a cigarette with a chair?
5. Is five more than two?
6. Do people sleep on a table?
7. Does milk come from a cow?
8. Does Coke come from a cow?
9. Do you catch fish with a bus?
10. Do you tell time with a watch?

Questionnaires often can be useful adjuncts as well. Wertz and colleagues[14] and Collins[15] modified the FCP. Called the Rating of Functional Performance, it differs from the FCP principally in its scoring system (1–5 equal-appearing interval scale), number of categories introduced, and the inclusion of spouse, friend, or caregiver as informant. The scoring ranges from 1 (Cannot do what is asked in the question) to 5 (No difficulty doing what is asked in the question and can do it as well as people who have not had a stroke). There are six categories in this rating: Recognition/understanding, Responding, Reading, Speaking, Writing, and Other, and 60 items.

The wife of Bill, one of our globally aphasic patients, recently completed the Rating of Functional Performance. She rated his overall ability as "4," patient can do what is asked in the question(s) most of the time, but every now and then he cannot or makes mistakes. She felt that his recognition and understanding of usual, familiar events, is essentially normal, for example, is aware of emotional voice tone, understands simple conversation, listens to radio or TV, and responds appropriately. But she said he was unable to make change. Under "responding." she reported that he often answered "yes," ". . . but very often changes after answering yes." She was not sure that he could read and understand newspaper headlines, but felt he read and understood letters from family members and friends. Nevertheless, when asked if he read and understood newspaper stories and magazine articles, she replied "Of current events I don't know, but he reads the records in our daily paper and reads articles of people he knows in our hometown paper." Although not precisely a rating of severity, her rating of "4" contrasts sharply with our rating of "2" (Usually cannot do what is asked in the question, but he has done it infrequently since his stroke), and the overall score of 6.50 (14th percentile) he achieved on the PICA.

The preceding discussion is included to illustrate several points, and we should consider that Bill and Marge had been married 40 years, had raised seven children who became successful adults, and loved and admired each other. First, our perceptions of a patient's ability are not always shared by the family. Perhaps they should not be. Where we see 10 responses, they see hundreds, perhaps thousands. Even success on only a few of them softens the harshness of the reality of the majority. Several studies, for example Linebaugh and Young-Charles,[16] reported a strong tendency for families to rate the abilities of aphasic patients higher than speech pathologists do, and they seemed very confident in their ratings. Speech pathologists may be just as confident, but certainty in our clinical judgments should be tempered with understanding and not arrogance.

Three other methods of assessing behavior in globally aphasic persons warrant mention here. The first, although not technically a measure of functional communication, purports to be sensitive to skills that remain intact in global aphasia. Edelman's[17] untitled test employs a 10-point, modified PICA scoring system to assess ability to follow whole body commands, relate to objects in the environment, respond to high affective content questions, and relate to the environment.

Houghton, Pettit and Towey[18] combined elements of several functional tests. The result is the Communicative Competence Evaluation Instrument (CCEI), which consists of 10 expressive and 10 receptive communicative competence behaviors. Five-minute video tape samples of each patient's behavior are made before and after treatment, and the behaviors are rated on a six-point scale. This procedure is designed to be used in conjunction with Towey and Pettit's[19] program to improve communicative competence in global aphasia.

Finally, Holland[20] apparently is the only authority to have written about in vivo measurement. She also developed a system for describing communicative behaviors in a variety of settings while rating form, style, conversational dominance, correctional strategies, and metalinguistics of verbal and nonverbal output, and includes ratings of reading, writing, mathematical ability, and similar skills. For a two hour period, Holland tallied the frequency of success and failure to communicate, and how patients chose to communicate. She found that when they were allowed to select their form, style, etc., there were more successes than failures.

Summary

The preceding section highlighted some procedures for measuring both severity of aphasia and communicative competence. The list is subjective, although some of the tests are objective. It is not this author's intention to suggest that all are equally sensitive. The selection of one or more over others will be influenced by severity, responsiveness, and time constraints. The only factor influencing selection is that they provide data that will significantly enhance our knowledge of the person's deficits and competencies, permit us to speculate about site and etiology of lesion, make educated guesses about prognosis, and allow us to direct our treatment toward appropriate, realistic targets.

Predicting Recovery

Implicit in our designations of aphasia as acute, evolutional, and chronic is the notion that global aphasia is not always global aphasia. Prognosis is dependent on severity of communication impairment, which in turn is dependent on lesion size and location. Lesion size and location frequently can be inferred by severity of aphasia and relative involvement of modalities. The severity of aphasia, and the relative involvement of modalities must be interpreted in light of the duration of the illness. We know that physiological recovery occurs most rapidly during the first month postonset and then slows gradually for the next year or so until performance is relatively stable. Therefore, predicting recovery very early postonset is less successful than predicting recovery late in the process. There are, however, several valid reasons for attempting to predict recovery soon after onset. First, it helps us allocate our treatment resources. Second, cautious predictions may hasten the family's healing process and permit them more realistic views of their future.

There are several general methods of predicting recovery. In the prognostic variable approach, the clinician compares a patient's biographical, medical, and behavioral profile against such variables as age, health, and etiology. These are believed to influence eventual recovery levels.

The behavioral profile approach compares performance on formal measures of communication with profiles of similar patients. Variations of this approach[21,22] have compared an individual patient's one month postonset score to Porch's normative sample at one and then at six months postonset, and compared an individual aphasic patient's scores between one and six months with recovery curves generated by a large sample of aphasic patients. One final variation proposed by Porch[21] bases prognosis in part on variability within and across subtests on the PICA. Variability scores, which are also called Peak Mean Difference (PMD) scores, above 400 suggest excellent prognosis, and those below 200 suggest a poor prognosis for recovery.

In the statistical prediction method, formal test performance data are used to generate statistical formulae. Instead of making comparisons to group performance, a prognosis is created using the individual's own language performance.

Treatment

Perhaps the most credible reason for testing is to determine treatment focus. It should be the last thing we do because we need the information that precedes it, and we need to know why, and for what, we are treating.

Some general features of successful treatment have emerged over the years. They suggest that the treatment that has the best chance of success is treatment that:

1. Allows the patient some success, but challenges him at the same time.

2. Gets the cleanest possible signal in, and establishes the conditions that allow for the best possible signal out.

3. Is organized in a hierarchy of difficulty.

4. Is relevant to the patient's needs, or to our attitudes about what a patient needs.

5. Is based on formal and informal tests.

6. Is designed so that it can be tested.

Somewhere between general and specific treatments for aphasia are those that set the stage for maximizing the person's potential to respond and benefit from treatment. Environmental treatment is one of those.

Environmental Treatment

Environmental treatment is treatment that establishes a positive communicative environment. Lubinski[23] has provided guidelines for doing so, which include educating staff, facing the patient, alerting the patient that communication is about to occur; speaking slowly and clearly in "adult talk"; talking about concrete topics; keeping related topics together; using short, syntactically complete utterances; pausing between utterances; and using nonverbal cues to augment communication.

Educating the Staff

The staff should be as informed about the aphasic person's condition as possible, through reports of evaluation, staff meetings, in-services, and reminders about how best to communicate with the globally aphasic patient. Towey and Pettit's[19] treatment program for global aphasia emphasizes communicative competence in nonlinguistic areas such as eye contact, head nods, facial expressions, reciprocity of affect, physical proximity, and posture. They suggest that the clinician train all staff members to identify those nonlinguistic but communicative behaviors that occur in communicative interactions. Part of this training is done through the use of videotaped recordings of a staff member interacting with a globally aphasic patient. The tapes are then reviewed by the staff person and a speech pathologist to identify thoughts and feelings experienced during the interactions, to increase empathic communication skills.

As a result of this program, the authors suggest that several globally aphasic patients made significant gains in communication, but not linguistic, skills.

Table 6–2 is an outline of guidelines for communicating with severely aphasic people. Clinicians, staff, and families have found them useful. The annotated guidelines are contained in Appendix 1.

Establishing Goals

Realistic goals should begin with a needs assessment. All patients need to communicate, but some patients feel the need more than others, and others are less dependent on speech. Part of our understanding of what those needs are will come from our data, but we need to rely on our family interview and our covert assessment of the patient as well. Goals will vary, but some realistic goals might include the following:

1. Improving auditory comprehension, supplemented with contextual cues, to per-

Table 6–2. Guidelines for Communicating with the Severely Aphasic Person

1. Simplify
2. Clue the person in
3. Allow time
4. Guess
5. Confirm
6. Be clear
7. Reduce extraneous variables
8. Respect

mit consistent comprehension of one-step commands in well-controlled situations.

2. Improving production of yes and no to consistent, unequivocal responses in controlled situations.

3. Improving ability to spontaneously produce several written responses, or approximations, of functional or salient words of daily living.

4. Improving production of several simple, unequivocal gestures.

5. Improving drawing so that several simple, unequivocal messages can be conveyed in this modality.

6. Ensuring that a small, basic core of communicative intentions can be conveyed in one or a combination of modalities.

It is realistic to expect that these goals can be attained. They should be minimal goals for all globally aphasic patients. Expanding this repertoire will depend on a number of factors, including availability of the patient, cooperation and motivation, and general health. Enhancing and improving upon them may not always be possible. If new goals beckon because a person has demonstrated his capacity to reach them, they should be welcomed.

Specific Treatments for Global Aphasia

Visual Action Therapy

Helm and Benson[24] developed a treatment program for global aphasia called Visual Action Therapy (VAT). In this program, the patient is trained to associate ideographic forms with particular objects and actions, and to carry out a series of tasks in association with these drawings. No verbalization is used during the training.

Helm-Estabrooks, et al[25] reported a significant, positive effect from VAT treatment. They also point out several advantages to nonverbal, gestural training. First, gestural communication may be used independently of vocal communication; second, hand gestures for manual communication require less refined motor control than the articulatory movements required for speech communication; limb movements, unlike facial movements, have more predominantly unilateral control, because the left arm and hand are innervated by right hemisphere pyramidal pathways that are presumably uncompromised in right hemiplegic global patients having exclusively left hemisphere lesions; finally, the hand and arm, unlike the buccofacial apparatus necessary for speech, is visible to the initiator and can be visually monitored.

The authors used Visual Action Therapy to treat eight globally aphasic patients who had not responded to traditional therapeutic intervention. When all training was completed, the authors grouped pre- and post-treatment PICA scores for ten subtests: two pantomime tasks and two auditory comprehension tasks, which they labeled group one and predicted would improve; two reading subtests (group two), which they predicted might improve; and four verbal subtests (group three), which they predicted would not improve. Their analyses revealed significant pre- and post-treatment effects for group one, with a significantly larger effect for the gestural subtests than for the auditory subtests, and no significant effect for groups two and three.

The primary purpose of VAT is to train globally aphasic patients to produce representational gestures for visually absent stimuli through the manipulation of real objects. Despite its gestural focus, their treatment seemed to generalize to some other modalities. The authors suggest that their findings might be explained, and offer four hypotheses:

1. Patients may employ internal verbal monitoring during the training program.
2. VAT may improve general attentional skills.
3. VAT may improve visual spatial and visual search skills.
4. VAT may reintegrate some of the conceptual systems necessary for linguistic performance.

The only replication of the study is an unpublished master's thesis by Conlon,[26] which suggests that the results may not be replicable.

Voluntary Control of Involuntary Utterances (VCIU)

Helm and Barresi[27] developed a program designed to capitalize on, and bring under volitional control, spontaneous utterances that were potentially appropriate in a variety of situations.

Helm and Barresi used VCIU to treat the verbal output of three aphasic subjects. All three were severely impaired in verbal output, all three had moderately intact auditory comprehension, and none had responded to other treatments. The program steps, from identification of potentially useful words to conversational use, are not reported. The authors state that their subjects made significant gains, as measured by the BDAE. All improved so much that they moved to another form of treatment more suitable to their current language functioning.

The Equivocal Response

Establishing an unequivocal "yes" or "no" response is frequently the most important link to establishing communicative interaction. Responses may be gestural or verbal, but the clear imperative is that they are unequivocal. The following strategy seems to be effective with most patients.

1. Shaping the response

   a. First, make it very clear to the patient what is required. You might begin by saying "We need to work on 'yes' and 'no.' I'm going to say the word, and I want you to watch and listen while I say 'yes' (accompanied by gesture) [pause], and 'no' (with gesture)." Begin with two 3 X 5 cards, with "yes" printed on one and "no" printed on the other. Present either card, point to it, and very clearly say the word accompanied by the appropriate gesture. Pause five seconds, repeat the word and gesture. Repeat five times in succession. Repeat the procedure for the opposite response.

   b. Physically assist the patient with five repetitions of "yes" (head nod).

   c. Physically assist the patient with five repetitions of "no" (side to side head movements) while clinician says the word.

   d. Present four, then three, then two "yes–no" stimuli with physical assistance while clinician says the word. Pause approximately 5 seconds between responses. If incorrect, responses must always be corrected.

   e. Request gestured "yes" responses to two simple unambiguous questions while clinician assists with gestures and says the word. Same two opposing questions, with "no." Work on these until they are stabilized.

   f. Request five repetitions of gestured "yes," then "no." Facilitate with physical or verbal cues if necessary.

   g. Request alternating "yes," then "no," at approximately five second intervals, facilitating if required.

2. Stabilizing the response

   a. Request gestured response to simple questions, facilitating if required.

   b. Permit only "yes" or "no" response (verbal or gestural) while playing the card game "21."

   c. Establish a performance baseline, then begin treatment of personal, environmental and informational questions.

Gestural Communication

Gestural communication is frequently as impaired, or nearly so, as other modalities in global aphasia. Nevertheless, globally aphasic patients may benefit from pantomimed instruction and combined pantomime and verbal instructions. We try to incorporate gestural training in our treatment early in recovery. We assess spontaneous gestural ability informally and formally, and a part of each session is devoted to training these gestures.

We begin with one gesture, accompanied by its verbal equivalent. That gesture is drilled until it is intact, then a second gesture is added. At this level, we alternate between the two gestures with fewer repetitions of each until the patient can alternate gestures successively through the final step. At this point, a third gesture is added and the process repeated until all three gestures are reliable.

When the patient has learned several gestures, uses them in response to questions, and recognizes the need for them, they are incorporated into a program of total communication. Specific steps for such a program are contained in Table 6–3.

Playing Cards

Many globally aphasic individuals respond to playing cards when they do not respond to other stimuli. Many can sequence cards, match according to suit and number, and respond appropriately to commands such as "Pick up the Queen of Hearts" even when several foils are present. Unfortunately, as in many other tasks, the person who is destined to remain chronically, globally aphasic frequently is unable to move beyond the third step. For those who promise greater auditory comprehension, the program contained in Appendix I has proved to be a useful adjunct to treatment.

Writing

The writing of even a single word, or the first letter or two of an important word, can be strikingly communicative. We devote a part of each treatment session to writing drill, generally following the outline in Table 6–4.

The approach of Haskins[28] is similar, and may be more useful for some globally aphasic individuals.

1. Clinician points to letters of the alphabet as the sound is produced, and increases the number of letters in sequence as success is achieved.
2. Clinician points to printed words after synthesizing the sounds of the words into a whole, e.g., g-o, c-a-t, beginning with two sounds and gradually increasing the length of the words.
3. Client points to the letter after clinician names it, or client traces the letter after it is named.
4. Client points to printed words after the clinician spells them, beginning with short, unrelated words that have varied spellings, and gradually increases the complexity by selecting words with similar spellings.
5. Client points to printed words after the clinician names them, beginning with four short, common words and increasing the display to ten more abstract words as the patient improves.

Table 6–3.   Strengthening the Gestural Response

1. Clinician gestures and says the word simultaneously.
2. Clinician says word, clinician and client gesture simultaneously (clinician assistance with gesture may be required).
3. Client imitates gesture.
4. Client imitates gesture after enforced delay.
5. Client gestures in response to auditory stimulus.
6. Client gestures in response to auditory stimulus after enforced delay.
7. Client gestures in response to written stimulus.
8. Client gestures in response to written stimulus after enforced delay.
9. Client writes word in response to gestural and auditory stimulus.
10. Client gestures in response to appropriate stimuli.

Table 6-4. Communication with Writing

1. Tracing of single words with necessary assistance.
2. Copying of single words.
3. Prolonged exposure (as long as the patient needs it) of the target word, with several repetitions of the auditory analogue.
4. Brief presentation of auditory and lexical stimulus, with written response.
5. Brief presentation of auditory and lexical stimulus, with imposed delay (5 to 15 seconds), then a written response.
6. Writing to dictation, with a return to previous levels at any point if necessary.
7. Writing to pictured presentation.
8. Writing in response to question, e.g., "What would you write if you were thirsty?", or "Write this person's name."

6. Client copies letters of the alphabet, beginning with printed capital letters, then small printed letters, and eventually transcribes these to cursive letters if improvement permits.

7. Client writes letters of the alphabet to dictation, beginning with the alphabet in serial order, then in random order.

8. Client writes words to dictation. These words should be words that have been practiced in previous sequences by tracing, pointing, etc.

Communication Boards

Communication boards seem to be the first thing nursing staff and other hospital personnel think of when they discover that a patient is unable to speak or gesture meaningfully. For some reason, the ability to point to pictures, or to point to words, or to spell words with an alphabet board is thought to be an isolated skill unrelated to speaking, gesturing, or comprehension of language. Clinicians, of course, wish that was true. Many of us have found, however, that with appropriate training some globally aphasic patients can use a communication board effectively, provided the message is simple and the listener is insightful and demonstrates patience. Alphabet boards, or boards that contain only single words or ideas, are generally not effective for the globally aphasic person. Some, however, make more effective use of boards containing both the picture and its written equivalent. Presentation of both stimuli seems to enhance the saliency of the stimuli. Additional enhancement may be provided by constructing individualized communication boards containing words and/or pictures that are particularly useful to that person, pictures of wife, children, familiar household objects, and personal objects. Pictures of these items can be taken with a polaroid camera and affixed to a board covered with acetate or acrylic.

Whichever type of board is chosen, training in its use is essential. Training should begin with a format similar to that used for natural language learning, in which initially only the target word is exposed. The clinician should repeat the stimulus, perhaps in sets of five, until the client can point unfailingly to the named item. When that level is achieved, the item should be presented again, this time with approximately a 15 second delay.

The next step is to present one foil, and again ask the patient to point to the target. This foil should be maximally differentiated from the target, and should not be an item presented anywhere else on the communication board. It may, in fact, be an object, or an amorphous picture.

When the client can successfully point to the desired object, the foil should be removed, and two items on the communication board exposed. The clinician should present only the previously trained item first, in sets of five. When the client is successful consistently, present the second item, again in sets of five. Do not alternate between items at this point. Gradually reduce the number of presentations, first to four, then three, then two. At this point, let the client know clearly that the next item will be the foil. Again, as with the previously trained item, gradually reduce the number of presentations. At this point, begin alternating between items, with two presentations for each one. Allow the patient plenty of time to respond, and be certain that the item is presented clearly.

The same procedure should be followed for each of the items to be in the client's core vocabulary. Performance often begins to falter, even after prolonged and intensive training, when five or more items are exposed, and there may be at least a temporary ceiling on the number of items that can be used on one board. One alternative is to use several boards, one containing pictures of family, one containing pictures of family and friends, and one containing pictures of familiar household and personal objects.

This type of training is a tedious process, but one that should not be hurried. It may be best to limit this training to only part of each session.

Several other treatments with at least possible application to global aphasia follow. They include the use of drawing, blissymbolics, visual communication, and computerized visual communication. Some have had their efficacy studied and demonstrated, and some of have not, but all are promising. At least one study reported the successful acquisition of a blissymbol lexicon by globally aphasic patients.[29] Two of the four subjects with global aphasia trained with blissymbols were able to use them to communicate with relatives. Gardner, et al.,[30] found that even severely aphasic persons can appreciate and discriminate visual humor in the form of uncaptioned cartoons, and this may indicate preservation of rudimentary visual symbolic functions.

The use of drawing in the treatment of aphasias ranging from moderate to severe has recently been gaining in popularity. Studies by Morgan and Helm-Estabrooks,[31] Lyon[32] and Lyon and Sims[33] have suggested their promise more than demonstrated their efficacy, but continued study of the technique seems to be a worthwhile pursuit. For example, Morgan and Helm-Estabrooks[31] treated two patients with an experimental program called Back to the Drawing Board (BDB). Both were right-handed patients who had suffered left-hemisphere lesions. Both patients were described as having severely limited verbal expression when the study began. One patient was initially described as globally aphasic.

Drawing may be an inefficient, time-consuming procedure, particularly when too much detail is required in the drawings. That seems to be a legitimate criticism, however, only when other means of communication are available to the patient.

Steele et al.[34] documented their efforts to computerize a manual, visually representative, alternative communication system (VIC) for severely aphasic individuals. They described a person who had suffered a massive left intracerebral hemorrhage. His residual deficits included severe right hemiplegia, moderate right visual field deficit, and global aphasia. Performance on the BDAE ranged from the 1st to the 30th percentiles when "0" scores were excluded; overall performance on the PICA was at the 9th percentile. Gestural performance was at the 6th, verbal at the 2nd, and graphic at the 24th percentile. The authors document the patient's performance on functionally analogous tasks in English and in a computerized symbol-learning task (C-VIC) in which the patient is asked first to select an item from a field of objects in response to a spoken word or presentation of a C-VIC symbol, and in the second task to speak the names of the objects. In the C-VIC task the patient uses the computer entry system called the "mouse." The authors report that the mouse is a "fairly simple pathway to operating the interface," and that they ". . . pick it up quite quickly." Performance on both tasks demonstrated the superiority of C-VIC over natural language performance.

The authors also investigated "abstract naming" with C-VIC. Employing a multiple-baseline design, they measured the ability of the patient to infer the object name from a trainer's pantomiming of the object. Their results revealed two primary effects: (1) performance on each subgroup improved with treatment, to exceed criterion, and (2) performance generalized from treated stimuli to untreated stimuli. In fact, on the fourth subgroup, performance reached criterion and remained for three consecutive sessions, even though the person had not been trained on these stimuli.

The preceding examples demonstrate the depth of innovation of investigators who would improve communication in severely aphasic individuals. Not surprisingly, they all seem to be capitalizing on the intactness and potential of the right hemisphere. This is not surprising when one considers that in 1969 Geschwind anticipated some of these recent developments: "It is my belief that the major hope for the eventual effective rehabilitation of the type of aphasic patient for whom we can do so little now lies in the possibility that language is present but inaccessible in the minor right hemisphere" (p 1209).[35] We hope that possibility becomes reality.

APPENDIX

Guidelines for Communicating with the Severely Aphasic Person

1. SIMPLIFY

Handle only one idea at a time; use short sentences with simple, common words; speak more slowly, but naturally; and don't speak to the patient as if he were a child.

2. CLUE HIM IN

Be sure you have his attention; use gestures and pointing where possible; facial cues may also help him. Use redundant wording, for example "Are you hungry enough to eat dinner?" Repeat and reword the idea until he understands.

3. ALLOW TIME

Allow the patient additional time to understand and to respond; be patient, unhurried, and accepting of his speech attempts.

4. GUESS

Determine the subject by asking increasingly specific questions.

5. CONFIRM

Make statements about what you think he means to make sure you understand.

When he responds to a question, ask the opposite also. If the response doesn't change, you're not communicating.

6. BE CLEAR

Say "I'm sorry, I don't understand you" when necessary. Don't leave abruptly when attempts fail.

7. REDUCE EXTRAVENOUS VARIABLES:

A noisy environment, additional activities, such as television or radio, and talking with more than one person at a time.

8. RESPECT

He is usually an intelligent adult who is quite aware of his surroundings even though language function is impaired. Include him in the conversation, and don't treat him as though he is not there, or deaf, or mentally retarded.

References

1. Selnes OA, Niccum NE, Rubens AB: CT scan correlates of recovery of auditory comprehension. In Brookshire R (ed): *Proceedings of the Conference on Clinical Aphasiology*, 1982. Minneapolis: BRK Publishers.
2. Hanson W, Metter E, Riege W, et al. Comparison of Regional Cerebral Metabolism (PET), Structure (X-Ray CT) and Language in Categories of Chronic Aphasia. In R Brookshire (ed): *Proceedings of the Conference on Clinician Aphasiology*, 1986. Minneapolis: BRK Publishers.
3. Sarno MT, Levita E: Some observations on the nature of recovery in global aphasia. *Brain and Language.* 1981; 13:1–12.
4. 21. Porch BE (1967). *Porch Index of Communicative Ability.* Palo Alto, CA: Consulting Psychologists Press.
5. Mayo Speech and Language Evaluation Battery. Unpublished manuscript, 1972.
6. McNeil MR: The nature of aphasia in adults. In Lass JJ, McReynolds LV, Northern JL, et al. (eds): *Speech, Language and Hearing*: vol II. *Speech and Language Pathology.* Philadelphia: WB Saunders, 1982.
7. DiSimoni F, Keith R, Darley F: Practicality of shortening the Porch Index of Communicative Ability. *J Speech Hear Res* 1975; 18:491–497.
8. Holtzapple P, Pohlman K, LaPointe L, et al. (1989). In T. Prescott (ed) *Clinical Aphasiology.* Boston: Little, Brown, & Co.
9. Goodglass H, Kaplan E: *Boston Diagnostic Aphasia Examination,* Philadelphia: Lea and Febiger, 1983.
10. Kertesz A: *The Western Aphasia Battery.* New York: Grune and Stratton, 1982.
11. Raven J: *Coloured Progressive Matrices.* London: HK Lewis, 1962.
12. Sarno M: *The Functional Communication Profile.* New York: New York University Medical Center, Institute of Rehabilitation Medicine, 1969.
13. Holland A: *Communicative Abilities in Daily Living.* Baltimore: University Park Press, 1980.
14. Wertz RT, Collins M, Weiss D, et al: The Veterans Administration cooperative study on aphasia: A comparison of individual and group treatment. *Journal of Speech and Hearing Research.* 1981; 24:580–594.
15. Collins MJ: Unpublished data, 1980.
16. Linebaugh C, Young-Charles H: Counselling needs of the families of aphasic patients. In Brookshire R (ed): *Proceedings of the Conference on Clinical Aphasiology*, 1978. Minneapolis: BRK Publishers.

17. Edelman GM, Assessment of understanding in global aphasia. In Rose FC (ed): *Advances in Neurology: Progress in Aphasiology.* New York: Raven Press, 1984.

18. Houghton PM, Pettit JM, Towey MP: Measuring communicative competence in global aphasia. In Brookshire R (ed): *Proceedings of the Conference on Clinical Aphasiology,* 1982. Minneapolis: BRK Publishers.

19. Towey MP, Pettit J: Improving communicative competence in global aphasia. In Brookshire R (ed): *Proceedings of the Conference on Clinical Aphasiology,* 1980. Minneapolis: BRK Publishers.

20. Holland A: Observing functional communication of aphasic adults. *J Speech and Hear Dis* 1982; 47:50–56.

21. Porch BE: *Porch Index of Communicative Ability.* Palo Alto, California: Consulting Psychologists Press, 1983.

22. Porch BE, Collins MJ: Unpublished data, 1973.

23. Lubinski R: Environmental language intervention. In Chapey R (ed): *Language Intervention Strategies in Adults.* Baltimore: Williams & Wilkins, 1981.

24. Helm N, Benson F: Visual action therapy for global aphasia. Paper presented at the Academy of Aphasia, Chicago, Illinois, 1978.

25. Helm-Estabrooks N, Morgan A, Helm-Estabrooks N: Back to the drawing board: A treatment program for nonverbal aphasic patients. In Brookshire R (ed): *Proceedings of the Conference on Clinical Aphasiology,* 1987. Minneapolis: BRK Publishers.

26. Conlon K: Unpublished Master's Thesis, University of Wisconsin-Madison, 1988.

27. Helm N, Barresi B. Voluntary control of involuntary utterances: A treatment approach for severe aphasia. In Brookshire R (ed): *Proceedings of the Conference on Clinical Aphasiology,* 1980. Minneapolis: BRK Publishers.

28. Haskins S: A treatment procedure for writing disorders. In Brookshire R (ed): *Proceedings of the Conference on Clinical Aphasiology,* 1976. Minneapolis: BRK Publishers.

29. Johannsen-Horbach H, Cegla B, Mager U, et al: Treatment of chronic global aphasia with a nonverbal communication system. *Brain and Language.* 1985; 24:74–82.

30. Gardner H, Ling P, Flamm L, et al: Comprehension and appreciation of humorous material following brain damage. *Brain.* 1978; 98:399–412.

31. Morgan A, Helm-Estabrooks N: Back to the drawing board: A treatment program for nonverbal aphasic patients. In Brookshire R (ed): *Proceedings of the Conference on Clinical Aphasiology,* 1987. Minneapolis: BRK Publishers.

32. Lyon JG: Drawing: An augmentative means of communication for the functionally nonverbal aphasic adult. Paper presented at the Third Annual Southeastern Aphasiology Conference, Fort Walton Beach, Florida, 1984.

33. Lyon J, Sims E: Drawing: Evaluation of its use as a communicative aid with aphasic and normal adults. Paper presented at the Second International Aphasia Rehabilitation Conference, Goteberg, Sweden, 1986.

34. Steele RD, Weinrich M, Kleczewska M, et al: Evaluating performance of severely aphasic patients on a computer-aided visual communication system. In Brookshire R (ed): *Proceedings of the Conference on Clinical Aphasiology,* 1987. Minneapolis: BRK Publishers.

35. Geschwind N: Problems in the anatomical understanding of the aphasias. In Benton A (ed): *Contributions to Clinical Neuropsychology.* Chicago: Aldine, 1969.

7

Acquired Dyslexias

Wanda G. Webb

Introduction

In a highly technical society such as ours, most of us are inundated daily with written material. Signs are posted everywhere, many without ideographs. There are numerous forms to fill out and written directions to follow for almost every activity. If desired, all of our leisure hours could be spent reading, with the monumental number of books, magazines, and other publications available. Thus, the person with an acquired dyslexia, or reading disorder, is at a serious disadvantage in this "age of literacy."

Retraining reading following the onset of an acquired dyslexia clearly is the purview of the speech–language pathologist. In 1969 Benson and Geschwind[1] pointed out that this therapy must be highly individualized and requires considerable ingenuity on the part of the clinician. The speech–language pathologist also should take into account research from teaching reading to normals and to developmental dyslexics, and should have knowledge about the normal processes of reading. Information from these areas is often lacking in clinical training, making the task of retraining reading seem even more difficult. However, treatment of reading disorders can be both challenging and rewarding, especially with a highly motivated client. The ideas and information presented here are designed to provide background information and a core of treatment principles and suggestions to make the task a little less formidable.

Pathophysiology

Normal Reading Process

To understand what may go wrong in the process of reading, one should have a model of what occurs in normal reading. Marshall[2] provides a flow diagram and explanation of an information processing model of reading, as shown in Figure 7–1. The model conceives that early visual analysis (EVA) extracts visual features from the stimulus array and then these are fed through three distinct reading routes employed in the assignment of linguistic form. These routes are the *phonic route,* the *direct route,* and the *lexical route.*

THE PHONIC ROUTE

In the use of this route, the features that aid letter recognition are fed from the EVA to letter representations (LR) and abstract letter identities are assigned. Words are assumed to be segmented into their component letters and then entered into the grapheme parser (P). At this stage the string of letters is segmented into graphemic chunks that will map onto a single phoneme in real words (or regularly spelled nonsense words). When a grapheme combination is an exception to a rule, it will be misparsed. Following the parsing, the output is sent to the GPC, phoneme correspondence rules, and each grapheme is associated with the single phoneme that is its most frequent realization. This phonological code is then entered into the blender (B) where it is assigned an articulatory code with specified phonetic values for coarticu-

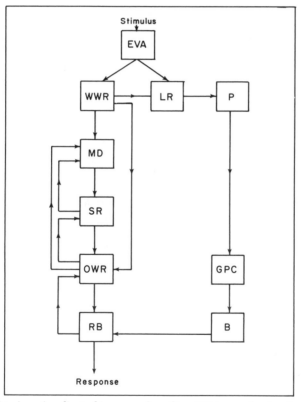

Figure 7-1.   Mechanisms implicated in normal reading. EVA = early visual analysis; WWR = whole word representations (visual); LR = (abstract) letter representations; P = (graphemic) parser; MD = morphological decomposition; SR = semantic representations; OWR = output word representations (oral); GPC = grapheme–phoneme conversion; B = blender (phonological); RB = response buffer. (Reprinted with permission from Marshall, J.C.: On some relationships between acquired and developmental dyslexias. In Duffy FH, Geschwind N (eds): *Dyslexia: A Neuroscientific Approach to Clinical Evaluation,* Boston: Little, Brown, 1985.)

lation. In turn, this pattern is entered into the response buffer (RB) from which the articulatory system is triggered when oral output is necessary.

Readers depending totally on the phonic route would be able to read words and nonwords with regular phonological correspondences, but irregular words would be much in error, often "regularized." Semantic interpretation then would be determined from what the reader thought the word was. The disorder called *surface dyslexia* has features that indicate reading is primarily dependent on the phonic route.

THE DIRECT ROUTE

The EVA may also feed a global mechanism titled WWR or whole word representations. Parallel processing of visual stimulus information, such as word length and overall configuration, helps to locate representations of the words. This generates an arbitrary code that serves to find the phonological realization of the word in the OWR or oral word representations. Access to meaning is accomplished through a feedback loop from OWR to semantic representations.

Readers depending solely on the direct route have access only to their "sight vocabulary." Regular and irregular words may be read equally well. However, the interpretation of homophones may cause difficulty since access to the lexical route is limited. Semantic categorization and classification may be very impaired, and nonsense words often cannot be read accurately.

THE LEXICAL ROUTE

Using this pathway, WWR is fed to MD or morphological decomposition. This mechanism segments the whole word into its potential base form and potential affixes. The MD does not appear to have access to the full lexicosemantic knowledge base because words will be incorrectly segmented through rule generalization. The segmented form of the word is next passed to the semantic representations (SR) for a syntactic–semantic interpretation. If it was a correct segmentation, the form is then passed to the OWR for phonological assignment. If the initial morphological parsing was incorrect and a match cannot be made, it will be returned to the MD for alternative parsing. When a correct parsing (one that can be matched in the SR) is found, it is sent to the OWR and then to the response buffer (RB).

When reading using the lexical route only, a person should be unable to read nonsense words aloud. Words with inflectional or derivational structures are often misread.

Using only the lexical route may manifest itself also in difficulty reading functor words and as frank semantic substitutions. Patients with *phonological alexia* and patients with *deep dyslexia* are believed to be depending primarily on the lexical route.

Schneider and Shiffrin[3] have shown that most readers learn to use both automatic and controlled processing in reading. Automatic processing implies a learned association in long-term memory that occurs with consistent training. It operates in parallel with other simultaneous processes and does not require attention. In non-brain-injured persons, most of skilled reading, in terms of word identification and access to meaning, is probably through more automatic processing. Controlled processing becomes necessary for new words or for comprehension of difficult text.

Neurological Substrate of Reading

The neuroanatomical sites for control of the processes described above have been defined primarily through studying patients with brain lesions that impair reading. As will be discussed under the nature and differentiating features of the dyslexias, there are several fairly distinct classifications of acquired dyslexias. The brain lesion data from these disorders implicate certain areas of the brain as having primary responsibility for understanding the written word.

It is well agreed that reading, like all primary language functions, is a left hemisphere function. The area that seems to be more directly related to reading than any other is the area called the angular gyrus. This structure lies in the large association area at the junction of the temporal, parietal, and occipital lobes.

Because of the reading problems associated with lesions of Wernicke's area in the temporal lobe, it is also agreed that this area is involved in the processing of written as well as auditory language. The lower portion of the frontal lobe around Broca's area seems to have some function in reading, especially in the processing of grammatical aspects. The occipital area is obviously involved in the early visual analysis.

Although it is generally accepted that these areas of the dominant hemisphere are responsible for reading, the localization for the separate components of the normal reading process are not known nor are the association pathways. As technology allows more specific brain-activity mapping, perhaps these mysteries will one day be solved.

Nature and Differentiating Features of Acquired Dyslexias

As is typical with acquired language disorders, the symptomatology of acquired dyslexia is varied. Two approaches have been taken in attempts to classify these disorders and to differentiate among patterns of break-down.

Traditional Classifications

A traditional approach to classification has been emphasized by Benson[4] and affirmed by earlier research by such authors as Goldstein,[5] Geschwind,[6] and Hécaen and Kremin.[7] This traditional approach breaks reading disturbance into two main categories: alexia (or dyslexia) without agraphia and alexia (or dyslexia) with agraphia.

The patient with *alexia without agraphia,* or "pure" alexia, shows greatly compromised reading comprehension, with oral language normal or nearly normal. The ability to copy is usually impaired and may tend to worsen over time. Written acalculia and color anomia are often present. A right homonymous hemianopsia is almost always present, but a right hemiparesis is rare. A visual agnosia for objects and/or colors occasionally accompanies the syndrome.

The patient with alexia without agraphia often is noted to read in a "letter by letter" fashion. Each letter of the word is named, often aloud, before the word is identified. Comprehension of words spelled aloud is usually good.

Alexia with agraphia is the second traditional classification but can be subdivided into aphasic alexia and agraphic alexia.[8] Aphasic alexia refers to the reading disorder that is a part of the aphasia. The two most frequently cited reading disturbances are those accompanying Wernicke's aphasia and accompanying Broca's aphasia. The reading problems tend to parallel the overall language disorder. In Wernicke's aphasia, part of speech is not an important predictor, although the patient may read function words somewhat better than contentives. Paralexic errors are frequent, like the paraphasic errors of oral language. The degree of reading disturbance usually parallels auditory comprehension deficit, although case studies have shown that there may be a strong modality bias in Wernicke's patients.[9,10]

Broca's aphasia shows reading disturbance similar to that referred to as the "third alexia," anterior alexia or frontal alexia.[11] As in their speech, word class and frequency show an important effect, with concrete nouns being read more accurately than abstract nouns or function words. The Broca's patient may comprehend more than would be expected because comprehension of the contentives may be good. Sentences in which the meaning is derived from syntax may be very difficult. These patients tend to read with a whole word or "gestalt" attack rather than a letter-by-letter or syllable approach. Comprehension of words spelled aloud is impaired.

Agraphic alexia is implicated when reading and writing are impaired in the absence of a significant aphasia. This has also been referred to as a parietotemporal alexia.[4] There is difficulty with identification of letters and words as well as a significant impairment of writing in all aspects of written tasks. Often, but not always these patients will show elements of the Gerstmann syndrome: agraphia, acalculia, impairment of finger identification, and right-left disorientation. Hemianopsia is sometimes present and apraxia is often found to accompany it.

Psycholinguistic Classifications

Since 1973 when Marshall and Newcombe[12] published an article on the psycholinguistic approach to studying acquired dyslexias, there has been great interest in looking for patterns of breakdown in reading. Primarily assessed through oral reading tasks, three major classifications or disorders have resulted from these studies: phonological alexia, deep dyslexia and surface dyslexia.

Phonological alexia is characterized by an inability to read pseudowords and some difficulty with low-frequency words.[13] High frequency words are likely to be read correctly. Errors are usually visual errors, i.e., the words identified are visually similar to the target words. Spelling may or may not be impaired, and aphasia may be absent. It is assumed that the patient with phonological alexia is impaired in the ability to use the letter-to-sound conversion rules of the language.

The patient with *deep dyslexia* makes predominantly semantic errors in oral reading, i.e., the identified word is semantically related to the target word in some way.[14] Visual and derivational errors (e.g., *baker* → *"bakery"*) also are made. Function words are misread much more often than contentives, and verbs are more difficult than adjectives, which are more difficult than nouns. The person with deep dyslexia also is unable to read pseudowords.

The syndrome of *surface dyslexia* is distinguished by poor ability to use grapheme-to-phoneme conversion rules, though there is a heavy reliance on these rules.[15] Errors are phonologically similar to the target, and there is great sensitivity to spelling regularity. There is little sensitivity, however, to word meaning; and the patient may match the meaning to the word he has identified, even though it may not fit in context.

Thus, there are various ways to look at the acquired dyslexias and to classify them. Classifications interrelate and dyslexic individuals may exhibit features of more than one category. It is important to note that all of the acquired dyslexias affect the comprehension of written material in some way, and this is the clinician's primary interest. Though assessment may be accompanied by the use of many oral reading tasks, the extent or severity of the dyslexia is measured by the effect on reading comprehension. In all of the acquired dyslexias, comprehension is impaired whether it be from inaccuracy of word identification, difficulty with comprehension of meaning carried by syntax, inability to remember and analyze what was read, or just because reading is so slow and laborious.

Evaluation

Prior to beginning evaluation, it is vital that the clinician obtain a "literacy history" through interviewing the client or family regarding reading skills and interest. It is not feasible to teach the client skills that were not obtained premorbidly. Furthermore, it is more difficult to succeed with treatment if the client has little motivation or interest in relearning reading.

It is important also that the client have a full language evaluation assessment of all modalities. Beyond the language skills, there are factors that influence comprehension, such as knowledge base and cognitive resources of the reader, that should be estimated. Questions must be answered regarding such things as attentional abilities and ability to access information not directly given in the text (i.e., inference). If the patient can participate, testing of higher level cognitive functions is often recommended.

In many cases of acquired dyslexia, the initial evaluation would consist of a standard aphasia battery for a CVA patient or a battery of tests used to assess the cognitive – linguistic functioning of a person with a closed-head injury. Most aphasia batteries include tests of written comprehension. Some measure of reading comprehension should be included in all screening or testing of brain-injured individuals who were premorbidly literate. A screening could include a test of paragraph comprehension such as the one included in the Minnesota Test for Differential Diagnosis of Aphasia.[16] Note that the research of Nicholas, Machennan, and Brookshire[17] has shown that multiple sentence reading test items from five of the most widely used aphasia batteries were often answered correctly by both normal and aphasic subjects who had not read the passages questioned.

The patient also should be asked to read aloud. The same passage may be used, or passages specifically meant for oral reading, such as the Gray Oral Reading Paragraphs,[18] could be utilized. Number of errors, types of errors, and fluency should be noted.

In cases in which reading may be targeted as a treatment modality, the clinician should gather more in-depth information than a screening or the aphasia battery subtests can yield. It is not enough to know that a person cannot read even single words or does not answer paragraph comprehension questions correctly after reading. The clinician must have a good idea of what is interfering with word recognition or comprehension of meaning.

The evaluation of the acquired dyslexias has not been given much emphasis in commercially available tests for brain-injured adults. *The Reading Comprehension Battery for Adults*[19] (RCBA) is one of the few tests available with subtests that were carefully designed according to research findings concerning reading. It uses silent reading in all tasks because it is designed for measuring comprehension. It is a very useful battery though the testing of contextual material is limited, and the clinician may want more information prior to beginning therapy.

The *Woodcock Language Proficiency Battery*[20] also contains useful measures and is normed on adult readers. Again, the clinician may want additional information for designing a reading treatment program.

Most of the clients who have any difficulty at the single word level should be evaluated with a task that uses reading words aloud from word lists. Johnson[21] suggests that these lists be constructed to include high frequency nouns, CVC words organized according to vowel patterns, words with regular grapheme-to-phoneme correspondence which have consonant clusters in the initial and final position, words which have the potential for letter reversals and transpositions, and word lists organized according to semantic groups (e.g., fruits, clothes, jewelry). Rothi and Moss,[22] who designed and reported on a reading battery called the Battery of Adult Reading Function, use word lists divided into regular words (follow regular phoneme–grapheme conversion), rule-governed words (e.g., marriage, debt), irregular words (tomb, shoes), functor words, and nonsense words.

The client should be asked to read the words aloud, and all responses should be transcribed. A miscue or error analysis then may be performed and errors or miscues may be categorized. Types of errors frequently noted among readers with acquired dyslexia are visual confusions (bear → bean), semantic confusions (plane → jet), derived errors (baker → bakery), and errors of grapheme-to-phoneme conversion (Pete → pet). No response and successful and unsuccessful corrections also should be noted.

After such an analysis, the clinician should be able to determine if particular types of words are easier for the client to read. Following the analysis of the *Battery of Adult Reading Function,* the clinician may be able to determine which "reading routes" are intact and which are not utilized.

For the person who can read at the sentence level but becomes very confused or nonfunctional when asked to read more than a paragraph, a reading test such as the RCBA and a measure of single word reading will probably guide the clinician well in planning treatment. For those patients who can read at a simple paragraph level, however, the literature on the treatment of children and adults with developmental dyslexia is relatively convincing that the clinician should evaluate the patient's comprehension and oral reading of *text.*[21,23] To implement a more valid and helpful assessment, the clinician should have on hand many examples or reading passages at different grade levels. It is recommended that each one be about 500 words in length, as research has shown that the quality of the reading errors begins to change after the first 200 words, when the reader begins to develop meaning.[23] Therefore, it is preferable to ignore the errors that occur in the first 200 words of the text. The passage should be complete in itself, i.e., a story, a textbook chapter, an article, etc. A story should have a strong plot and an identifiable underlying theme. All material should use natural rather than stilted language. (For example, instead of "He was persistent in his attempts until he finally succeeded," choose "He kept trying until he finally did it.") A wide variety of material should be on hand as it is imperative that the reading material be something that the patient can understand and relate to, but it must be material that is new to him or her. The most efficient way to gather such materials would probably be to enlist the aid of a curriculum librarian at an educational institution. The lengthier passages will be harder to find for the lower grade levels. It is preferable to use adult literacy training materials.[24,25,26]

After selecting passages for use in assessment, the clinician should prepare for using them by reading each selection aloud and writing down what can be recalled after each reading. The important items relating to the characters, events, setting, plot, and theme should be noted. If possible, someone else should be asked to do this also and the notes compared. What is needed is a good sense of what is relevant to the average reader from that passage. Each passage should have a list or outline of the expectations to be used in evaluating the patient's retelling of what has been read.

The client is asked to read the passage aloud. This is tape recorded and then an error or "miscue" analysis is later done. This should include the type of error analysis done with single words, but it should go beyond that type of analysis. It should document omission, insertion, and reversal of words as well as repetition of a word or phrase when it is done apparently for reflection or for getting a "running start."

According to Weaver,[23] the miscue analysis procedure may be concentrated on trying to determine the reader's strategies and the use of context. She suggests that the following questions be asked about each error or miscue.

1. Did the miscue go with the preceding context? A miscue that resulted in a meaningful sentence should be acceptable even if it changed the original meaning.
2. Did it go with the following context?
3. Did it preserve the essential meaning. Consider as to whether it had a major effect on understanding of the whole.
4. Was the error corrected?
5. Was it either corrected or meaning-preserving. If the answer is yes, you are answering essentially that no significant loss in comprehension resulted.

Following the reading, the client should be asked to retell what was read, pretending the clinician has never read it. The client obviously must have a degree of intact verbal skill for this task. It is not necessary, however, that verbal language skills be normal. If there are too many word substitution errors or speech is too sparse, the retelling will not be helpful. A question-and-answer format with multiple choice questions might be necessary. For clients who can participate in the retelling, it still may be necessary to ask some guided questions following the retelling concerning characters, events, plot, theme, and/or setting. It is not a time to focus on insignificant details. The clinician may probe further and ask the more verbal client to use advanced reasoning by hypothesizing, explaining cause/effect relationships, or relating the story to themselves and situations they have experienced.

There will be some clients who do not comprehend well simply because they are reading aloud and are struggling too much with the verbalization or are accustomed only to silent reading. For this patient it will be necessary to do an oral reading for the miscue analysis and retelling as well as to select another comparable passage for silent reading and retelling. Memory and interpretation would then be assessed primarily from the silent reading.

While the miscue or error analysis provides the clinician with information about how well the reader seems to comprehend during reading, the retelling gives an indication of how well the reader can remember and interpret what was read. The miscue analysis is to ascertain whether or not the reader is reliably using the preceding context to predict what will come next and the following context to correct or confirm what was just read. If the retelling shows poor use of those strategies with a resultant disruption of meaning, the patient will need training to develop these and other strategies.

The desire and motivation to relearn to read also must be assessed by the clinician before beginning treatment. The patient who does not care whether (s)he is able to read the newspaper or a book may not need as thorough an evaluation of contextual reading and may need only assessment of functional skill. A patient must be strongly motivated and willing to work very hard to try to learn to read again. The patient who wants to return to school or to a job in which much reading is required must make this commitment.

Treatment

There is a burgeoning literature of clinical descriptions of cases of acquired dyslexia and consequent hypotheses concerning the reading process and brain function. There is not, however, a vast literature on treatment of the acquired dyslexias. Most of the clinical research done in this area comes from single case studies which indicates, perhaps, how variably the disorder manifests itself.

Treatment for acquired reading disorders is usually a long, arduous process and, as previously indicated, the client must be motivated strongly and committed to the objectives. To regain ability to read, the client must *read* as much as possible; therefore, a commitment of time and effort is essential.

The clinician working with the acquired dyslexias does have information from previous research on the disorder and on normal reading processes. This research provides the basis for several principles of treatment that should be followed. These principles can be summarized as follows.

1. Accurate comprehension of what is read is the principle goal, not accurate oral reading.
2. In selecting or designing the vocabulary or content, the properties or features of words that are known to have an effect on recognition and comprehension should be considered. These features are length, part of speech, frequency of occurrence, concreteness, imageability[27] and familiarity. Gernsbacher[28] has shown that experiential familiarity has a strong effect on recognition.
3. The patient's interests and functional needs should be of priority in selecting training material rather than what is readily available in the clinical setting.
4. Reading should be physically facilitated by making certain the print size is large enough, the material is placed in the visual field correctly, and there are no distractions.
5. Difficulty level for contextual reading can be advanced in two major ways: (1)

increasing length and (2) increasing vocabulary as well as syntactical complexity. The clinician should consider controlling one or the other as much as possible to be able to analyze reading comprehension failures.

6. If phonemic decoding is chosen as a useful objective, consonants rather than vowels should be targeted.

7. Reading comprehension should be a generative process for understanding.[29] There should be a cognitive interaction with the material. The clinician must facilitate this by the design of the treatment tasks and the selection of stimuli.

Specific Treatment Tasks

The Severely Impaired Reader

For the person demonstrating very poor reading comprehension even at the single word level, the basic goal is *survival reading skill*. If possible this patient should understand a reading vocabulary containing functional vocabulary for signs, foods, TV, emergency procedures, etc. Darley[30] lists a suggested lexicon which may be taught as single words and then combined easily for following printed directions.

Matching activities are a good starting point for this patient. If attention to visual detail is lacking, then the client may first match line drawings, gradually decreasing the number of different features in the foils. When the patient is able to do this, words may be matched, again gradually increasing the similarity of all choices. Words may then be matched to an auditory stimulus or a visual stimulus (picture) depending on the individual's strengths. The number of choices or foils should gradually be increased.

These words may then be matched to a verbal description of the item, action or concept ("Which one would be on the door of the bathroom you would use?" "Which one is a cold drink?" "Which one would you call if you saw someone breaking into your neighbor's house?"). A specific functional vocabulary of 10–20 words should be selected for these tasks maintaining that vocabulary throughout all levels of matching.

Every opportunity should be given for cognitive and functional interaction with this vocabulary. If real-life experiences can be designed to use the targeted words, it should be done. The vocabulary should continue to be increased as the patient reaches 90% comprehension when a wide variety of choices are given. By this point, the client who has the verbal ability should be able to read the words aloud without cues. If possible, (s)he should explain what the word's meaning is and/or in what kind of situation you would find it. If the client can write, copying and, later independently writing the words should be done. Pictures and signs can be labeled by the client with appropriate words.

Rothi and Moss[22] have designed a treatment program to improve recognition and oral reading of single words. The techniques used depend on which "reading route" the clinician wants the patient to learn to use. Their treatment protocols are based on assessment results using the *Battery of Adult Reading Function*. In brief, they suggest the design of activities for strengthening use of each route as summarized below:

1. *Phonic Route.* Select tasks that use nonwords or words that have direct gra-

pheme-to-phoneme correspondence. Phonological comparisons or decisions are the objective of the activities.

2. *Lexical Route.* Stimuli should be real words that require a lexically based phonological analysis and not a semantic analysis. Limit the exposure time to 500–600 seconds with a tachistoscope or as long as it takes to say it if exposing by hand.

3. *Direct Route.* Real words that do not require a phonological analysis, but rather a semantic analysis should be utilized. When exposing by hand, flash the word as quickly as possible or use 350 msec or less on a tachistoscope.

If the more severely involved client is able to develop a fairly extensive single word functional reading vocabulary, (s)he may be able to go further and begin to combine words for reading phrases and sentences. The function words (noun determiners, verb auxiliaries, prepositions, and conjunctions) will need to be memorized as sight vocabulary words. They should be taught by accompanying them with appropriate words that the person already knows, thus creating a phrase (*the* school, men *and* women, *will* drive, come *in*).

Matching tasks as discussed above will assist in learning the recognition and function of these words in phrases. The client, if possible, should be reading the phrases aloud to try to increase the fluency of reading. The clinician reading the phrases aloud while the client listens and looks at the phrases is facilitory also.

The Moderately Impaired Reader

The client who can read at the sentence level, even though poorly, is a better candidate for improving reading because there is obviously better underlying skill. This person should be reading contextual material in therapy. The initial assessment should provide information on the grade level at which the patient can read at an instructional level, i.e., comprehension is at about 45–55% without help from someone. The readability of any text that isn't graded can be determined individually by using the Bormuth Close Readability procedure.[23]

When this procedure is used the patient is asked to fill in blanks put in the reading material by omitting words. The value is that the client may choose the material to be read and then actively participate in determining whether it is too difficult to use in training. If the client's other language deficits prevent such participation, the clinician can choose the reading material. If it is ungraded, one of the readability formulas made for teachers' use in determining difficulty level may be used.[31]

The client should begin reading passages of more than 200 words, and reading should be assessed as to understanding of what has been read. The person may read silently and aloud, so that the clinician can hear the errors. Depending on the degree of language impairment, various assessment strategies may be used. The client may be asked to retell what has been read, answer written questions using multiple choice, or answer verbally presented questions. These questions should not relate only to details. They should help guide the individual in relating what has been read to his/her own experiences. The questions also should require the patient to make use of cognitive–linguistic processes, such as association, deductive reasoning, sequencing, and analysis.

The client who can read aloud at the contextual level will give the clinician much insight into the use of contextual cues for confirming and predicting. If the reader does not seem to be using contextual information, have him stop at errors that change meaning and analyze whether the error fits with the context. Explain why it does not and have the client read it correctly. This client also may be asked to stop reading at designated points in the text, depending on how much can be read before comprehension begins to fail, and analyze what has been read up to that point. Some may retell it, others may write it down and some may have to be questioned. The main point of the exercise is to teach that the reader must use previous context in reading to be able to understand what will follow. It also should be noted that as one gets into the body of the material, part of the later context should confirm what has been read previously. The reader must learn to monitor when those do not match.

If memory is a limiting factor, as in closed-head injury, the client may need to take notes as (s)he reads. Most paragraphs can be summarized in one to two sentences unless there is a great deal of factual information in them. Listing might then be used. The reader must learn, however, to differentiate important details from inconsequential details.

Another good approach for training monitoring and comprehension of context is to use material that involves following directions. There are workbooks available that approach the language of directions for reading. Activities designed for auditory-comprehension training often can be adapted. Although readability must be considered, directions found on the packages for the use of many household items or work-related items can be gathered and used for functional training. Again, the self-monitoring of reading in terms of what makes sense with the context and, in this case, the outcome is one of the primary objectives.

The research of Gardner, et al.[32] on aphasics' understanding of semantic and syntactic errors in reading resulted in a useful treatment task for improving monitoring. Sentences that contain syntactic and/or semantic errors are given to the patient to read and find the errors. Some patients can be asked to correct the errors. Syntactic errors have been shown to be more difficult for aphasics to identify. The reader who can find the more subtle syntactic errors of subject – verb agreement or pluralization is probably reading closely and becoming able to comprehend meaning at a deeper level than surface semantics.

Some dyslexic individuals may need therapy time concentrated on comprehension of meaning carried by different syntactical constructions and the accompanying semantic indicators. The embedding of clauses beginning with such words as "unless", "except", and "instead of" may present challenges that need extra treatment time.

The Mildly Impaired Reader

The mildly impaired reader may be extremely frustrated with reading. Although (s)he can read context at the appropriate grade level, reading may be slow and laborious. These patients may reread material continuously because they cannot synthesize or remember what has been read. They may falter when a new unknown word is in the context and they cannot figure it out. They may read every word correctly, but read most texts in an arduous, one-word-at-a-time fashion. If they are willing to devote the time and effort, these patients can usually improve their reading. They may never regain, however, the automaticity and ease with which they read premorbidly.

A clinical report[33] has noted that techniques used in speed reading training may assist these patients in increasing comprehension and speed. In this training much of the emphasis is on searching for the main idea and skimming unimportant details. Treatment tasks to train rapid scanning may need to be used. Ann Arbor Publishers has several programs available (e.g., *Letter Tracking, Thought Tracking*) that target purposeful scanning. Scanning the phone book for certain names or scanning context for particular facts are good training tasks.

Emphasis on using the strategies of confirming and predicting, as used with the moderately impaired reader, is increased for the mildly impaired person. The reader scans the material for a sense of what it concerns, finds the main idea as (s)he reads, skims unimportant details, and continually interacts cognitively with what is read to keep up with the meaning of the context. Initially, it may mean stopping and discussing the context or making notes, but it should gradually become the *method* the reader uses automatically. It is probable that some people who use a lot of reading in work or school will need to continue to use note-taking to reinforce and organize what was read. Outlining the material is a good strategy for some, especially for academic tasks.

The student who wants to return to school or the adult who wants to return to a job with heavy reading requirements presents a difficult challenge for the clinician. For the closed-head injured patient and often for the vascular lesioned patient, organizational strategies are of the utmost importance. They often do not know how to think about what they've read in order to glean information even after they've taken notes and summarized the information. One organizational method suggested by Raphael[34] for answering questions concerning reading material is the QAR or Question Answer Relationship strategy. She suggests providing the learner with experience in using three different sources of information by describing them as (1) *Right There* — the answer can be found explicitly stated in the text; (2) *Think and Search* — the answer is in the text but not directly stated; and (3) *On my own* — the reader must search his/her own knowledge for the answer. Thus when the client is reading with specific purpose or questions to answer, the QAR strategy will help organize the search of material.

For readers who seem to use a word-by-word reading approach resulting in very decreased reading rate, speed reading techniques suggest rapid fixation or perception exercises to force the reader to take in more information or more words at one visual fixation. Flash cards can be used or a tachistoscope or tachistoscopic program on a computer can be utilized. Many of these exercises can be found in speed reading texts such as Lewis' *How to Read Better and Faster*.[35] There is now some controversy in reading rate training for normal readers concerning the use of tachistoscopic programs versus using full pages of text that are moved or scrolled at various rates. Both methods probably should be assessed if available. This kind of drill will need to be practiced intensively if the patient is to progress.

Word Identification: Phonics

The reader should always use a strategy that allows for continued flow of reading. If a word cannot be pronounced but this failure does not reduce overall comprehension of the passage, the reader should just continue rather than struggle. This would be true, for example, if the word were a character's name or the name of a particular city or animal. If "what's-its'-name" or "blank" could be inserted and the meaning unchanged, reading should continue. On the other hand, if the difficult words are more frequently those that carry more linguistic weight, then the reader needs a way to approach finding out what the word is.

It is generally acknowledged that the consonants facilitate word recognition much more than vowels do. Therefore in pronunciation efforts, it seems more productive to concentrate on consonants. There are also far too many exceptions for vowel pronunciation. Thus the patient can sound out the consonants more expediently while guessing at the vowels. Then by trial and error (s)he may find a word that fits with the context.

Clients with milder impairment and retained ability for new learning may be able to learn a few phonic rules to assist in pronunciation of new words. May and Elliott[36] conclude that only a very few phonic rules are consistent enough or cover enough words to warrant spending valuable time when teaching children to read. These consistent rules are:

1. The "c rule." When *c* comes just before *a, o,* or *u,* it usually has the /k/ sound. Otherwise it usually has an /s/ sound.
2. The "g rule." When *g* comes at the end of words or just before *a, o,* or *u,* it sounds like /g/. Otherwise it has the /dz/ sound. *Get, give, begin* and *girl* are important exceptions.
3. The VC pattern. In either a word or syllable, a single vowel letter followed by a letter, digraph, or blend usually represents a short vowel sound.
4. The VV pattern. In a word or syllable containing a vowel digraph, the first letter of the digraph usually represents a long vowel sound and the second is usually silent. This is fairly reliable for *ee, oa, ay, ea,* and *ai* but not as reliable for others.
5. The VCE pattern. In one-syllable words containing two vowels, one of which is a final *e,* the first vowel usually represents a long vowel and the final *e* is silent.
6. The CV pattern. When there is only one vowel letter in a word or syllable and it comes at the end, it usually represents a long vowel.
7. The "r rule." The letter *r* usually modifies the short or long sound of the preceding vowel.

If these are the only rules thought to be consistent enough to teach children, then it seems that we might limit our teaching to brain-injured patients also, at least initially. In therapy each rule would be slowly introduced with many examples and opportunities to practice sounding out words using the rules and the consonant grapheme–phoneme conversion that should be concurrently emphasized.

Use of Computers and Other Equipment

Computers can be a valuable asset in retraining reading. Mills[37] cites three different models of training when using computers: (1) dependent, in which the clinician is at the patient's side assisting, (2) clinic independent, and (3) home independent. Obviously the behavioral prerequisites increase as level of independence increases.

Computers may be used for training attention, vocabulary building drills, sentence comprehension, paragraph comprehension, and rapid scanning or perception activities. Commercially there are more and more software programs available that target reading both for the normal and impaired learner. These will be found most often through educational software companies though there are programs that target aphasic populations. Strickland[38] et al cite other functions such as using software programs that assess readability or informally assess reading grade level.

Card readers, such as the Language Master from Bell and Howell, can be useful in providing drill activity early in reading training. The client can look at the word and picture or at a sentence and hear it at the same time.

The clinician may want to use a tape recorder at some point in training. Contextual material may be recorded by the clinician and the client can follow along in reading practice before reading it independently.

Compensatory Strategies

Though we live in the "literacy age," there are patients who cannot read functionally but can carry on a routine without that skill. For others, who need or want methods to compensate for reading, many books are now recorded on tape and are available for loan at the public library. Friends may also record books on tape for the patient.

The student or person working may need the assistance of a "reading partner." This individual would be available to help with reading difficult material and would verify or correct comprehension.

Conclusion

The challenge of working with the acquired dyslexias is an enjoyable one. There is much to be learned about better ways to facilitate reading both for the developmental and the acquired dyslexias.

For the present, the speech–language pathologist can best prepare for treating clients with these disorders by learning how normal reading takes place, how reading is taught to non-brain-damaged learners, and how the brain injury affects the learning and reading process. Armed with this information and plenty of creativity, the speech–language pathologist can, in most cases, target functional reading with optimism.

Suggested Readings

Adamovich BB, Henderson JA, Auerbachs: *Cognitive Rehabilitation of Closed Head Injured Patients.* San Diego: College Hill Press, 1985.

Coltheart M: Functional architecture of the language processing system. In Coltheart M, Giuseppe S, Job R (eds): *The Cognitive Neuropsychology of Language.* Hillsdale, N.J.: Lawrence Erlbaum, Associates, 1987.

LaPointe LL: Aphasia Therapy: Some Principles and Strategies for Treatment. In Johns DF (ed): *Clinical Management of Neurogenic Communicative Disorders.* 2nd ed. Boston: Little, Brown, 1985.

LaPointe L, Kraemer I: Treatment of alexia without agraphia. In Perkins W (ed): *Current Therapy of Communication Disorders:* Language Handicaps in Adults. New York: Thieme-Stratton, 1982.

Singer MH (ed): *Competent Reader, Disabled Reader:* Research and Application. Hillsdale, N.J.: Lawrence Erlbaum, 1982.

Strickland DS, Feeley JT, Wepner SB: *Using Computers in the Teaching of Reading.* New York: Teachers College Press, 1987.

Weaver C: *Reading Process and Practice.* Portsmouth, NH: Heinemann Educational Books, 1988.

Ylvisaker, M: *Head Injury Rehabilitation: Children and Adolescents.* San Diego: College Hill Press, 1985.

References

1. Benson DF, Geschwind N: The alexias. In Vinken PJ, Bruyn GW (eds): *Handbook of Clinical Neurology: Disorders of Speech, Perception, and Symbolic Behavior*, vol. 4, Amsterdam, North-Holland, 1969.
2. Marshall JC: On some relationships between acquired and developmental dyslexias. In Duffy FH, Geschwind N (eds): *Dyslexia: A Neuroscientific Approach to Clinical Evaluation*, Boston: Little, Brown and Company, 1985, 55–66.
3. Schneider W, Shiffrin RM: Automatic and controlled information processing in vision. In LaBerge D, Samuels SJ (eds): *Basic Processes in Reading: Perception and Comprehension*, Hillsdale, N.J.: Lawrence Erlbaum, 1977, 127–154.
4. Benson DF: *Aphasia, Alexia, and Agraphia*, New York: Churchill Livingston, 1979.
5. Goldstein, K: *Language and Language Disturbance*, New York: Grune and Stratton, 1948.
6. Geschwind N: Disconnexion syndromes in animals and man, I and II. *Brain* 1965; 28:237–294; 585–644.
7. Hécaen H, Kremin H: Reading disorders resulting from left hemisphere lesions: Aphasic and "pure" alexias. In Whittaker H, Whittaker HA (eds): *Studies in Neurolinguistics, vol. 2*, New York: Academic Press, 1977.
8. Friedman RB, Albert MC: Alexia. In Heilman K, Valenstein E (eds): *Clinical Neuropsychology*. New York: Oxford University Press, 1985.
9. Hier DB, Mohr JP: Incongruous oral and written naming: Evidence for a subdivision of Wernicke's aphasia. *Brain and Language* 1977; 4:115–126.
10. Kirshner HS, Webb WG: Alexia and agraphia in Wernicke's aphasia. *Journal of Neurology, Neurosurgery and Psychiatry* 1982; 45:719–724.
11. Benson DF: The third alexia. *Archives of Neurology* 1977; 34:327–331.
12. Marshall JC, Newcombe F: Patterns of paralexia: A psycholinguistic approach. *Journal of Psycholinguistic Research* 1973; 2:175–186.
13. Beauvois MF, Dérousné J: Phonological alexia: Three dissociations. *Journal of Neurology, Neurosurgery, and Psychiatry* 1979; 42:1115–1124.
14. Coltheart M: Deep dyslexia: A review of the syndrome. In Coltheart M, Patterson K, Marshall JC (eds): *Deep Dyslexia*. London: Routledge and Kegan Paul, 1980.
15. Deloche G, Andrewsky E, Desi M: Surface dyslexia: A case report and some theoretical implications to reading models. *Brain and Language* 1982; 15:12–31.
16. Schuell H: *The Minnesota Test for Differential Diagnosis of Aphasia*. Minneapolis: University of Minnesota Press, 1965.
17. Nicholas LE, MacLennon DL, Brookshire RH: Validity of multiple-sentence reading comprehension tests for aphasic adults. *Journal of Speech and Hearing Disorders*, 1986; 51:82–87.
18. *Gray Standardized Oral Reading Paragraphs*. Indianapolis: Bobbs-Merrill, 1967.
19. LaPointe L, Horner J: *Reading Comprehension Battery for Adults*. Austin, Texas: Pro-Ed, 1979.
20. Woodcock R: *Woodcock language Proficiency Battery*. Allen, Texas: DLM Teaching Resources, 1984.
21. Johnson D: Remediation for dyslexic adults. In Pavlidus GT, Fisher DF (eds): *Dyslexia: Its Neuropsychology and Treatment*. New York: John Wiley, 1986.
22. Rothi LG, Moss SE: Alexia/agraphia in brain damaged adults. Paper presented at the convention of the American Speech–Language–Hearing Association, Washington, DC, 1985.
23. Weaver C: *Reading Process and Practice: From Socio-psycholinguistics to Whole Language*. Portsmouth, NH: Heinemann Educational Books, 1988.
24. *Laubach Literacy*. New York: New Readers Press, (no date).
25. Boning R: *Specific Skills Series*. Baldwin NY: Barnell-Loft, 1978.
26. *Reading Skills Builders*. Pleasantville, NY: Readers Digest Services, Education Division, (no date).
27. Paivio A, Yuille J, Madigan S: Concreteness, imagery and meaningfullness values for 925 nouns. *Journal of Experimental Psychology* 1968; 76 I, part 2.
28. Gernsbacher MA: Resolving 20 years of inconsistent interactions between lexical familiarity and orthography, concreteness and polysemy. *Journal of Experimental Psychology: General* 1984; 113:256–281.
29. Wittrock M: Reading comprehension. In Pirozzolo FJ, Wittrock M (eds): *Neuropsychological and Cognitive Processes in Reading*. New York: Academic Press, 1981.
30. Darley FL: *Aphasia*. Philadelphia: W.B. Saunders, 1982.
31. Vacca RT, Vacca JL: *Content Area Reading*, 2nd ed. Boston: Little, Brown, 1986.
32. Gardner H, Denies G, Zurif E: Critical reading at the sentence level in aphasia. *Cortex* 1975; 11: 60–72.
33. Webb WG: Intervention strategies in mild reading disorders associated with aphasia. Paper presented at the annual convention of the American Speech–Language–Hearing Association, Toronto, 1982.
34. Raphael TE: Teaching learners about sources of information for answering comprehension questions. *Journal of Reading* 1984; 27:303–311.

35. Lewis N: *How to Read Better and Faster.* New York: T.Y. Crowell, 1978.
36. May FB, Elliott S: To Help Children Read: Mastery Performance Modules for Teachers in Training. Columbus, Ohio: Charles C. Merrill, 1973.
37. Mills RH: Dependent and independent use of microcomputers in aphasia rehabilitation. In Hagen C (ed): *Topics in Language Disorders: Approaches to Poststroke Treatment* 1987; 8, 1:72–85.
38. Strickland DS, Feeley JT, Wepner SB: *Using Computers in the Teaching of Reading.* New York: Teachers College Press, 1987.

8

Acquired Neurogenic Dysgraphias

MALCOLM R. MCNEIL
CHIN-HSING TSENG

Introduction

Writing is one major expressive communication channel that is parallel, rather than subordinate, to speaking. Disorders of writing invariably reflect the neurological dysfunctions of a complex cognitive system. We define acquired neurogenic dysgraphia as the family of writing disorders resulting from central or peripheral neurological damage. Implied in this very general definition is the exclusion of psychiatric and affective disorders, such as schizophrenia or depression, from those conditions more clearly attributable to CNS insult or disease. We will limit our treatment of this topic to those neurogenic dysgraphias that occur in adulthood. Our goal is to present the current paradigm(s) governing the theoretical and clinical literature on neurogenic dysgraphia. Our emphasis on the neuroanatomically based classification systems is dictated by historical precedence and the utility of the systems for helping organize a disparate body of literature.

Among the various communication disorders that result from either focal or diffuse CNS lesions, acquired dysgraphia is the one type that has received the least attention from researchers and clinicians responsible for their study. Several reasons may account for this inattention. First, speech is often better appreciated as the major functional communication channel, thus speech disorders are the primary targets for assessment and treatment. Second, writing is often considered as secondary to speech in terms of its order of acquisition and its neural organization (e.g., the view of P.M. Marie, 1906).[1] Therefore, the common attitude is that writing problems derive from speech impairments[2] and usually parallel those of speech especially in word retrieval and syntax.[3] Finally, the investigations of normal writing have received little scientific attention until recently.[4-8] Without tests of pathological writing on normal subjects and without normal reference data, the evaluation of writing disorders will remain subjective and will continue to lead to uninterpretable experimental results and imprecise or inaccurate clinical decisions.

From a task-analysis perspective, normal writing can be performed only with a large ensemble of intact skills: calligraphy, orthography, visual–spatial orientation, and linguistic capacities.[9,10] For instance, Keenan and Brassell[11] reported the effects of education on handwriting and its differentiation from aphasia. They reported substantively more misspelled words (54.4% vs. 6.7%) and substantively fewer changed sentence meanings (0.0% vs. 33.3%) in the poorly educated group than in the educated group. Holtzapple[12] also found important effects of illiteracy on aphasic test performance. The effects of writing with the nondominant hand and the confusion of these effects with pathologic writing was demonstrated by Hansen, McNeil, and Vetter.[7] Even the level of meaningfulness (voluntariness vs. automaticity) ascribed to the task can affect performance. Goldstein[13] explained that:

> In the usual writing of an individual very much accustomed to write, the automatic part is very much in the foreground when the person performs writing for everyday communication. Writing of isolated words on dictation is less automatized, still less than of isolated letters. If we are asked to write a definite letter, our attitude is much more voluntary than when we write the same letter within a word. Even the form of the letter differs. This concerns words too. The same words may be pronounced much more fluently in sentences than when isolated. (p. 126)

With so many sources of variability even in neurologically intact adults, it can be imagined that the underlying mechanism of dysgraphic performance is not always easy to determine. In addition to the various mechanistic causes of dysgraphia, several neuroanatomically or neurophysically based models have been and continue to be proposed. To date, and without exception, these models have failed to gain the needed evidence to support their adoption. Although it is generally agreed that no single brain center or pathway can be called the dysgraphia center, these models continue to guide the classification schema used and the behaviors used for classifying. There has, however, persisted a belief among many that Exner's area (an area close to the hand region of the motor cortex) houses the writing capacities.

Pathophysiology

Localization: A Cortical Center for Writing?

Since the late nineteenth century, academic battle has been waged among the opponents and proponents for a single brain center for writing. In 1881, Exner postulated that the writing function resided in the foot of the left second frontal convolution.[14] This idea was not accepted without challenge by his contemporaries (e.g., Wernicke and Dejerine). This challenge was waged on the basis of several assumptions: First, written language is a later acquired skill on both phylogenetic and ontogenetic scales; second, writing movements are nothing more than the visual copying of the oral language; and finally, writing can be achieved only through a combination of many skills all of which appear to be localized in disparate locations of the brain.

Hecaen and Angelergues[15] conducted a clinical–anatomical study in which the severity of functional disturbances in seven communication domains was correlated with the locus of the lesion. A five-point equal-appearing interval scale, with a score of zero representing intact writing, was used to quantify the deficits. They found that no single lobe could be totally responsible for writing disturbances. They stated:

> Writing disturbances due to impairment of one lobe manifest themselves clearly only among temporal (1.35) and parietal (1.13) lesions. When the lesion affects two lobes, agraphia is most noticeable when the parietal lobe is involved (parieto-temporal lesion, 2; parieto-occipital lesion, 2; and fronto-parietal lesion, 1.18); but the degree of agraphia is always more marked among massive lesions and predominates in posterior impairment (3.66 compared to 2.83). [The numbers in parentheses are the average scale values for severity of the writing deficits.] (p. 241)

Furthermore, they claimed:

> The degree of writing disturbances is coupled in a preferential fashion with the parietal factor but the temporal factor remains important, and the occipital and rolandic factors are not negligible; the frontal factor is non-existent. (p. 243)

Hecaen and Angelergues' work, the reports of Russell and Espir,[16] and several more recent brain–behavior correlational studies are important for settling the issue of the existence of a specific CNS writing center. These studies provide empirical evidence refuting the strict localizationist view. Perhaps, due to the failure to find a single writing center, proponents of strict localization realize that the mapping of the writing function(s) onto the brain is not a binary matter. Instead, it has been proposed that writing disorders are manifested in a qualitatively different way according to the locus of lesion. Thus far, the left/right, the anterior/posterior, and the cortical/subcortical distinctions have been suggested to reflect specialized features of dysgraphia and perhaps the specialized processes that support the writing functions in the central nervous system.

Left vs. Right Hemisphere

If there is a golden rule of behavioral neurology, it is that language is lateralized to the left hemisphere in most humans.[17,18] In addition, for as yet unknown reasons, most people are also left hemisphere dominant for limb movements.[18] Writing, a limb motor act involving linguistic formulation, is thus thought to be mediated, if not controlled, primarily by the left hemisphere. The essential elements of the writing disturbance known as paragraphia (neologism, agrammatism, etc.) are frequently observed in the writing of left hemisphere-damaged patients. Other defects such as the inability to form letters and the difficulty in using either script writing or block printing, but not both, also have been identified in the writing of some persons with left hemisphere lesions.

In recent years, the role of the right hemisphere in psycholinguistic processing has gained support.[19] The dysgraphia literature also has documented a number of cases of writing disturbances resulting from right hemisphere damage.[20,21] Although all of these discoveries seem to discredit our golden rule (at least as far as writing is concerned), most theorists and clinicians prefer to modify, rather than abandon the rule. That is, the critical part of the language functioning, namely symbolic formulation and manipulation, is still believed by most to be the domain of the left hemisphere. Only such auxiliary processes as spatial perception[20] and subconscious (or automatic) operations[22] required for a successful writing act are said to be realized in the right hemisphere. Therefore, the right hemisphere-damaged individuals present alignment problems, such as unusual left or top margins and line slopes, awkward grapheme configurations (often with extra strokes), left agnosia or neglect, and other deviant spatial features.[20]

One interesting consequence of the right hemisphere's role in processing visual–spatial information is the speculation that right brain-damaged patients might have difficulty processing nonalphabetical written languages (e.g., Chinese *Hanji* and Japanese *Kanji*). That is, persons with right hemisphere damage might suffer a character formulation problem for the appreciation of "picture-like" (iconic) script. The findings of Tzeng, Hung, Chen, Wu and Hsi,[23] however, do not support this hypothesis. These researchers presented a case of a Chinese right hemisphere patient who, although he could not copy geometric configurations satisfactorily, could copy pseudo-characters that followed the legitimate orthographic rules of the language. This finding suggests some caution regarding the use of the term "spatial–perceptual defects" when written language processing is discussed.

Even if adequately defined and objectified, the spatial–perceptual deficits known to accompany right hemisphere lesions do not provide an adequate account of the role of right hemisphere writing and dysgraphia. In fact, it has been proposed that right hemisphere may be involved substantially in one mode of lexical writing, namely, the direct access of word spelling from the word engram without a phoneme–grapheme transformation procedure.[21] Damage to the right hemisphere may result in a particular type of dysgraphia called, by some, *lexical dysgraphia* (see discussion below).

Anterior vs. Posterior

Benson and Geschwind[17] divide the agraphia associated with aphasia into *anterior* or *posterior* types, according to the lesion location. This anatomically based classification parallels a common typology found in the spoken language-based aphasia typology literature. Misspellings, agrammatism and some abnormal mechanical anomalies (due to the nonpreferred hand's lack of experience and practice in writing movements) are said to be the predominant characteristics of the writing produced by anterior lesioned persons. On the other hand, well-formed letter configurations are seen more often in individuals with posterior lesions who show frequent spelling errors, word order abnormalities (verbal paragraphias), and word omissions. Kaplan and Goodglass[24] also made an interesting distinction between the writing in Broca's aphasia (anterior) and that in Wernicke's aphasia (posterior): block printing being more common in the Broca's type, whereas cursive writing was more frequently used by the Wernicke's aphasic.

Cortical vs. Subcortical

In contrast with cortical lesions, to which most attention has been paid, subcortical lesions have been associated only recently with speech and language deficits. The thalamus has received the most intensive investigation among the subcortical structures suspected of playing a significant role in language functioning. Lesions in this structure (in the left hemisphere) are often associated with a transient aphonia, fluent aphasia, anomia with perseveration, verbal memory deficits, and contralateral motor neglect.[25]

As the same linguistic mechanisms subserve writing that subserve spoken language, it would not be surprising to observe writing disturbances in patients with subcortical lesions. Even though it may not be surprising to evidence dysgraphia with subcortical lesions, little effort has been made to analyze systematically the writing disturbances seen in patients with subcortical lesions and compare them with dysgraphias of cortical origin. One recent article by Margolin and Wing[26] provided some initial effort in this direction, although the emphasis was on the "components of motor control of writing" related to cortical and subcortical functions, respectively. Their case of cortical dysgraphia (supposedly an apraxic dysgraphic) was characterized by frequent but inconsistent letter malformations, better performance on copying than other writing tasks, and superior block printing to cursive writing. In contrast, Margolin and Wing's subcortical patients, all with Parkinson's disease and presumed basal ganglia involvement, showed micrographia (abnormally small writing).[27] An analysis of the spatial–temporal characteristics of the handwriting produced by these subcortical patients revealed a significant increase in movement time and decrease in letter height for grapheme output. Margolin and Wing[26] hypothesized that the increase in movement time appeared to be an attempt to compensate for an underlying diminution in force. In other words, the Parkinsonian patients with micrographia "were able to access an intact graphic motor pattern but could not generate the proper neuromuscular activity to produce a letter of adequate size" (p. 282). On the other hand, the explanation proposed for their case of cortical dysgraphia was "a deficit at the level of the graphic motor pattern" in addition to visual perceptual deficits. Deficits in other subcortical structures including the caudate nucleus and internal capsule,[28] the putamen and internal capsule,[29] and the corticocerebellar pathways[30] also have been proposed.

Gerstmann's Syndrome

Gerstmann's syndrome is characterized by four behavioral signs that are necessary and sufficient for the diagnosis. These signs are: finger agnosia, right–left disorientation, acalculia, and dysgraphia. Although the existence of the syndrome continues to attract fervent debate, the most controversial issue surrounding the syndrome is the presence of a single unifying mechanism for these seemingly disparate components. Some researchers have proposed a left parietal lesion reflecting a disorder of spatio–temporal sequencing to account for these signs. Our present purpose is to determine whether the dysgraphia in Gerstmann's syndrome has a specific clinical profile. Benson and Geschwind[17] concluded that the apraxic dysgraphia (a type of dysgraphia discussed below, in which the patient has difficulty forming letters) is often associated with this syndrome. However, from Roeltgen's[31] analysis of the documented Gerstmann's dysgraphic cases in the literature, it is apparent that any kind of dysgraphia may occur with this syndrome.[31,32]

Confusional States

Patients with various confusional states have been reported to demonstrate attentional disturbances as their primary clinical feature. The etiology for these confusional states varies from head injury to metabolic–toxic encephalopathy, especially of rapid onset.[33] Interestingly, writing by the confused patient has been reported to be more defective than speech.[34] Further, in a study designed to compare communication functions among four patient groups (aphasia, general intellectual impairment , apraxia of speech, and confusion) writing to dictation ranked third in impairment in the confused patient group, but was less impaired in the other groups.[35] Chedru and Geschwind[34] in an attempt to dismiss the idea of "pure dysgraphia" (not associated with any other neurological signs), documented the writing disturbances in 33 of 34 acutely confused patients. They summarized the dysgraphia associated with confusional states as follows:

> The writing disorder could involve the motor and the spatial aspect of writing as well as spelling and syntax. It was the most constant and the most striking linguistic disorder seen in these patients. It disappeared when the confusion cleared. The spelling disorder had the following features: high error rate in consonants and of small grammatical words in their entry, high rate of omission and substitution, high involvement of the last letters of the words. (p. 343, 1972)

It appears that these authors suspected that previous researchers might have misidentified (at least in some cases) dysgraphia associated with confusional states as "pure" dysgraphia.

Although we have tried to summarize the neuroanatomical–dysgraphic correlates from several perspectives, it is still unclear whether or not a particular dysgraphic feature or pattern of features can be mapped onto a specified cerebral pathway or center. While the interpretation of these data are as yet unclear, it is even less clear whether this effort would be productive enterprise if such cartography were possible. Somewhat independent of this enterprise, one conclusion seems to have emerged: Writing is a highly complex cognitive function supported by many interrelated skills that are housed in, or mediated through, a number of functional CNS structures.

Nature and Differentiating Features

Modularity in Writing

The last 15 years have witnessed a growing enthusiasm for the application of information processing models to the functional localization of neuropsychological and neurolinguistic symptoms. Dyslexia, for instance, has become a classical testing ground for a variety of reading and neurolinguistic theories.[36-38] The two well-known transcoding pathways in reading, phonemic mediation and direct access, seem to have been crystallized.[39] The basic assumption behind this enterprise is simply borrowed from faculty psychology; that is, human cognitive functions reside in the brain in such a way that componential skills or capacities are independently operating within certain temporal limits.[40] For theoretical and clinical scientists, this concept of modularity of mind has not only reinforced the well-accepted neuropsychological notion of "selective impairment" (of higher cognitive functioning) but also is consistent with the centers and pathways neurological models governing the study of all neurogenic speech and language disorders. Because of this componential theory, studies of dysgraphia also have moved to a stage of micro-level analysis. Strub and Geschwind[32] succinctly express this view:

> Writing is a high-level, complex, cognitive process and a series of steps-each a distinct neuropsychologic function- is required for its successful execution. . . . The individual

functions are carried out in separate brain regions and, because of this, a focal cerebral lesion can disturb the writing process in a selective fashion, depending upon the location and extent of the damage. (p. 304)

Roeltgen and Heilman's[41] model of writing and its disorders is an elaboration based on this assumption, and thus can be viewed as exemplary of such theorization under this academic fashion. This model is interesting in its attempt to map the cognitive modules subserving the writing act onto the cortical topography. Several sources of clinical findings provided the empirical basis for this clinicoanatomical correlative model. Therefore, in order to understand better this theoretical proposal, we need to examine the clinical symptomatology in greater detail.

Clinical Symptomatology

In this section we describe the more salient clinical features associated with various types of dysgraphias. The differential signs are discussed under the various categories of dysgraphia as these categories are commonly used. Note that the terminology used by different authors has different theoretical motivations. Therefore, the definitions given here are only samples taken from the recent literature and these definitions may not be exclusive of one another. Likewise, the specific graphic characteristics associated with each dysgraphia type rarely are exclusive of the other categories.

PURE DYSGRAPHIA

As mentioned earlier, the existence of this syndrome has been questioned.[34] Theoretically, a writing disorder can be said to be "pure" or "isolated" if it is not associated with any aphasic, alexic, apraxic, or spatial/constructional deficits.[42] In addition, general intellectual functioning and peripheral neuromuscular execution are said to be normal in pure dysgraphic patients. Laine and Marttila[28] described a subcortically lesioned subject whose spontaneous writing contained a number of paragraphias and misspellings, but his automatic writing, copying, and letter formation were not impaired. Interestingly, his oral spelling was better than writing, whereas written spelling was better with higher frequency of occurrence items. Inasmuch as the neurobehavioral profile of this individual corresponded to the above conditions, this case was labelled pure dysgraphia. Auerbach and Alexander[43] also reported a parietal lobe lesioned subject with a similar clinical picture. They, however, speculated that the writing impairment might be secondary to a general difficulty in visually guided hand movements (i.e., optic ataxia).

APRAXIC DYSGRAPHIA

One way to categorize writing abnormalities is to divide them into letter (or grapheme) malformations and misspellings. The selective impairment of letter formation has been thought to be the major deficit of the apraxic dysgraphic. The "grapho motor patterns" generated by some motor programs are said to be damaged from focal lesions.[44] Roeltgen and Heilman[45] described the writing characteristics of an apraxic dysgraphic person as follows:

. . . he could neither write his name nor write words or letters dictated to him. When asked to write with his right (preferred) hand, he would correctly grasp the pen or pencil

Table 8-1.   Expected Performance of Various Dysgraphias on Writing Words to Dictation

	SPELLING				
DYSTRAPHIA	*Nonword*	*Irregular Word*	*Amgibuous Word*	*Semantic Paragraphia*	*LETTER FORMATION*
Phonological	−	+	CR(high) = CR(low)		
Deep	−	+		present	
Lexical	+	−	CR(high) < CR(low)		
Apraxic		+			−
		(using anagrams)			(improved with copying)

Key: + = good; − = poor; CR = correct percentage; high = highly ambiguous words.

and would produce meaningless scrawl. When asked to write words, he would frequently *say* the correct letters and then write approximately one meaningless scrawl for each letter said. He also could not print with either hand or write with his left hand. Because of his severe reading deficit, he was unable to spell using anagram letters. . . . His copying was much better than writing: He was able to copy most words with few errors. (p. 37)

This patient was reported to demonstrate no limb apraxia as evidenced by relatively intact pantomime, performing correctly on 12 of 15 commands.

Recently, Crary and Heilman[46] attempted to extract a "letter imagery" component in apraxic dysgraphia. According to these authors, the distinctive aspect of this letter imagery deficit lies in the fact that the patient could spell words correctly orally and with anagram letters but could correctly produce only half of the letters formed with toothpicks. In contrast with her normal performance in object/color imagery recognition tasks, her letter imagery recognition was very poor. This letter imagery deficit they considered as part of "apraxic dysgraphia." Additional descriptions of apraxic dysgraphia and its phenemonology have been reported by Baxter and Warrington;[47] Fukazawa;[48] Heilman, Coyle, Gonyea, and Geschwind;[49,50] and Valenstein and Heilman.[51]

PHONOLOGIC DYSGRAPHIA

This type of dysgraphia, along with lexical dysgraphia (see below) are hypothesized by researchers to be two distinct syndromes resulting from damage to the two written word retrieval routes.[36] Patients with phonological dysgraphia can spell irregular words correctly but have difficulty in producing orthographically legitimate nonwords (or pseudowords).[52,53] Shallice[53] described a patient who could repeat and read aloud, but not spell the nonwords. Since the spelling difficulty in this patient could not be explained by auditory imperception and was restricted to nonwords, it was hypothesized to originate from the inability to convert phenomes to graphemes.

DEEP DYSGRAPHIA

From what has been described in the literature about this syndrome, it appears that deep dysgraphia is a variant of phonological dysgraphia. The profiles of the two types look similar except that the deep dysgraphic subject shows more frequent occurrences of semantic paragraphias.[54] Bub and Kertesz[55] presented a subject who had good comprehension of written and oral words, showed telegraphic speech, and performed well in the automatic writing and copying tasks. She made many semantic errors in writing words to dictation (e.g., "happy" written as "funny") and had great difficulty generating the nonwords according to the orthographic rules. In writing words to dictation, she was poorer on function words than nouns, and was better at spelling concrete words than abstract words, regardless of the regularity of these words. Table 1 summarizes the differential features detected through the "writing words to dictation" task for the four types of dysgraphia discussed so far.

Other diagnostic categories such as spatial dysgraphia, aphasic dysgraphia (anterior and posterior), Gerstmann's syndrome dysgraphia, confusional dysgraphia, and the micrographia in Parkinson's disease have been discussed in the section on Pathophysiology.

LEXICAL (SURFACE) DYSGRAPHIA

This type of writing disturbance is manifested in the individual's inability to spell irregular words that do not follow the ordinary sound-letter transformation rules. The person does not randomly generate letters to dictated words, and productions tend to approximate the phonetic shape of the target word using known orthographic rules.[56] Beauvious and Derouesne[57] described a patient who could write nonwords to dictation with 99% accuracy, but wrote the irregular real words in the same task with only 38% accuracy. In the cases where a number of spellings seemed to be legitimate according to the orthographic rules (homophones), the patient made fewer errors when a reduced number of plausible spellings were present. This patient's clinical picture fits well with the theoretical expectation of the dual spelling pathway hypothesis. From an analysis of written transcripts, Sartori[58] has hypothesized that Leonardo Da Vinci, the great Italian Renaissance scholar, was a victim of this writing disorder.

The Roeltgen and Heilman Model

No other contemporary theorists have been more explicit about the neuropsychological components and their interrelations for a complete handwriting act than Roeltgen and Heilman.[41] Although their model is not explicit with regard to the details of motor control and of perceptual–motor links in writing, it provides a current, multifaceted, and representative view of writing and its disorders. Figure 8–1 shows their box diagram from which it is apparent that different subsystems, such as linguistic and motor components, are presumed to be functionally independent and therefore can be selectively impaired. The model is briefly summarized in Roeltgen and Heilman's own words as follows:

> The model contains certain postulated pathways. Following auditory analysis, auditory input is mapped onto auditory word engrams (component 3). In order to spell, these auditory word engrams may be translated using sound to letter (phoneme-grapheme) conversion (phonological system, pathway 7, 8) or mapped onto visual word images (lexical system, pathway 4, 5). Semantics or meaning may be incorporated into the spelling systems either directly (pathway 11, 13, 5) or indirectly (pathways 11, 12, 4 or 11, 12, 7). Output from these linguistic systems provides letter sequences for words that are spelled or written. For oral spelling the output of these systems maps onto the auditory word en-

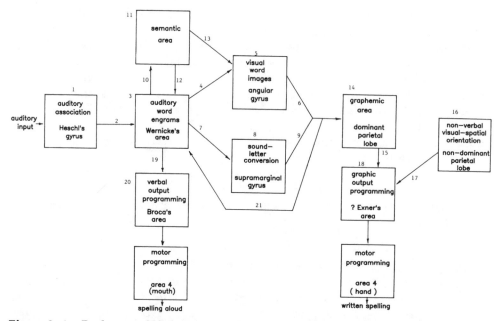

Figure 8–1. Roeltgen and Heilman's (1985) neuropsychological model for writing and oral spelling. The neuropsychological component is noted in the upper portion of each box. The lower portion contains a probable anatomical substrate for that function. (Adapted from Roeltgen and Heilman, 1985.)

grams (pathways 6 or 9, 21, 3). The auditory word engrams, or more specifically, letter engrams, provide encoding of the motor output for producing oral letters (pathways 3, 19, 20). For writing, the output of the spelling systems maps onto the graphemic area (pathway 6 or 9, 14). This system encodes the motor output for producing written letters (pathway 14, 15, 18). In order to produce correctly formed written letters (graphemes), output from the system for nonverbal, visual spatial-orientation interacts with graphic output programming (pathway 16, 17, 18). (p. 209[11])

Three features of this model should be noted: first, there are two parallel linguistic spelling subsystems that have been discussed earlier; second, there are also two spelling output systems; finally, there is a direct interconnection between the semantic storage and the visual image of words. These features illustrate the prevalent belief that word spellings can be accessed either by phonic mediation or lexical transcoding, that oral spellings and written spellings are executed through different motor control systems, and that the physical identity of a word may be represented separately in both visual and auditory formats. In fact, the first assumption was said to be confirmed by the distinct clinical patterns of phonological (including deep) dysgraphia and lexical dysgraphia.

The second assumption has received support from the documented cases of dissociation of oral and written spellings.[44,59] The third assumption was supported by the clinical observation that some Wernicke's aphasic patients (whose "auditory engrams" for words were supposedly damaged) showed relatively intact ability to spell. Note that the focus of this model is on the spelling processes. The interaction of these spelling processes with other oral language processes is not discussed. While the assumptions of modularity and selective impairment are essential tenets of the model, it does not make explicit predictions about dissociations. However, it would not be difficult for the model to account for the dissociation of oral and written expression (e.g., naming) observed in some patients.[60,61]

Roeltgen and Heilman[41] accounted for the various aspects of the dysgraphias by identifying differentially the origin of the restricted functional deficits in their information flow chart. Table 8–2 outlines the damaged pathways associated with different categories of dysgraphia.

At this point, it is appropriate to point out that Roeltgen and Heilman's model is only a tentative "neuropsychological" model. That is, it is a working hypothesis based on the documented clinical profiles of a limited number of cases (fewer than 50). This limitation should caution us to examine both the confidence one has in the validity of the model as well as its generalizability. This model also has made an attempt to integrate the anatomical data and to provide the typography of dysgraphias. However, because of the inherent methodological weakness of this approach, we present the neuroanatomical correlates postulated by the model with great reservation.

In addition, several other factors should be kept in mind when examining the model and its supporting data. First, in many (if not most) cases reported as support of the model, there appeared to be accompanying aphasic and (limb) apraxic signs. Reading disturbances may or may not have been associated with dysgraphia. It is, we believe, safe to conclude that the cases of isolated dysgraphia appear to be very rare. Most importantly, the damage to any "pathway" in Roeltgen and Heilman's model of writing and spelling has never been documented as "complete." That is, consistent with the case made by McNeil[62] and McNeil and Kimelman[63] for the auditory modality, the presumably defective process or function causing the clinical profile associated with a particular type of dysgraphia *does* function occasionally. For instance, Shallice's[53] patient with phonological dysgraphia successfully produced nine (of 60) nonwords. Similarly, Beauvois and Derouesne's[57] patient with

Table 8–2. The Damaged Pathways Associated
with Different Types of Dysgraphia

Type	Damaged Pathway*
Phonological dysgraphia	7, 8, 9
(in Wernicke's aphasia	7, 8, 9 + 3
Deep dysgraphia	7, 8, 9 + 11
Lexical dysgraphia	4, 5, 6
Semantic dysgraphia†	11 or 12, 13
Apraxic dysgraphia	14
Spatial dysgraphia	16, 17, 18
Oral spelling impairment	3, 19, 20

* See Figure 8–1, Roeltgen and Heilmann's model for writing and
oral spelling.

† Semantic dysgraphia is observed in patients who can spell and
write semantically incorrect but correctly spelled dictated homophones.

lexical dysgraphia did correctly spell the irregular words more than one-third of the time. This kind of "incomplete impairment" is a rule rather than an exception in the clinical dysgraphia literature. It is not, however, clear how Roeltgen and Heilman's model could reconcile this performance variability.

One additional consideration is that the consistency of errors that dysgraphic patients make has never been examined other than in the context of test–retest measures on formal aphasia diagnostic batteries. The omission of this piece of information necessarily jeopardizes, or at the very least proposes a threat to the reliability and hence the validity of, the differential classification of the dysgraphias. Any model that is critically reliant upon a clinical classification that has unknown reliability will remain open to concern for the soundness of its empirical bases.

Summary

For students of neurological and behavioral sciences, the nature of dysgraphia is easily clouded by the confusing terminology and many idiosyncratic classification systems. Since the 1860s, when the term "agraphia" was first introduced by M. Benedikt and J. Ogle, there have been more than a dozen ways of classifying the writing disorders.[1,14,64] This state of confusion can be attributed to the equivocal views on the dissociability of dysgraphia from aphasia, the structure of component skills required for performing a successful writing act, the neural substrates for these skills, and the possibility for these skills to be selectively impaired due to brain damage. In the previous two sections, we have tried to provide a concise review of different perspectives on these issues. By reviewing the Roeltgen and Heilman[41] model, we have provided a reasonable summary of the state of the art. With this framework, and the many obligatory qualifiers that must accompany our current understanding of neurogenic dysgraphia, an appreciation of the sophistication of the process and the disorders of neurogenic dysgraphia can be realized. Armed with this information, a discussion of the clinical assessment and treatment of the many forms of acquired neurogenic dysgraphia can be undertaken.

Evaluation

Reasons for Assessing Acquired Dysgraphia

As with the evaluation of any cognitive, linguistic or communicative function, the procedures used in the evaluation will reflect the philosophy of the test's authors relative to the nature of the hypothesized deficits as well as the purpose(s) for which the test was constructed. The philosophical decisions involve those discussed earlier in this chapter under Nature and Symptomatology. The purposes for developing (and eventually administering) a test of handwriting parallel those purposes for the assessment of the other features of neurogenic speech, language, cognitive, and sensorimotor disorders.[65] The purposes for assessing handwriting might be summarized as:

1. The detection or confirmation of a suspected deficit relative to a normal or premorbid standard.
2. The localization of the structural or chemo–electric lesion causing the observed writing deficit.

3. The differential diagnosis of the writing deficits according to their cognitive, linguistic, or sensorimotor origin or by their broad pathologic category such as aphasia, dementia, schizophrenia, confusion, hemipareses, etc.

4. The prediction of change in, or recovery of, writing functions as a consequence of treatment or physiologic change. Within this purpose treatment candidacy would be decided.

5. The classification by syndrome within a diagnostic category such as Broca's or Wernicke's aphasia or apraxic vs. surface dysgraphia.

6. The classification by severity of the deficit within the category or syndrome.

7. The focus of treatment.

8. The measurement of change as a result of treatment, no treatment, or additional pathology.

9. The setting of treatment termination criterion.

While the specific writing tasks (e.g., copying vs. writing to dictation), the stimuli used to elicit the response (e.g., copying letters vs. copying sentences) and the analysis procedures (e.g., counting misspelled words vs. measuring intergraphemic distance) used to assess writing may differ for these different purposes, a single task can often serve more than one purpose. Multiple test purposes have been designed into some of the standardized and published aphasia tests.

Published and Experimental Dysgraphia Tests

Unlike tests for auditory or reading processing and comprehension, there are no standardized and published tests solely for the evaluation of writing associated with neurogenic disorders. Writing is usually assessed as part of a larger battery of tests and when these tests appear inadequate for the purposes of the clinician, a hierarchy of informal–unstandardized tasks is recommended for its assessment.[66] Most standardized writing tests typically used for the assessment of aphasia and related disorders possess several subtests. These subtests reflect the philosophy of author of the test relative to the mechanisms believed to account for various characteristics of the writing and the test purposes that the author has in mind. One difficulty with most writing assessment tools is that the test creator has not been explicit in either theory or purpose. This leaves for the consumer the responsibility of deciding the theory to which the tasks, stimuli, and analyses best fit and the test purposes best served by these procedures.

These limitations notwithstanding, the assessment of writing employed in one of the most widely used tests for aphasia serves to illustrate the general hierarchy of tasks and stimuli, along with the procedures used for performance evaluation. A brief description of the writing portions of the Porch Index of Communicative Ability (PICA),[67] along with a moderately detailed analysis of the test's fulfillment of the various testing purposes is presented below.

The Boston Diagnostic Aphasia Examination (BDAE)[68] and the Western Aphasia Battery (WAB)[64] are two other frequently used aphasia batteries that posses a number of subtests used for the assessment of dysgraphia. Because of the number and severity of the psychometric problems inherent in the published version of the BDAE,[69] it will not be discussed. Because of space constraints, and psychometric limitations of the graphic portions of the test that are similar to those of the BDAE, the value of the WAB for the various purposes of assessment will not be discussed in great detail.

WESTERN APHASIA BATTERY

WAB subtests are divided into the standard tasks used by most examiners and found in most graphic sections of published aphasia batteries. The first three involve writing: name and address, connected sentences about a picture, and a single low frequency of occurrence sentence to dictation. If performance is high on these three tasks, the following four tasks are not administered: Writing the name of a named object or the name of the actual object, writing the alphabet and numbers from recall, writing dictated letters and numbers, and copying words. The usefulness of the WAB for differential diagnosis was addressed by Kertesz.[64] He reported that the writing scores discriminated all pathological groups [eight categories of aphasia (total N = 225), a small group of recovered aphasic subjects (N = 18), and a large group (N = 69) of nondominant hemisphere damaged individuals] from a small group of normal controls (N = 22).

Horner, Lathrop, Fish et al[70] reported the results of a discriminant function analysis with the written picture description task of the WAB using 10 left hemisphere stroke subjects, 8 right hemisphere stroke subjects and 10 Alzheimer dementia subjects. Given the very small number of subjects in each group it is difficult to place a great deal of confidence in the result. Nonetheless, 70% of the left hemisphere group, 63% of the right hemisphere group, and 20% of the Alzheimer dementia group were classified correctly. Overall, only 50% of the subjects were classified correctly. The authors concluded that the WAB graphic scoring approach was unable to classify patients into their true etiologic groups.

PORCH INDEX OF COMMUNICATIVE ABILITY

PICA[67] has six subtests that assess graphic abilities. A very important and unique feature of the PICA is that it uses the same 10 common objects (toothbrush, cigarette, pen, knife, fork, quarter, pencil, matches, key, and comb) across all 18 subtests. Several of the graphic tasks parallel verbal (spoken) and gestural (including pantomimic) subtests so that direct comparisons between spoken and written language modality performance can be made. The writing tasks involve describing the function of each of the 10 objects using complete grammatical sentences (subtest A), writing the name of each object (subtest B), writing the name of each object after it is spoken (subtest C), writing the name after it is spelled orally, segmenting the letters by syllables (subtest D), copying the name of each of the objects (subtest E), and copying geometric shapes and nonmeaningful sequences of letters (subtest F).

As with the other subtests, the method of evaluating the performance is accomplished with a 16-point multidimensional scoring system. This scoring system attempts to quantify the severity of aphasic and communicative performance along the dimensions of accuracy, responsiveness, completeness, promptness, and efficiency of the response. The theory on which the PICA graphic subtests was designed is consistent with the general philosophy and purposes for which the entire test battery was developed. That is, the PICA is best described as a test of information processing in which the systematic manipulation of tasks reveals deficits at various levels of processing and degrees of severity. Based on the particular conceptual framework that the author had for the selection of tasks, scoring system, and standardization procedures, the PICA graphic subtests address several of the purposes for testing. These include: detection/confirmation, lesion localization, differential diagnosis, prediction, severity classification, treatment focus, and measurement of performance change.

The detection or confirmation of a writing deficit on the PICA can be made by comparing the scores achieved to the normative data provided by Duffy and Keith.[71] It is important to keep in mind that education and employment are variables that are likely to influence writing performance.[12,70,71] Any reference data will need to account for these biographical variables. The degree to which the discriminant function analyses discussed below under differential diagnosis separates normal from pathological writing, is also evidence for the PICA's ability to detect or confirm the presence of acquired neurogenic dysgraphia.

Porch[72] presented a model and its rationale along with some preliminary case studies for inferring the localization of lesions from PICA test results. While a strict lesion location–behavioral deficit model is quite antithetical to the information-processing model on which the test was constructed, Porch predicted that lesions affecting the graphic subtests would be localized to the inferior-posterior parietal/posterior temporal lobes and to the superior-anterior occipital lobe. No studies have followed this preliminary report. Therefore, to date, the predicted correlation of PICA graphic performance with lesion location remains a model waiting to be tested. It might be noted, however, that these predicted lesion locations are not consistent with the great body of literature confirming the presence of dysgraphia in subcortical, frontal, mid and anterior temporal regions and with all forms of aphasia resulting from lesions in areas other than those proposed by Porch.

Graphic performance on the PICA also has been used for differential diagnosis. Watson and Record[73] reported that disturbances on graphic subtests E and F were the first clinical symptoms observed for differentiating dementia from left hemisphere damaged aphasic and bilaterally lesioned aphasic persons. These deficits were attributed to "a high-level visual perceptual deficit." They reported several unique characteristics on these two writing tasks. These included: Difficulty with horizontal or vertical lines, as in crossing t's; double letters; incomplete letters; letter reversals; inability to associate two written words; reading words and visualizing the image; lack of distinction between the letters "TVN" on subtest F; poor closure on figures; and inappropriate responses. While these authors provided some interesting observations, the degree to which the graphic subtests of the PICA differentiated demented subjects from left hemisphere damaged aphasic persons remains unclear. Using discriminant function analyses designed to quantify the differentiation of subjects belonging to various pathological populations, Metzler and Jelinek[74] correctly classified 100% of a group of 20 right hemisphere patients and 95% of a group of normal subjects on the PICA graphic subtests A through E. The variables that were selected in the discriminant function analysis were: (1) test time for each of the 5 subtests; (2) metathetic errors; (3) stroke, grapheme, syllable, and word perseverations; (4) stroke, grapheme and word omissions; (5) undotted i's and uncrossed t's. All of these variables were significantly different between the two group ($P < 0.10$) except word perseverations. Neither length of time since onset nor the hemispheric lobe involved predicted performance on any of the variables.

In a second discriminant function study, Porch, Friden and Porec[75] were able to classify correctly 100% of persons feigning aphasia from aphasic subjects using 14 subtests of the PICA, with four of the graphic subtests (A, B, D, and E) among them. Recent work by Brauer, McNeil, Duffy, et al[76] has demonstrated that graphic subtests A and B, along with five other subtests plus total test time were able to correctly classify 100% of the normal subjects in their study and 94% aphasic subjects.

Using standard PICA scoring, Brauer[77] has also shown that graphic subtest A, along with subtest I and IX were the critical variables in a PICA discriminant function analysis that correctly classified 55% of a group of learning disabled (LD) adults from a group of aphasic adults. Fifty-four percent of the aphasic group were correctly classified. None of the LD subjects were misclassified as aphasic, but four percent of the aphasic subjects were misclassified as LD. Likewise, 76% of the LD subjects and 60% of the normal control subjects were correctly classified by discriminant function with graphic subtest B being one of the four classificatory variables. In a three-way discriminant analysis among the LD, aphasic, and normal subjects, graphic subtests A, B, C, and F, along with total test time provided the most accurate classification of subjects. Overall, only 43% of the subjects were correctly classified in this three-way analysis; however, only two percent were misclassified overall. In all of these discriminant analyses using the PICA, graphic subtest performance provided a substantial proportion of the differentiating power.

Selinger, Prescott, and Katz[78] sought to evaluate the "mechanical" (biomechanical and sensorimotor) influences on PICA graphic performance (subtests A through E) for eight aphasic individuals. This was motivated by a need to assess, in as pure a form as possible, the linguistic aspects of the writing. These researchers used a microcomputer as the graphic output modality. A comparison of the handwritten performance with the computer-generated performance revealed that there were no significant differences in PICA scores between the two graphic output modes. However, the computer method took significantly longer than the handwritten method (mean = 45.37 vs. 27.13 minutes). These authors concluded that the "Concern that the mechanics of writing tend to mask the actual language abilities of the subjects are not supported by these findings." They further speculated that once brain damage is incurred, it may be easier to express written language in the manner that is first learned, even in persons who are skilled typists. Additionally, they concluded that the motoric and visual–spatial aspects of the writing that are purported to be critical for the differential diagnosis of neurogenic dysgraphias would be sacrificed with the typed assessment procedures.

The ability of the PICA to accurately predict future performance has received a great deal of experimental attention and scientific debate.[79-81] While this research has not reached an asymptote, it is clear that performance on the writing subtests of the PICA contributes to the overall ability of the test to statistically predict performance.[82] Performance on the writing subtests alone do not appear to offer sufficient predictive power. Porch,[67] however, has stated that graphic performance (presumably subtests A–D) shows slow change during early periods following onset in aphasic subjects, but shows a more rapid, positively accelerated curve at times further from onset. Porch[67] stated that copying words and geometric forms are believed to ". . . improve more quickly or are lost later than the other subtest skills." McNeil[83] reported that the average of all of the PICA graphic subtests recovered relatively (by percentile) more rapidly than gestural or verbal subtests for three aphasic subjects with an arteriovenous malformation etiology. Taken together, these scattered and preliminary findings suggest, but do not yet provide, strong evidence for the predictive power of PICA graphic performance.

By virtue of the quantifying nature of the scoring system, the PICA offers a relatively sensitive method for classifying writing deficits by their severity. Although the various mechanisms (e.g., sensory, motor, linguistic) for dysgraphia are not clearly differentiated within the scoring system, these attributes are considered to some degree in many of the individual scores. With the exception of no contextual writing sample, the PICA graphic tasks are typical of those found in all published tests used for the assessment of dysgraphia and, in this aspect of content validity, the test appears to offer a reasonable estimate of the severity of dysgraphia.

The PICA offers the greatest structure of any published aphasia test for focusing treatment.[84] This structure is derived from the scoring system, which gives some insight into the disordered processes involved in the dysgraphia, and from the tasks used to separate deficits attributable to visual–spatial, motoric, and various levels of linguistic and information processing variables. Because the same 10 objects are used for each of the subtests, comparisons across subtests can be made based on the task requirements that are not biased by the stimuli used to elicit the behaviors nor to different scoring procedures from subtest to subtest. This provides the ideal framework for making many appropriate decisions regarding treatment planning and its implementation. It should be noted that the PICA does not offer an adequate sample of contextual writing so as to perform pragmatic, discourse, or more sophisticated linguistic level analyses. This, according to some aphasiologists is a serious limitation to its treatment planning utility for some aphasic patients as well as for demented, closed head injured, and right hemisphere damaged individuals.

The measurement of performance change is sensitively detected and quantified using the 16-point multidimensional scoring system of the PICA for the tasks that it samples. This ability to measure subtle changes in performance as a result of treatment or progressive pathology makes the PICA a more attractive tool for this purpose than any other published test for many clinicians. Even with this degree of sensitivity, the PICA does not describe or quantify many features of handwriting with sufficient precision and confidence so that it can be used to fulfill many of the purposes of assessment.

Graphic performance on the PICA, as with the other published tests, does not provide information on classifying aphasia by syndrome. This is not surprising, as this modality has not traditionally been part of the centers and pathways models for determining aphasia type. In addition, the PICA graphic subtests have not been investigated as criteria for determining treatment candidacy or treatment termination.

NEUROGENIC DYSGRAPHIA BATTERY (EXPERIMENTAL)

The description of an experimental neurogenic dysgraphia battery that follows is offered as an example of the complexity of tasks and analysis procedures that have been developed and are required for the adequate assessment of dysgraphia. This battery represents a composite of the literature on the tasks and analysis procedures required for the development of a neurogenic dysgraphia battery that will meet many of the purposes of assessment outlined above. Many of the tasks and scoring procedures are consistent with, although not derived directly from, the dysgraphia model of Roeltgen and Heilman presented earlier in the chapter. The purpose for presenting these tasks and the analysis procedures in this chapter is to illustrate the complexity of the enterprise and, in the absence of an adequately standardized and published test for neurogenic dysgraphia, to provide the rudiments of such a battery.

The first data from this experimental test battery were reported by Hansen and McNeil[6] and Hansen, McNeil and Vetter.[7] In this version, there were eight subtests in the battery: Subtest 1 (Elicited: Picture Description) required the subjects to write, for two minutes, as much as they could about what they saw happening in the "cookie theft" picture from BDAE. Subtest 2 (Automatic: Name and Address) required the subject to write his/her own name and address. Subtest 3 (Writing to Dictation: Sentences) required the subject to write each of five different sentences presented from a taped recording. Subtest 4 (Writing to Dictation: Words) required the subject to write each of 20 words presented from a taped recording (25% frequently occurring and orthographically regular, 25% infrequent and regular, 25% frequent and irregular, and 25% infrequent and irregular). Subtest 5 (Writing to Dictation: Graphemes) required the subject to write each of five graphemes presented from a taped recording. Subtests 6 (Copying Sentences), 7 (Copying Words), and 8 (Copying Graphemes) used the same stimuli as subtest 3, 4, and 5 respectively, but required the subjects to copy instead of write from dictation. The same stimuli are used for the copying and dictation tasks. The methods of analysis utilized 11 features of the writing that were judged perceptually and nine features that required computer-assisted measurements.

Table 8–3 summarizes the various categories and subcategories of the perceptual measures. These measures attempt to account for many of the motoric and linguistic characteristics of the writing. Table 8–4 summarizes the categories used in the computer assisted measures. The computerized measures are, essentially, an attempt to quantify some of the spatial characteristics of the writing. These perceptually and computer derived measures are not, however, the entire corpus of measures that are currently being used. Several higher-level linguistic and spatial measures have been added to the list so that a total of 134 different variables are

Table 8–3. Major Categories of Perceptual Measures and Subcategories Used for the Analysis of Writing in the Experimental Neurogenic Dysgraphia Battery*

1. Grapheme formulation error: (substitution, addition, omission, reduplication, transposition, reversal, overlap, undotted i, uncrossed t.)
2. Grapheme errors detected:
3. Grapheme errors corrected:
4. Graphemes capitalized:
5. Word omissions:
6. Word substitutions:
7. Word additions:
8. Word deletions:
9. Illegible words:
10. Number of graphemes per word:
11. Number of words per sentence:

* Hansen and McNeil[6]; Hansen, McNeil, and Vetter.[7]

Table 8-4.   Major Categories of Computer-assisted Measures Used for the Analysis of Writing in the Experimental Neurogenic Dysgraphia Battery*

1. Top margin Distance:
2. Left margin width:
3. Right margin width:
4. Grapheme height:
5. Intergraphemic distance:
6. Interword distance:
7. Line slope:
8. % Graphemes deviating from slope:
9. Number of graphemes per deviation from slope:

* Hansen and McNeil[6]; Hansen, McNeil, and Vetter.[7]

currently used across the eight subtests to describe the various aspects of the graphic productions.

Current research involves a detailed statistical evaluation of the battery for redundancy of information, an evaluation of the battery's psychometric properties (various validity and reliability attributes), and the battery's effectiveness in differentiating various pathological populations. As stated above, the research on this battery is as yet too incomplete for the recommendation of its clinical use or its service as a model for other batteries. It does, however, serve to highlight the complexity of the task involved in the assessment of neurogenic dysgraphia and the dire need for such a tool.

In these initial studies with this experimental battery, Hansen and colleagues[7] reported some comparisons of normal geriatric controls writing with their dominant and nondominant hands. In addition to providing normal reference data for the battery prior to its use with various neurogenic populations, the motivation for these studies stemmed from the hypothesis that everything that a neurologically abnormal subject does may not be attributable to his neurologic differences. In other words, since many neurogenic populations write with their nondominant hand, it is difficult to determine whether any observed differences are due to the special characteristics of the lesion or the pathology or to the use of a unpracticed writing hand. In the Hansen and McNeil study,[6] the 20 measures summarized in Tables 8–3 and 8–4 were computed for the writing produced with both the dominant and nondominant hands on the spontaneous writing task for 50 normal geriatric subjects. There were no significant differences between the writing produced with the two hands for any of the measures. Great variability in writing was observed on this task, both within and between subjects. Further, correlation coefficients computed comparing the various measures were, with one exception, small and predicted less that 50% of the variance in the two data sets. These low correlation coefficients were interpreted to suggest that individuals were not consistent from one hand's production to the other. For example, individuals who wrote small or produced large intergraphemic spaces with one hand would not predictably make small letter and large intergraphemic spaces with the other. This finding of no difference between hands was surprising given that five normal judges were able to sort the writing sample by the hand believed to have produced it with 93% accuracy (range = 83–100%).

A study of interhand performance of the same 50 normal subject's sentence dictation writing, reported by Hansen, McNeil, and Vetter,[7] found significant differences between the two hands on one of the eight perceptual measures and on four of the eight computer-assisted measures. Writing with the nondominant hand yielded significantly more grapheme errors detected, a greater percentage of graphemes deviating from the slope of the written line, a greater number of graphemes per deviation from the slope (longer oscillations), larger grapheme height, and greater intergraphemic distance. A greater number of detected errors might be expected since more errors in writing would be expected because of the use of the unpracticed nondominant hand. Because these subjects were selected on the bases of normal higher cognitive, linguistic, and perceptual abilities that support handwriting, all of the differences found with the computer-assisted measures were hypothesized to occur as a result of reduced motoric control in the use of the unpracticed nondominant hand. From this, the authors cautioned in the attribution of a neuropathological substrate for these behaviors in neurologically disordered persons until clear differences from normal performance can be found. It is essential that future research describe the performance of various neurologically impaired samples on the same protocol, with the same analysis procedures in order to provide data useful in differentiating normal variations in writing from writing disorders that have neuropathologically predictable substrates.

Indeed, while writing performance has received the least attention of any modality in the assessment of language and communication among the neurogenic populations, it has been shown to be a critical modality for many of the purposes of assessment. No area of neurogenic language and communication research is in greater need of valid, reliable, and standardized assessment procedures than the area of dysgraphia. The adoption of tasks and scoring procedures from the experimental literature on dysgraphia will not substitute for a well-standardized and psychometrically sound assessment battery. Using "informal," "unstructured," "observational," or "custom designed" assessment techniques that have not stood the rigor of psychometric design and standardization will not provide the assurance of replicability, predictability, or comparability with other subjects that are needed for accurate detection, classification, lesion localization, and the various treatment-related issues. Continued research with the standardized and published tests currently available, along with continued research on experimental protocols such as the one sketched above, will eventually provide the tools needed in this most neglected area of neurogenic language and communication assessment.

Treatment

While the literature on the nature and assessment of dysgraphia is thin, the literature on the treatment of dysgraphia is skeletal. In spite of the paucity of treatment data, several theoretical approaches to the clinical management of neurogenic dysgraphia can be culled from an amalgamation of the theoretical and the treatment literature.[85] One approach is a rather utilitarian one in which the behaviors observed are evaluated against some internal standard of the clinician, and a direct assault is made upon the behavior believed to account for the discrepancy between the observed and the expected. Typically the clinician hypothesizes about the origin of the identified behavior. Following the traditional model of neurogenic dysgraphias, the hypotheses involve the attribution of the deficit to a specific visual–spatial, motoric, linguistic, or other cognitive (e.g., memorial or attentional) origin. If a more current information-processing model is imputed, then the hypotheses might involve the attribution of the deficit to a specific subcomponent of the phonological route or to a subcomponent of the lexical–semantic route.

Particularly important for this discussion is the fact that models of normal writing can serve as legitimate heuristics for many neurogenic dysgraphias. In other words, what we know about the processes of writing from the study of normal subjects under idealized or degraded conditions (e.g., without kinesthetic or visual feedback or under conditions of divided attention) will have relevance for the understanding and treatment of the disordered writing. In addition, what we know about all aspects of all of the neurogenic disorders will influence our management of dysgraphia. As Hatfield[86] described, there is a clear correspondence between reading and writing and, since more work has been done on reading, familiarity with the relevant constructs is essential to understanding dysgraphia. It takes little expansion of logic to realize that a full account of spelling, semantics, phonology, lexical storage and access, limb motor control, attention, memory, and a myriad of other legitimate areas of inquiry are necessary for the development of a theory of handwriting and its disorders and for the application of this theory to clinical management. Therefore, a parochial view of writing will impede the development of a theory of dysgraphia and will delay a full accounting of the relevant variables and procedures needed for its most efficacious treatment. Even if such a theory were developed and available, it would be beyond the scope of this chapter to even review its outline. It will suffice to be aware that cognitive (including linguistic) and motor processes never operate in isolation. Writing errors are rarely if ever attributable to a simple mechanism.

Following the observation of the deficit and the application of the theoretical model, one of three strategies is usually adopted. The behavior is: (1) retrained directly or indirectly, (2) compensated for by strengthening a system capable of assuming the same function, or (3) conveyed and practiced through an alternative system or modality. The clinician needs to make three decisions before instituting one of these treatment strategies: (1) target a behavior or a process for remediation including the context in which this treatment is to be administered[1] (see Appendix at end of the chapter). (2) decide on the technique(s) to be used to manipulate or influence the behavior in some direct or indirect way so as to effect change in the specific observable writing behavior; and (3) specify the exact measurement techniques to be used to decide whether to change or terminate treatment. This final process involves specifying the single subject design that will allow the differentiation of any change in the specified behaviors that are to be measured that are due to the treatment versus those that are due to the myriad of other factors that could cause change. If the efficacy of a particular technique can be applied with a reasonable degree of confidence based upon its previously documented efficacy, then step number three can be simplified or perhaps even eliminated.[87,88]

Dysgraphia Treatment Literature

A cursory review of the aphasia treatment efficacy literature[89-93] provides ample evidence that dysgraphia associated with aphasia *can* be improved with therapy. However, of necessity, these general efficacy studies do not provide sufficient detail to the rationale or structure of this treatment to be of much value to the clinician. The following review of eight treatment studies provides some insight into the rationale and methods for the successful and unsuccessful treatment of writing associated with aphasia. It is hoped that these sketches will illustrate the current notions about treating aphasic writing disorders, and will provide a model for other clinicians. Like the general efficacy studies, these studies, mostly reported as single subject studies, provide evidence that treating dysgraphia *can* be effective, especially if a careful analysis of the mechanisms causing the specific deficits are addressed.

Positive Treatment Results

Pizzamiglio and Roberts[94] provided what is perhaps the first experimental dysgraphia treatment study and the first objective data to suggest that writing can be treated efficaciously. They trained two groups of 10 aphasic adults to write a sentence-completion task and to do a graphic picture-naming task. A teletype typewriter, capable of providing feedback of wrong spellings, was used as the training device. One group received daily treatment while the other received treatment every other day. A significant between-group difference was found in the number of sessions required to meet criterion (90% correct for three consecutive sessions) and in the number of correct responses. On both dependent measures, the group receiving *daily* treatment required fewer sessions to criterion and had a greater mean increment in correct responses per session. No significant between-group differences in a one week maintenance probe was found.

Mills and Kaufman[95] reported the effects of treating an aphasic man for a letter-writing-to-dictation impairment using a gestural signing technique. The patient was reported to have had substantive impairments across language modalities, with inordinately well-preserved graphic copying abilities, visual reception skills, and letter-naming ability. Following 60 weeks of multimodality stimulation therapy, including the use of reauditorization and tracing practice (the Fernald Approach) along with the pairing of the sound of the letter with a key word (the phono-visual approach), graphic (as well as overall) performance evidenced minimal change on the PICA. Guided by the transcoding model (defined as "transposing certain prescribed units of one code system into the relevant units of another code system")[96] proposed by Weigl and Fradis[97] for writing to dictation, these authors devised tasks that focused on auditory-to-visual transcoding using an alternate (and intermediate) perceptual code. The alternate code utilized finger spelling. The transcoding was accomplished through a series of steps linking the sign to the visual characteristics of the letter, linking the sign and the letter name, and linking the sign and the grapho-motor code. The goal was to write, without cues, letters to dictation. This patient learned the alternate code and improved on the linking tasks. In addition, this skill appeared to generalize to all of the PICA graphic subtests.

Hatfield[86] provided an illustration of how theory can influence the selection of the treatment task and the behavior measured. Treatment was provided for four patients. One patient was diagnosed as a "surface dysgraphic" and three patients were labeled as "deep dysgraphic." While the attribution of the changes that occurred in the patient's writing following the treatment cannot be ascribed to the treatment itself because of a lack of proper experimental (clinical) controls, the nature of the treatment based on this theoretical distinction is of interest. Treatment for the three deep dysgraphic patients involved choosing a small number of function words and gradually working through the prepositions, the auxiliaries, and the pronouns. It was assumed that the process of phoneme-to-grapheme conversion had broken down in these patients, and direct attempts to rehabilitate this process were reported to have failed. These patients could write some words to dictation and were spontaneously observed to write contentive homophones for functor words which they could not write (e.g., they wrote inn/in). Therefore, a content homophonic or quasi-homophonic (link) word (e.g., Don/on, history/his or hymn/him) corresponding to the target word was dictated first in isolation, then in a sentence containing the target function word. The task was to write the function word under the link word. The goal was to spontaneously write functor words. Hatfield's subjective impression of the effects of the treatment was that it was effective at improving these patients' written agrammatism.

Treatment for the single surface dysgraphic patient had two goals. The first used a didactic method of teaching the spelling rules of "doubling the consonant" in order to preserve the quality of the vowel. The second involved a cueing technique for the reacquisition of the spelling of three groups of words with vowels or diphthongs (i.e., two different ways of writing the phoneme /e/ (e.g., pain, pane), two different spellings of /i/ (e.g., meat, meet), and three different spellings of /ou/ (e.g., road, rode, rowed). A "key-word" (a well known word which the patient could reliably write) was given for the different spelling patterns (e.g., the word "boat" was the key word or mnemonic for the group "road, oak, soak, foam"). The author reported between 20% and 30% improvement on both tasks.

A recent report by Hillis and Caramazza[98] provides a sophisticated example of the direct influence that a specific dysgraphia model can have on the selection of treatment stimuli, tasks, and evaluation procedures. Unlike the inadequate pretest–posttest design used for evaluating the effects of treatment in most of the other writing treatment studies, the employment of a single-subject multiple-baseline experimental design allowed the evaluation of the effectiveness of the treatment technique. Similar to Hatfield, these researchers reasoned that since their patient had a selective disorder of spelling that could be attributed to the "graphemic buffer," strategies for teaching specific spelling of words or specific morphological rules would be futile. As their subject could select accurately the spellings of appropriate morphological forms of words from sentence frames and thus demonstrated an intact graphemic lexicon, they chose to exploit his ability to recognize correct spellings. They attempted to train the types of words likely to be in error by enhancing the subject's ability to self-correct by searching his production for incorrect spellings. They contrasted the two possible treatment approaches by differentially measuring the effects of training specific spellings of words (corrections provided by the clinician) and by measuring the effects of training self-correction (search) strategies. With some surprise, both techniques improved spelling, although the specific spelling training did not generalize to untrained words in written narratives, while the self-correction strategy did. They reported that the self-correction technique was so successful that the subject was able to return to his previous employment, which the dysgraphia had prevented previous to treatment.

Behrmann[99] reported the effects of a "homophone" retraining program with a "surface dysgraphic" patient. Based on extensive pretreatment testing, the authors concluded that this subject had a selective impairment of the lexical processing of homophones and irregular words in writing but not in reading. The treatment involved the pairing of the written homophone with its pictorial representation in order to link the orthography with the word's meaning so as to provide direct lexical access. As with the Hatfield[86] study, the pretest–posttest case study does not allow, with any degree of confidence, the attribution of the observed changes to the treatment. However, Behrmann reported significant improvement in writing-treated homophones and generalization to untreated irregular words. Minimal generalization to untreated homophones was reported.

Negative Treatment Results

Schwartz, Nemeroff, and Reiss[100] reported no significant differences in overall PICA score between a group of eight aphasic individuals treated with writing tasks for 20 sessions and a group of six matched aphasic subjects treated on a variety of multimodality language tasks including writing the names of pictured objects. While the groups did not differ significantly from each other on the PICA posttest, the group receiving the writing therapy only, improved significantly from their pretest performance, while the other group did not. The specific writing tasks were (1) writing the alphabet from memory, (2) writing the names of mono-syllabic pictured objects, (3) writing mono-syllabic words to dictation, (4) writing mono-syllabic words to dictation after each had been said three times by the experimenter, and (5) writing mono-syllabic words to dictation, after each had been put into a sentence by the experimenter.

Selecting subjects for treatment because they were believed to be negatively influenced by their emotional reactions to their own speech and language errors, McNeil, Prescott and Lemme[101] designed a study to evaluate the effects of systematic training in general muscle relaxation through the use of electromyographic biofeedback. Using a pretest–posttest experimental design (with a stable baseline) with four aphasic/speech apraxic patients, they reported improvement in several language modalities, but the changes evidenced on the PICA graphic subtests did not reach statistical significance.

Specific Treatment Procedures

While the literature on the efficacy of treating neurogenic dysgraphia is sparse, a number of treatment protocols and suggested hierarchies have been proposed. Without exception, these treatment tasks are unaccompanied by sufficient data on their effectiveness to allow them to be recommended for use without careful vigilance of their effectiveness for each patient for whom they are employed. As a model or a heuristic, these tasks and procedures can be helpful. While they might be helpful for the structure of a treatment regimen and a reasonable place to start for the beginning clinician, their ordering and adaptation to individual patient's strengths and weaknesses is necessary. As LaPointe[102] stated:

> Failure to underscore the importance of hand-tailoring the goals and techniques of therapy to the individual would be folly. On the other hand, the attitude that specific suggestions or examples of therapy tasks cannot, or must not, be given has left beginning clinicians with the queasy and dually frustrating feeling of being both impotent and emptyhanded. (p. 206)

If these cautions are appropriately heeded, the following specific suggestions offered by LaPointe[102] should be tried with confidence. In addition to these specific suggestions for treatment, the availability of a number of treatment workbooks[103-106] provides a variety of tasks that appear to be well developed both conceptually and technically.

A condensation of the writing tasks provided by Haskins[107] illustrates a typical hierarchy of tasks: (1) Trace letters named by clinician. (2) Connect dot-to-dot to form letters. (3) Copy printed letters. (4) Write alphabet in serial order from dictation. (5) Point to orally spelled printed word from closed set (manipulating homographs). (6) Point to printed word from oral presentation of the word (manipulated by pointing to a series of words. (7) Simultaneously trace and spell words orally following clinician oral presentation of the word. (8) Print copied word (manipulated with an imposed delay between stimulus and response). (9) Write words to dictation. (10) Write names of specified word categories. (11) Formulate and write short sentences using previously practiced words.

LaPointe[102] provided a series of seven tasks for the treatment of writing (six of which are presented in Table 8–5). He divided the enterprise into the general *task*, the stimulus *input*, the *stimuli*, and the *output*, which in this instance is always graphic. This particular series illustrates the interplay between the stimulus modalities, the difficulty level of the task itself, and the difficulty level of the stimuli used to evoke the response.

Conclusion

Attempts to categorize writing disorders and relate them to the location of lesions thought to have caused them have been documented and summarized in this chapter. A brief review of the assessment and treatment literature on dysgraphia was also provided. From this summary it is evident that acquired neurogenic dysgraphia has never been afforded the status of being a particularly essential or enlightening window into the mystery of language processing and language breakdown. This conclusion is reflected in the neglect of dysgraphia in the major aphasic taxonomies, the lack of standardized psychometric tests and instrumental procedures evaluating dysgraphia, and the paucity of treatment research on the topic. Although recent interest in spelling processes involved in both reading and writing may signify the coming of a new era of dysgraphia research, caution must be exercised to avoid too narrow a focus on spelling processes and the biases that may accompany the reposing on a single explanation or theory. To manage the total communication of the neurogenic patient, a complete account of language production, including that of writing and the performance factors that influence it, needs to be presented.

We have attempted to summarize the current relevant state of knowledge on

Table 8-5.   Specific Hierarchy of Tasks Proposed by LaPointe[102] for the Treatment of Dysgraphia

Task	Input		Output	Stimuli
Copy geometric forms and letters		Visual	Graphic	X, >, T,], V, L, O, H, Z, #.
Copy words		Visual	Graphic	tie, car, bed, pills, comb, money, pants, chair, shoes, glasses.
Write single letters to dictation	(List 1)	Auditory	Graphic	i, n, w, h, d, b, u, g, p, m.
	(List 2)			o, y, f, e, s, c, l, r, a, t.
Write words, letter by letter	(List 1)	Auditory	Graphic	top, cat, bad, yes, sit, was, fat, run, pan, fan.
	(List 2)			ham, hot, wet, his, dog, bet, bus, let, tin, mop.
Write words to dictation		Auditory	Graphic	Same lists as above.
Write two-letter words and nonwords to dictation	(Words)	Auditory	Graphic	I'm, no, we, hi, do, be, up, go, in, my.
	(Nonwords)			ba, tu, ca, ye, sa, wa, bu, hu, fa, ru.
Write three-letter words to dictation	(Set 1)	Auditory	Graphic	not, wet, his, dog, bet, got, hit, bed, him, nod.
	(Set 2)	Auditory	Graphic	bad, top, cat, yes, sat, was, bus, he's, fat, run.

writing and its disorders. While this state of knowledge leaves us wanting in many domains, we hope that it has some factual and theoretic information that serve to guide the search for an understanding of acquired neurogenic dysgraphia along with its most efficacious management strategies.

APPENDIX

Context of Treatment

Following the decisions of whether to treat, what and how to treat, clinicians are faced with an important decision regarding the context in which the treatment is administered. Current trends in aphasia treatment are, with increasing frequency, emphasizing the need to program generalization into the treatment's design. In the minds of some clinicians, this generalizability *must* extend to the use of writing (or speaking and gesturing) for interpersonal communication. These clinicians have argued that treatment must incorporate (and in fact be governed by) pragmatic variables in order to enhance and ensure this form of generalization. Some have even argued that treatment directed at a process, in the absence of contextual influences, is doomed to failure with respect to generalizability. The definition of the goal as the function that the communique serves (interpersonal communication) may, however, be myopic. An analogy may serve to illustrate the point. The treatment of the skin lesion in syphilis will neither affect the cause of the lesion nor prevent additional lesions, even though interpersonal communication may be enhanced by the dermatological intervention. The emphasis on context in aphasia treatment may detract from the search for the lowest common denominator(s) that will explain the deficits and lead to specific and focused treatment approaches and techniques to identifiable problems. Nowhere is this threat of focusing on context to the exclusion of other treatment considerations more evident than in the aphasia treatment literature. One of Hatfield's[86] concluding remarks illustrates the importance of looking beyond the goal that the elimination of the deficit will serve. She stated:

> The value of so much attention to writing, especially of function words, for patients with such severe all-round verbal handicaps, might be questioned. In a brief justification it should be pointed out, firstly, that writing can consolidate and assist oral language and, secondly, that there are some cases . . . where the graphic modality is better preserved than the oral for certain function words. (p. 169)

In addition to this, it might be remembered that writing can be the goal of treatment for some patients, and, as yet, there are no models nor evidence that the contextual influences being discussed will affect graphic performance in a way that will lead to greater generalization.

References

1. Marcie P, Hecaen H: Agraphia: Writing disorders associated with unilateral cortical lesions. In Heilman KM, Valenstein E (eds): *Clinical Neuropsychology.* New York: Oxford University Press, 1979.
2. Goodglass H, Hunter MA: Linguistic comparison of speech and writing in two types of aphasia. *Journal of Communication Disorders,* 1970, 3:28–35.
3. Goodglass H: The syndromes of aphasia: Similarities and differences in neurolinguistic features. *Topics in Language Disorders,* 1981; 1:1–14.
4. Frith U: *Cognitive Processes in Spelling.* London: Academic Press, 1980.
5. Gregg N, Hoy C, Sabol R: Spelling error patterns of normal, learning-disabled, and underprepared college writers. *Journal of Psychoeducational Assessment,* 1988; 6:14–23.
6. Hansen AM, McNeil MR: Differences between writing with the dominant and nondominant hand by normal geriatric subjects on a spontaneous writing task. In Brookshire RH (ed): *Clinical Aphasiology,* 1986. Minneapolis: BRK Publishers.
7. Hansen AM, McNeil MR, Vetter DK: More differences between writing with the dominant and nondominant hand by normal geriatric subjects: Eight perceptual and eight computerized measures on a sentence dictation task. In Brookshire RH (ed): *Clinical Aphasiology,* 1987. Minneapolis: BRK Publishers.
8. Kao HSR, VanGalen GP, Hoosain R: *Graphonomics.* Amsterdam: Elsevier Science Publishers, 1986.
9. Benson DF: *Aphasia, Alexia, and Agraphia.* New York: Churchill Livingstone, 1979.
10. Taylor J: The sequence and structure of handwriting competence: Where are the breakdown points in the mastery of handwriting? *Occupational Therapy,* 1985, 205–207.
11. Keenan JS, Brassell EG: Factors influencing linguistic recovery in aphasic adults. *Journal of Speech and Hearing Disorders,* 1974; 39:1–12.
12. Holtzapple PA: The influence of illiteracy on predicting recovery from aphasia. In Brookshire RH (ed), *Clinical Aphasiology,* 1972. Minneapolis: BRK Publishers.
13. Goldstein K: *Language and Language Disturbances.* New York: Grune and Stratton, 1948.
14. Leischner A: The agraphias. In Vinken PJ, Bruyn GW (eds): *Handbook of Clinical Neurology,* Vol 4. Amsterdam: North-Holland Publishing, 1969.

15. Hecaen H, Angelergues R: Localization of symptoms in aphasia. In DeReuck A, O'Connor M (eds): *Disorders of Language*. London: Ciba Foundation, 1964.
16. Russell WR, Espir MLE: *Traumatic Aphasia: A Study of Aphasia in war wounds of the brain*. London: Oxford University Press, 1961.
17. Benson DF, Geschwind N: Aphasia and related disorders: A clinical approach. In Mesulam M-M (ed): *Principles of Behavioral Neurology*. Philadelphia: FA Davis, 1985.
18. Bradshaw JL, Nettleton NC: *Human Cerebral Asymmetry*. Englewood Cliffs, New Jersey: Prentice-Hall, 1983.
19. Zaidel E: Lexical organization in the right hemisphere. *INSERM Symposium*, 1978; 6:177–197.
20. Hecaen H, Marcie P: Disorders of written language following right hemisphere lesions: Spatial dysgraphia. In Dimond SJ, Beaumont J (eds): *Hemisphere Function in the Human Brain*. London: Elek Science, 1974.
21. Rothi LJG, Roeltgen DP, Kooistra CA: Isolated lexical agraphia in a right-handed patient with a posterior lesion of the right cerebral hemisphere. *Brain and Language*, 1987; 30:181–190.
22. Simernitskaya EG: On two forms of writing defect following local brain lesions. In Dimond SJ, Beaumont J (eds): *Hemisphere Function in the Human Brain*. London: Elek Science, 1974.
23. Tzeng OJL, Hung DL, Chen S: Processing Chinese logographs by Chinese brain damaged patients. In Kao HSR, van Galen GP, Hoosain R (eds): *Graphonomics*. Amsterdam: Elsevier, 1986.
24. Kaplan E, Goodglass H: Aphasia-related disorders. In Sarno MT (ed): *Acquired Aphasia*. New York: Academic, 1981.
25. Mateer CA, Ojemann GA: Thalamic mechanisms in language and memory. In Segalowitz SJ (ed): *Language Functions and Brain Organization*. New York: Academic, 1983.
26. Margolin DI, Wing AM: Agraphia and micrographia: Clinical manifestations of motor programming and performance disorders. *Acta Psychologica*, 1983; 54:263–283.
27. McLennan JE, Nakano K, Tyler HR, et al: Micrographia in Parkinson's disease. *Journal of the Neurological Sciences*, 1972; 15:141–152.
28. Laine T, Marttila RJ: Pure agraphia: A case study. *Neuropsychologia*, 1981; 19:311–316.
29. Tanridag O, Kirshner HS: Aphasia and agraphia in lesions of the posterior internal capsule and putamen. *Neurology*, 1985; 35:1797–1801.
30. Rosenbek JC, McNeil MR, Teetson M: Syndrome of neuromotor speech deficit and dysgraphia? In Nicholas LE, Brookshire RH (eds): *Clinical Aphasiology*. Minneapolis: BRK Publishers, 1981.
31. Roeltgen D: Agraphia. In Heilman KM, Valenstein E (eds): *Clinical Neuropsychology*. New York: Oxford University Press, 1985.
32. Strub RL, Geschwind N: Localization in Gertsmann syndrome. In Kertesz A (ed): *Localization in Neuropsychology*. New York: Academic, 1983.
33. Mesulam M-M: Attention, confusional states, and neglect. In Mesulam M-M (ed): *Principles of Behavioral Neurology*. Philadelphia: FA Davis, 1985.
34. Chedru F, Geschwind N: Writing disturbances in acute confusional states. *Neuropsychologia*, 1972; 10:343–353.
35. Halpern H, Darley FL, Brown JR: Differential language and neurological characteristics in cerebral involvement. *Journal of Speech and Hearing Disorders*, 1973; 38:162.
36. Ellis AW: Spelling and writing (and reading and speaking). In Ellis AW (ed): *Normality and Pathology in Cognitive Functions*. London: Academic, 1982.
37. Marshall JC, Newcombe F: The conceptual status of deep dyslexia: An historical perspective. In Coltheart M, Patterson K, Marshall JC (eds): *Deep Dyslexia*. London: Routledge & Kegan Paul, 1980.
38. Sasanuma S: Acquired dyslexia in Japanese: Clinical features and underlying mechanisms. In Coltheart M, Patterson K, Marshall JC (eds): *Deep Dyslexia*. London: Routledge & Kegan Paul, 1980.
39. Coltheart M, Patterson K, Marshall JC: *Deep Dyslexia*. London: Routledge & Kegan Paul, 1980.
40. Fodor JA: *The Modularity of Mind*. Cambridge: The MIT Press, 1983.
41. Roeltgen DP, Heilman KM: Review of agraphia and a proposal for an anatomically-based neuropsychological model of writing. *Applied Psycholinguistics*, 1985; 6:205–230.
42. Assal G, Chapuis G, Zander E: Isolated writing disorders in a patient with stenosis of the left internal carotid artery. *Cortex*, 1970; 6:241–248.
43. Auerbach SH, Alexander MP: Pure agraphia and unilateral optic ataxia associated with a left superior parietal lobule lesion. *Journal of Neurology, Neurosurgery, and Psychiatry*, 1981; 44:430–432.
44. Margolin DI, Binder L: Multiple component agraphia in a patient with atypical cerebral dominance: An error analysis. *Brain and Language*, 1984; 22:26–40.
45. Roeltgen DP, Heilman KM: Apractic agraphia in a patient with normal praxis. *Brain and Language*, 1983; 18:35–46.
46. Crary MA, Heilman KM: Letter imagery deficits in a case of pure apraxic agraphia. *Brain and Language*, 1988; 34:147–156.
47. Baxter DM, and Warrington EK: Ideational agraphia: A single case study. *Journal of Neurology, Neurosurgery, and Psychiatry*, 1986; 49:369–374.

48. Fukuzawa K: Impairment in the ability to operate the internal representation of Kanji and Kana characters in Japanese patients with pure agraphia. In Brookshire RH (ed): *Clinical Aphasiology*, 1986. Minneapolis: BRK Publishers.
49. Heilman KM, Coyle JM, Gonyea EF, et al: Apraxia and agraphia in a left-hander. *Brain*, 1973; 96:21–28.
50. Heilman KM, Gonyea EF, Geschwind N: Apraxia and agraphia in a right hander. *Cortex*, 1974; 10:284–288.
51. Valenstein E, Heilman KM: Apraxic agraphia with neglect-induced paragraphia. *Archives of Neurology*, 1979; 36:506–508.
52. Baxter DM, Warrington EK: Category specific phonological dysgraphia. *Neuropsychologia*, 1985; 23:653–666.
53. Shallice T: Phonological agraphia and the lexical route in writing. *Brain*, 1981; 104:413–429.
54. Coltheart M: Deep dyslexia: A review of the syndrome. In Coltheart M, Patterson K, and Marshall JC (eds): *Deep Dyslexia*. London: Routledge & Kegan Paul, 1980.
55. Bub D, Kertesz A: Deep agraphia. *Brain and Language*, 1982; 17:146–165.
56. Hatfield FM, Patterson KE: Phonological spelling. *Quarterly Journal of Experimental Psychology*, 1983; 35A:451–468.
57. Beauvois M-F, Derouesne J: Lexical or orthographic agraphia. *Brain*, 1981; 104:21–49.
58. Sartori G: Leonardo Da Vinci, Omo Sanza Lettere: A case of surface dysgraphia? *Cognitive Neuropsychology*, 1987; 4:1–10.
59. Kinsbourne M, Warrington EK: A case showing selectively impaired oral spelling. *Journal of Neurology, Neurosurgery, and Psychiatry*, 1965; 28:563–566.
60. Basso A, Taborelli A, Vignolo LA: Dissociated disorders of speaking and writing in aphasia. *Journal of Neurology, Neurosurgery, and Psychiatry*, 1978; 41:556–563.
61. Hier DB, and Mohr JP: Incongruous oral and written naming. *Brain and Language*, 1977; 4:115–126.
62. McNeil MR: Aphasia: Neurological considerations. *Topics in Language Disorders*, 1983; 3:1–19.
63. McNeil MR, Kimelman MDZ: Toward an integrative information-processing structure of auditory comprehension and processing in adult aphasia. *Seminars in Speech and Language*, 1986; 7:123–146.
64. Kertesz A: *Aphasia and Associated Disorders: Taxonomy, Localization and Recovery*. New York: Grune and Stratton, 1979.
65. McNeil MR: Current concepts in adult aphasia. *International Rehabilitation Medicine*, 1984; 6:128–134.
66. Collins M: *Diagnosis and Treatment of Global Aphasia*. San Diego: College-Hill Press, 1986.
67. Porch BE: *Porch Index of Communicative Ability*, vol II. Administration and Scoring. Palo Alto, California: Consulting Psychologist Press, 1971.
68. Goodglass H, Kaplan E: *The Assessment of Aphasia and Related Disorders*. Philadelphia: Lea and Febiger, 1983.
69. McNeil MR: Review of Boston Diagnostic Aphasia Examination (BDAE). In Mitchell JV (ed): *Tenth Mental Measurement Yearbook*. Lincoln: Buros Institute, 1989.
70. Horner J, Lathrop DL, Fish AM, et al: Agraphia in left and right hemisphere stroke and Alzheimer dementia patients. In Brookshire RH (ed): *Clinical Aphasiology*, 1987. Minneapolis: BRK Publishers.
71. Duffy JR, Keith RC: Performance of non-brain injured adults on the PICA: Descriptive data and a comparison in patients with aphasia. *Aphasia–Apraxia–Agnosia*, 1980; 1:1–29.
72. Porch BE: Profiles of aphasia: Test interpretation regarding the localization of lesions. In Brookshire RH (ed): *Clinical Aphasiology*, 1978. Minneapolis: BRK Publishers, p 78.
73. Watson JM, Records LE: The effectiveness of the Porch index of communicative ability as a diagnostic tool in assessing specific behaviors of senile dementia. In Brookshire RH (ed): *Clinical Aphasiology*, 1978. Minneapolis: BRK Publishers.
74. Metzler NG, Jelinek JEM: Writing disturbances in patients with right cerebral hemisphere lesions. In Brookshire RH (ed): *Clinical Aphasiology*, 1977. Minneapolis: BRK Publishers.
75. Porch BE, Friden T, Porec J: Objective differentiation of aphasic versus non-organic patients. Paper presented to the meeting of the International Neuropsychology Association, Santa Fe, New Mexico, 1976.
76. Brauer D, McNeil MR, Duffy JR, et al: The differentiation of normal from aphasic performance using PICA discriminant function scores. In Prescott TE (ed): *Clinical Aphasiology*. San Diego: College-Hill Press, 1988.
77. Brauer D: Differentiation of Learning Disabled, Aphasic and Normal Adults' Language Performance on Selected Aphasia Batteries. Unpublished Master's thesis, University of Wisconsin, 1988.
78. Selinger M, Prescott TE, Katz R: Handwritten vs computer responses on Porch Index of Communicative Ability Graphic Subtests. In Brookshire RH (ed): *Clinical Aphasiology*, 1987. Minneapolis: BRK Publishers.
79. Aten JL, Lyon JG: Measures of PICA subtest variance: A preliminary assessment of their value as

predictors of language recovery in aphasic patients. In Brookshire RH (ed): *Clinical Aphasiology,* 1978. Minneapolis: BRK Publishers.

80. Porch BE, Callaghan S: Making predictions about recovery: Is there HOAP? In Nicholas LN, Brookshire RH (eds): *Clinical Aphasiology,* 1981. Minneapolis: BRK Publishers.

81. Wertz RT, Deal LA, Deal JL: Prognosis in aphasia: Investigation of the high-overall (HOAP) and the short-direct (HOAP Slope) method to predict change in PICA performance. In Nicholas LE, Brookshire RH (eds): *Clinical Aphasiology,* 1980. Minneapolis: BRK Publishers.

82. Deal JL, Deal LA, Wertz RT, et al: Right hemisphere PICA percentiles: Some speculations about aphasia. In Nicholas LE, Brookshire RH (eds): *Clinical Aphasiology,* 1979. Minneapolis: BRK Publishers.

83. McNeil MR: Recovery from aphasia resulting from arteriovenous malformation: A report of three cases. In Nicholas LE, Brookshire RH (eds): *Clinical Aphasiology,* 1972. Minneapolis: BRK Publishers.

84. Porch BE: Therapy subsequent to the Porch Index of Communicative Ability. In Chapey R (ed): *Language Intervention Strategies in Adult Aphasia.* Baltimore: Williams & Wilkins, 1986.

85. Martin AD: The role of theory in therapy: A rationale. *Topics in Language Disorders,* 1981; 63–72.

86. Hatfield FM: Aspects of acquired dysgraphia and implications for re-education. In Code C and Muller DJ (eds): *Aphasia Therapy.* London: Edward Arnold, 1983.

87. McNeil MR, Kennedy JG III: Measuring the effects of treatment for dysarthria: Knowing when to change or terminate. In Rosenbek JC (ed): *Seminars in Speech and Language: Dysarthria: Nature and Assessment.* New York: Thieme-Stratton, 1984.

88. Yoder DE, Kent RD: *Decision Making in Speech and Language Pathology.* Toronto: BC Decker, 1988.

89. Basso A, Capitani E, Vignolo LA: Influence of rehabilitation of language skills in aphasic patients: A controlled study. *Archives of Neurology,* 1979; 36:190–196.

90. Butfield E, Zangwill O: Re-Education in aphasia: A Review of 70 Cases. *Journal of Neurology, Neurosurgery, and Psychiatry,* 1946; 9:75–79.

91. Hagen C: Communication abilities in hemiplegia: Effect of speech therapy. *Archives of Physical Medical Rehabilitation,* 1973; 54:454–463.

92. Vignolo LA: Evolution of aphasia and language rehabilitation: A retrospective exploratory study. *Cortex,* 1964; 1:344–367.

93. Wertz RT, Collins MJ, Weiss D, et al: Veterans Administration cooperative study on aphasia: A comparison of individual and group treatment. *Journal of Speech and Hearing Research,* 1981; 24:580–594.

94. Pizzamiglio L, Roberts M: Writing in aphasia: A learning study. *Cortex,* 1967; 3:250–257.

95. Mills RH, Kaufman E: Gestural signing: Treatment for a letter writing to dictation impairment. In Nicholas LE, Brookshire RH (eds): *Clinical Aphasiology,* 1978. Minneapolis: BRK Publishers.

96. Weigl E: Neuropsychological experiments on transcoding between spoken and written language structures. *Brain and Language,* 1974; 1:227–240.

97. Weigl E, Fradis A: The transcoding processes in patients with agraphia to dictation. *Brain and Language,* 1977; 4:11–22.

98. Hillis AE, Caramazza A: Model-driven remediation of dysgraphia. In Brookshire RH (ed): *Clinical Aphasiology,* 1987. Minneapolis: BRK Publishers.

99. Behrmann M: The rites of righting writing: Homophone remediation in acquired dysgraphia. *Cognitive Neuropsychology,* 1987; 4:365–384.

100. Schwartz L, Nemeroff S, Reiss M: An investigation of writing therapy for the adult aphasic: The word [sic] level. *Cortex,* 1973; 9:278–283.

101. McNeil MR, Prescott TE, Lemme ML: An application of electromyographic biofeedback to aphasia/apraxia treatment. In Brookshire RH (ed): *Clinical Aphasiology,* 1976. Minneapolis: BRK Publishers.

102. LaPointe LL, Aphasia therapy: Some principles and strategies for treatment. In Johns DF (ed): *Clinical Management of Neurogenic Communicative Disorders.* Boston/Toronto: Little, Brown, 1985.

103. Brubaker SH: *Workbook for Aphasia.* Detroit: Wayne State University Press, 1978.

104. Keith RL: *Speech and Language Rehabilitation: A Workbook for the Neurologically Impaired.* Danville: Interstate Printers and Publishers, 1980.

105. Keith RL: *Speech and Language Rehabilitation: A Workbook for the Neurologically Impaired.* Danville: Interstate Printers and Publishers, 1977.

106. Stryker S: *Speech After Stroke: A Manual for the Speech Pathologist and the Family Member.* Springfield: IL, Charles C Thomas, 1975.

107. Haskins S: A treatment procedure for writing disorders. In Brookshire RH (ed): *Clinical Aphasiology,* 1976. Minneapolis: BRK Publishers.

9

Right Hemisphere Syndrome

Penelope S. Myers
E. Louise Mackisack

Introduction

We are only beginning to understand the effects of right cerebral hemisphere damage (RHD) on communicative capacity. Management of RHD communication disorders is relatively new. Ten years ago, treatment was limited to the dysarthria that can occur with RHD lesions. Since that time, effort in the area of RHD communication deficits has been devoted largely to an exploration of the signs and symptoms themselves, and much has been learned in the process.

We are now beginning to address the underlying cause of the behaviors we observe. At present, treatment tasks tend to focus on these behaviors, not processes, and treatment goals stress compensation for deficits, rather than recovery of function. However, increased knowledge of the underlying functions comprised by RHD suggests some hypotheses about the interplay between processing disorders and impairment of symptoms of communication. Therapy that goes beyond compensation, that hopes to stimulate recovery, involves generating a set of working hypotheses or best guesses about the processes we hope to help the patient recover.

This chapter presents our best guesses. These characteristic deficits and remediation techniques that are the most salient will be presented in addition to a discussion of the presumed underlying processing disorders. The focus of this chapter will be on the effect of impaired right hemisphere (RH) processing on communication, and on evaluation and treatment techniques that address those impaired processes.

Pathophysiology

Damage to neural tissue in the RH arises from the same array of neuropathologies that can result in left hemisphere (LH) damage, i.e., cerebrovascular accident, tumor, head trauma, and various other disease processes. Although investigators now make an effort to be more specific in reporting site of lesion in RHD subjects, much less is known about localization of function in the RH than in the LH. In the past it was customary to attribute nondominant functions to the right or "minor" hemisphere without specifying site of function. Finally, the RH is thought to be more diffusely organized than the LH so that the distribution of function is more widespread and less focal than in the LH.[1,2]

Table 9–1 summarizes the presumed localization of function of the RH sensory, perceptual, and cognitive deficits that affect communicative ability in RHD patients. Listed deficits will be defined in later sections.

Aside from prosodic disturbances, communicative impairments are not included in the table since almost nothing is known about their localization. Based on hypotheses about left-side neglect, one can speculate, however, that like neglect, failure to use and respond to significant contextual cues during communicative events may be differentially affected by anterior and posterior lesions. Frontal areas may contribute to the search for relevant cues while posterior regions may contribute to their recognition as significant. More studies specifically addressing site of lesion are needed to arrive at more fully developed theories about localization of RHD communicative disorders.

Nature and Differentiating Features

RHD patients remind us that language is only one aspect of communication. Despite adequate linguistic skills, they are poor communicators. As in aphasia, site and size of lesion, age, and degree of lateralization all may affect the severity and prognosis for recovery from RHD communication deficit.

Communication impairments associated with RHD have been defined as a breakdown in the "expression and reception of complex, contextually based communicative events resulting from a disturbance of the attentional and perceptual mechanisms underlying nonsymbolic, experiential processing" (Ref. 18, p 446). While fundamental language processes are intact, attention to and perception to contextual information is compromised so that the individual's experience of events is altered.

The three main types of communication disorders associated with RHD can be

Table 9–1. Presumed Localization of Selected RH Impairments

Impairment	Presumed Localization in the RH
Left-sided neglect: impairment in directed attention	Reticular activating system, cingulate gyrus, frontal eye fields, and/or dorsolateral parietal cortex[3]
Acute Confusional States, including delusions and hallucinations	Posterior parietal cortex[4,5] Ventral temporal cortex[5] Frontotemporal cortex[6] Prefrontal cortex[5]
Prosopagnosia	Occipito-temporal cortex confined to the RH[7–9] Bilateral occipito-temporal cortex[8,10,11]
Reduplicative Paramnesia	Frontal cortex[12] Parietal cortex[13] Frontoparietal cortex[14]
Topographic Disorientation	Occipito-parietal cortex[8,14]
Impaired Prosodic Comprehension	Parietal and/or temporoparietal cortex[15–17]
Impaired Prosodic Production	Frontal cortex[16,17]

categorized as *linguistic, extralinguistic,* and *nonlinguistic* (see Table 9–2 for deficits in each category). When they exist, pure *linguistic* deficits are usually mild and, by themselves, represent the least of the patient's communication problems. The patient may suffer or appear to suffer from some word-finding problems and mild comprehension difficulty. It is extremely important that the clinician differentiate true language problems from those caused by inattention and visuospatial deficits, particularly in visual confrontation naming and even in auditory comprehension tasks where attention may be a factor.

Deficits in the *extralinguistic* category are usually the behaviors that first alert the observer to the person's communicative impairment. Essentially these deficits reflect a failure to adequately interpret cues and organize information in an efficient man-

Table 9–2.   Communication Deficits Associated with RH Impairment

Linguistic Deficits. May include mild problems in:
    Confrontation naming
    Word fluency
    Body part naming
    Auditory comprehension of complex material
    Oral sentence reading
    Writing: grapheme substitutions, omissions

Nonlinguistic Deficits. May include:
  Left-sided neglect
    Directed attention to the left side of space
    Recognition of stimulus significance
    Maintaining form in and including left-sided detail in visuoconstructive tasks
    Awareness of midline and kinesthetic sense of body position
    Anasognosia — recognizing physical limitations and impaired body parts as ones own
    Denial of illness
  Visuospatial Deficits
    Figure ground, figure integration, figure completion tasks
    Detecting the directionality and orientation of lines
    Mental rotation
    Visual recall of form
  Impaired Contextual Processing and Impaired Visual Associations
    Prosopagnosia
    Reduplicative paramnesia — geographic disorientation
    Topological disorientation

Extralinguistic Deficits. May include problems in:
    Distinguishing between significant and irrelevant contextual cues
    Integrating pictured and verbal story elements into a theme
    Interpreting implicit or intended meaning
    Grasping the figurative meaning of metaphor and idiomatic expression
    Over-personalization of external events
    Organizing information into an appropriate hierarchy
    Topic maintenance
    Demonstrating sensitivity to the communicative situation
    Impulsivity of response
    Recognizing the emotional valence of ongoing events
    Interpreting and producing affective facial expression
    Interpreting and producing the prosodic features of verbal messages

ner. They are among the most difficult disorders to treat, the ones for which compensation strategies are most often employed in treatment, and the ones for which generalization is the least likely outcome. It is hypothesized here that lack of success in treating extralinguistic deficits rests on the fact that most of the deficits are actually the result of processing disorders in the nonlinguistic area, and that this presumed underlying cause must be taken into account in their management.

The heart of the person's communication disorder is in the *nonlinguistic* area where specific attentional and perceptual deficits interfere with the recognition of salient cues, the integration of those cues into a meaningful pattern, and the ability to adequately interpret implied or implicit meaning. These deficits manifest themselves in the extralinguistic aspects of communication. Salient *extralinguistic* deficits are described below, and although the deficits are separated into individual symptoms, many of them share common features.

Extralinguistic Deficits

DIFFICULTY DISTINGUISHING SIGNIFICANT FROM IRRELEVANT INFORMATION

Patients may concentrate on insignificant detail and fail to apprehend the gist of a narrative or the main action in a given situation. For example, looking at a picture of a couple arguing over a missing boot that a dog, hidden behind a chair, is chewing, one patient began her description of the picture by looking at the window in the center of the picture showing the rain outside. She said:

> Two people are out in the rain with their umbrellas walking by a house which has a large door—a large window which you can see through to the out-of-doors. And there are draperies on the window. On the side there's a chair. On the floor is a single boot which the dog is worrying.

The tendency to focus on irrelevancies is found in response to verbal as well as to visual stimuli. Narratives and conversational exchange with RHD patients demonstrates their difficulty in synthesizing information, so that detail detracts rather than adds to the message.

DIFFICULTY IN INTEGRATION AND INTERPRETATION

The above example is a good demonstration of the documented tendency to use concrete labels to list, rather than integrate specific bits of information.[19-21] Failure to use interpretive concepts (i.e., mother versus woman) again may be based on failure to integrate features into an overall pattern. In nonverbal tasks, RHD subjects have been found more impaired than aphasic patients in organizing pictures by theme; that is, in integrating contextual features into a meaningful whole that suggests a common theme across pictures.[22] Finally, instead of paraphrasing narratives, RHD subjects tend to retell stories verbatim without the expected interpretation of events. Impaired performance on these tasks suggests a failure to infer implicit meaning, which very likely stems from a deficit in the ability to recognize, use, and integrate significant contextual features.

DIFFICULTY IN INHIBITING IMPULSIVE RESPONSES

When asked to generate a response to a complex question, RHD individuals often produce immediate answers without apparent thought or reflection. The shallowness of response reflects little concern about its accuracy or appropriateness and little regard for the listener's reaction. RHD speakers seem to be motivated less by the search for knowledge than by the production of a response. This characterization may help explain why they often refuse to admit to uncertainty or lack of knowledge. Asked to retell a story containing nonsensical elements, non-brain-damaged subjects react by questioning items that are at odds with the rest of the narrative. RHD subjects, on the other hand, include such elements without concern and posit logical explanations for their inclusion in the story.[23]

DIFFICULTY GRASPING FIGURATIVE AND IMPLIED MEANING

RHD patients tend to respond to the literal meaning of figurative language.[24,25] Examples of RHD explanations of common idioms include: "boxer" for "tight-fisted;" "hit someone" for "pleased as punch;" and "falling trees" for "he's out of the woods."[26] This tendency extends to general problems in recognizing the connotative aspects of language, and in this sense can interfere with overall appreciation of implied content. Failure to appreciate implicit or implied meaning, whether in verbal exchange or in pictures and ongoing events, is one of the hallmarks of RHD communication impairment.

DIFFICULTY IN TOPIC MAINTENANCE AND EFFICIENCY OF EXPRESSION

Mackisack, Myers, and Duffy[21] found that RHD subjects used almost twice as many words and twice as many nouns to describe pictures than did non-brain-damaged control subjects. RHD subjects were less efficient by virtue of their tendency to use more explicit versus interpretive concepts in their descriptions than controls. As noted above, they tend to focus on detail and fail to distinguish significant from insignificant information.

In addition, RHD subjects tend to overpersonalize and in so doing digress. Looking at the water overflowing from the sink in the "Cookie Theft" picture from the Boston Diagnostic Aphasia Examination (BDAE),[27] they may discuss a water shortage in their home town. Failure to attend to external cues may result in excessive reliance on personal or internal associations. Or perhaps overpersonalization is a strategy used to compensate for failure to apprehend the implicit meaning of events and conversational exchange. It is easier to reminisce than to interact when one is unsure of the nature of the conversation or uncertain of how to organize an opinion or explanation.

DIFFICULTY IN APPRECIATING THE COMMUNICATIVE SITUATION AND
LISTENER NEEDS

Asked to describe the "Cookie Theft" picture, one subject said,

> Well, it's on 8 1/2 by 11 inch paper overall covered by plastic. Looks like it may have been done with drawing pens and India ink on white paper. It's less than 20 lb. paper, else you wouldn't have used black to keep it from shining through.

Clearly, this person misinterpreted the nature of the clinician's request. Often, RHD clients appear not to care about their listener's needs or the adequacy of their own response to the situation at hand. They may assume too much knowledge or not enough on the part of the listener. Answers are offered without reflection or adequate search for the correct answer. Failure to make eye contact or to recognize the nonverbal cues that signal a listener's reaction may contribute to problems in this area.

RHD individuals may have difficulty interpreting the situational, facial and prosodic cues that signal the emotional content of a message. Looking at a picture of a woman desperately holding on to a man whose face is contorted into an expression of agony and panic, one patient said, "That looks like a mother and a father. And what I imagine they live real cheerful and cooperative and probably have a family. Sounds like their home might be interesting."

It is thought that unless limbic areas are involved, RHD does not impair the actual experience of emotion so much as its superficial expression and comprehension.[28] The patient may simply have difficulty in interpreting the environmental cues that signal emotional content (tone of voice, prosody, facial expression, and situational context).

In addition to these receptive difficulties, RHD individuals may be impaired in emotional expression through the use of the prosodic features of speech[29,16,17] and facial expression.[30] The patient may present with a flat affect and monotone speech, and in severe cases may appear to be clinically depressed.

Finally, patients may produce inappropriate affective responses, either hyereuphoric[31] or jocular. They may fail to recognize impaired body parts as their own (anosagnosia) and may not recognize or acknowledge their deficits in any area (denial of illness).

Nonlinguistic Deficits

The search for processing disorders underlying the array of extralinguistic impairments must begin with an exploration of their unifying features. The most striking feature common to this apparently disparate symptomatology is an attenuated responsiveness to intended or implicit meaning, whether it is conveyed verbally or nonverbally. We hypothesize that this breakdown in processing implicit meaning is based on the following nonlinguistic deficits:

1. Difficulty in recognizing and utilizing significant contextual cues.
2. Difficulty in integrating these significant cues into an overall pattern.

These difficulties stem from fundamental impairments in specific types of attentional and perceptual processing which the RH appears to mediate. Behaviors associated with these nonlinguistic deficits are described below.

Directed Attention.   One of the most frequently occurring signs of RHD is left-sided neglect, a disorder in which the individual does not respond to input from the left side of the midline, regardless of the sensory capacity to do so. Left-sided neglect interferes with the exploration of contralateral and occasionally ipsilateral space, and awareness of sensory information, particularly on the left side. The directly observable consequences of neglect are failure to attend to the left side of space, impaired localization of stimuli, impaired use of margins and punctuation in writing, failure to look to the left side of a page in reading, and incomplete drawings and internal representations (recalled images). It is thought that the type of neglect (motor versus sensory) may differ according to site of lesion[3,5] (see Table 9–3).

Neglect has far-reaching consequences for communication, not only because it disrupts the intake of information from the left, but also because it attenuates the patient's capacity to integrate concrete sensory and perhaps even abstract information. RHD individuals with neglect are usually more severely impaired in all aspects of communication than are those without neglect.

Current theories tie neglect to a particular type of attention, sometimes called "directed attention," in which the RH is thought to predominate.[3,5,32] Directed attention has been described as the capacity to determine "the distribution of attention within extrapersonal space" (Ref. 5, p 53). It involves attending to stimuli in the external environment, specifically through recognition of stimulus significance and orientation to a significant stimulus with the intention of acting on it. Research with primates and humans suggests a complex neural network for the representation of directed attention (see Table 9–1). It is distinguished by the heightened activity of the RH in all tasks involving directed attention, regardless of the hemi-space location of the stimuli. What is important in light of impaired RH processing and subsequent communication disorders is the possibility that the RH may be responsible for the recognition of significant environmental features.

Thus, depending on site of lesion, and the presence of left-sided neglect, attentional deficits in the RH patient not only may interfere with the ability to maintain or focus attention, but also with the ability to determine what to attend to — that is, in the capacity to recognize the boundaries of relevant space, to recognize significant features within that space, and to "intend toward" or act upon those features.

Confusion.   Deficits in attention also can result in some forms of confusion, particularly if multimodal or tertiary association areas of the cortex are affected. Although

Table 9–3.   Deficits Associated with Left-Sided Neglect

Sensory Neglect	*Definition:*	Disturbance in the distribution of attention such that there is a failure to attend and respond to stimulation presented in extra-personal or egocentric contralateral space.
	Signs:	Extinction to bilateral simultaneous stimulation Events in contralateral space are poorly processed May include deficits in response to events ipsilateral space Representation of the midline shifts to the right
Motor Neglect	*Definition:*	Disturbance in the inner representation of motor programs for the exploration and manipulation of contralateral space.
	Signs:	May impair intention to interact with and explore external space Disrupts the inner representation of motor sequences for exploring and manipulating contralateral space Impairs constructional abilities and scanning

Adapted from Mesulam.[3]

rare, deficits from damage at these sites can include in delusions, hallucinations, and acute confusional states not unlike those associated with toxic metabolic encephalopathies.

Specific forms of confusion can occur with RHD. Individuals may not attend adequately to the environmental cues that tell them where they are so that they are convinced they are in another location, resulting in a disorder called *reduplicative paramnesia*.[12] They may not know to whom they are talking because of a facial recognition deficit *(prosopagnosia)*, or how to get to their destination *(topographical disorientation)*. These deficits can be considered problems in retrieval of meaning,[11] that is, the person suffers not only from failure to attend to significant features that signal the identity of his location or friends, but also from difficulty in calling up the contextual associations needed to recognize familiar faces and landmarks.

PERCEPTUAL DISORDERS

Attention can be considered the first step in the process of assigning meaning to events. Equally important is the ability to accurately perceive them. We view perception as a process of creating representations about the world that are subject to certain rules of transformation. The visuoperceptual deficits in RHD are not usually characterized by problems in distinguishing surfaces and edges from one another, but rather by an impairment in the rapid recognition and synthesis of features into a form that is more than the sum of its parts. RHD individuals are notably impaired in identifying pictures of objects broken into parts even though they can match them to target.[19] The elements are "seen," but not integrated. This failure to see the pattern of meaning contained in collections of objects extends to ongoing perception of events. One patient, a former professor, described the problem by saying that in order to know he was in a classroom he had to consciously and carefully analyze each feature (desks, lectern, etc.) in the room.

The visuospatial deficits associated with RH damage have been described as stemming from a common problem in the ability to evaluate distinct elements in the context of an overall framework.[33] Of note is the fact that some people with left-neglect make perceptual errors on the right as well as on the left and that even the right side of their drawings often are characterized by spatial disorganization. The elements are there, but the form is lacking. This feature resonates with a similar theme in narrative production and comprehension in which the ability to integrate information into an overall form to preserve coherence of structure is impaired. Apprehending and conveying meaning on the more symbolic level thus may have its roots in the impaired perceptual capacity to integrate visual and spatial features contained in the visual array into a coherent pattern.

Summary

The search for meaning and knowledge may be sacrificed in RHD as a result of perceptual and attentional deficits. Impaired capacity to distinguish the significant from the irrelevant, to integrate those elements with one another, and to generate a pattern of meaning may so reduce the ability to respond to the environment that RHD individuals are forced to rely excessively on analysis where insight is called for. In so doing, their search for understanding is replaced by a self-conscious search for solution without the capacity to judge or evaluate the product of their efforts.

The extralinguistic deficits in RHD reflect an impaired capacity to use contextual cues to evaluate and interpret meaning. Such cues can include the nature and tone of the communicative exchange, the facial expression of the listener, the verbal cues that create the gist of a narrative, and the visual cues that suggest the underlying pattern of meaning in a complex array of objects and people. Impaired attention and perception are at the core of problems in interpretation. Evaluation and treatment must necessarily concern itself with the overt behaviors of communicative failure, but should address the underlying cause as well.

Evaluation

At present there is no single commercially available instrument that can be used to evaluate the linguistic, extralinguistic and nonlinguistic deficits associated with RHD communication impairment. A variety of subtests from published tests in addition to informal testing is recommended.

Initial Contact with the Patient

The initial contact with the patient should focus on establishing rapport. While client/clinician trust is crucial to success in treating any disorder, it is particularly important in treating RHD deficits. RHD persons may suffer from denial of some or all of their impairments, and this may impede any effort at treatment. They may be aware of their deficits, but afraid to admit to them for fear they will be considered mentally unbalanced or confused. Families and friends are often so relieved that patients can speak that they initially ignore other communication problems. This insensitivity to communicative impairment may lead RHD individuals to believe they are functioning normally in that realm even when they are not. Alternately, families may note impaired prosody, facial recognition, and/or geographic location difficulties, for example, and react to patients as if they are more confused than they actually are, leading patients to fear for their mental health. The interview is a good place for the clinician to allay fears by assurance that they are not unbalanced, but may be experiencing some specific and predictable deficits.

The interview should be taped and include open-ended questions that address orientation, awareness of illness and of specific impairments, concept of the future, and some personal history. The interview should then be assessed for content and style. The section on extralinguistic testing includes parameters for evaluating the quality of the patient's response to the interview.

The initial contact should also include a narrative description of a pictured scene such as the "Cookie Theft" picture from the Boston Diagnostic Aphasia Examination (BDAE).[27] It should be placed to the right of the individual's midline. The picture description provides further information about the person's verbal expression, intelligibility, prosody, visual perception, and attention. It also can be used to begin to demonstrate and explain some observed deficits to the patient. Given reassurance that their deficits are neither unusual nor inexplicable, most will admit to some or all of their problems.

The initial interview and picture description should be followed by evaluation of potential linguistic, nonlinguistic, and extralinguistic deficits.

Linguistic Testing

If a linguistic disorder is suspected, a standard aphasia battery should be used. Even if language appears normal, it is useful to use standardized tests to assess visual confrontation naming, word fluency, auditory and written paragraph comprehension, and reading and writing skills. Writing should be explored for deficits in punctuation, use of margins, and content. If necessary, an in depth look at reading comprehension can be accomplished through any standard reading battery. Though not a linguistic function, per se, mathematical skills can be assessed using subtests from any of the commercially available cognitive test batteries.

Nonlinguistic Testing

The purpose of tests in the nonlinguistic category is to establish the presence or absence type of neglect, visuospatial difficulties, specific forms of confusion, and attentional disorders.

MOTOR NEGLECT

Tests for the motor aspects of neglect should include spontaneous and copy drawings (in that order) of symmetrical objects to check for overall form and for differences in the amount of detail included on the left versus the right. A line bisection task helps establish the RHD person's sense of midline, particularly if they begin by successfully reading anchor letters on both sides of the line and still fail to cross the midline accurately. In people with neglect, one expects the bisection to shift to the right; the further to the right, the more severe the problem. A cancellation test helps determine the severity of neglect. The clinician can count the number of lines left uncrossed by the person and check to see if his approach to the task is systematic. Albert[34] and Mesulam[31] present more complete procedures for these tasks.

SENSORY NEGLECT

Tests for sensory neglect should include tests for extinction to double simultaneous stimulation in the visual, auditory, and tactile modalities. These tests are usually conducted by neurologists as part of their examination. In addition, it is important that a physician test the patient for homonymous hemianopsia to determine the presence of visual field cuts.

VISUAL PERCEPTION

Tests for visual perception usually include tests for scanning and tracking as well as standard visuoperceptual test batteries. A test that is frequently given is the Hooper Test of Visual Organization[35] because it specifically measures the individual's capacity to integrate visual information at the perceptual level, a skill that may have consequences for integration at a higher level.

ATTENTION

The RHD person's ability to maintain attention can be assessed informally during all testing. Short-term and immediate memory can be assessed using standard methods (i.e., digit span, story retelling) found in tests of language or cognitive function.

CONFUSION

Specific forms of confusion, such as reduplicative paramnesia and prosopagnosia, can be assessed informally. The interview should tell if the patient thinks he is somewhere else (i.e., a field hospital during World War II). Prosopagnosia can be assessed using photographs of familiar people, including the patient himself.

Extralinguistic Testing

Assessment of extralinguistic functions should include tasks designed to evaluate the person's capacity to:

1. Identify and see the relationships among salient cues.
2. Synthesize these cues into a coherent, organized, and meaningful pattern.
3. Integrate and interpret verbal and nonverbal information.
4. Maintain topic and produce efficient responses.
5. Recognize and use the pragmatic and prosodic aspects of communication.
6. Recognize and produce appropriate emotional response.

INTERPRETATIVE SKILLS

Picture description and story interpretation tasks are helpful in determining whether the patient has difficulty in distinguishing relevant from irrelevant information and in interpreting implicit meaning. One can begin with simple materials (straightforward action pictures) and move on to more complex materials in which the gist or meaning must be gleaned from a more subtle interplay of contextual features. Stimulus complexity in this case does not refer to the amount of information and detail, but rather to the degree to which the meaning is obvious and explicit versus implied and implicit. The clinician should check to see if the individual uses interpretive concepts or merely lists items in a picture using concrete labels. (See Table 9-4 for a list of some interpretive concepts for the "Cookie Theft" picture.) Does the patient respond to the intended meaning or merely to the explicitly presented one? For example, asked to retell a complex story, do patients basically repeat it verbatim

Table 9-4. Sample "Cookie Theft" Concepts

Two	*Asking for cookie
Children	Has finger to mouth
Boy	*Saying "shhhh"
*Brother	*Laughing
Standing	*Mother
*Falling over	Woman
On the floor	*Washing
*Hurt himself	Faucet on
Reaching up	Standing
*Taking (stealing) cookies	Water
*Handing to sister	*Feet getting wet
Girl	*In the kitchen
*Sister	Lawn

Adapted from Myers.[19]

* Interpretive concepts.

or paraphrase it, using their interpretive capacities? Or, confronted with a picture of an isolated girl, head bent upon her knees in front of a large darkened wall, does the patient state that she is merely resting or that she looks depressed, sad, or lonely? In this example, the picture is visually simple, but its interpretation requires awareness of the photographer's intended meaning in positioning the small figure of the girl against the large black wall. The ability to accurately interpret rests on the perceptual capacity to attend to and integrate salient contextual features contained in narratives and in pictured scenes such as this one.

The person's ability to see relationships among items also can be assessed nonverbally using tests such as the Raven's Progressive Matrices[36] and the Synthesis-Analysis subtest from the Woodcock–Johnson Psycho-Educational Battery.[37] Verbal tests of the ability to assess saliency and relationships include tasks in which the client is asked to explain analogies or the similarities and differences among items. For these purposes the clinician can use appropriate subtests from tests such as the *Detroit Test for Learning Aptitude.*[38]

ORGANIZATIONAL SKILLS

Organizational skills and topic maintenance can be evaluated using an opinion task. The patient can be asked to state and support his opinion on some topic of current interest, and the taped response can be evaluated using a rating scale. Ratings can include the degree to which the response is integrated, complete, efficient, related, and coherent. Does the opinion flow from a set of reasons sufficiently stated that do not wander from the topic? Is detail supportive or detracting? Are the statements related to each other and to the topic, and do they make sense within the laws of nature?

PRAGMATIC SKILLS

The initial interview provides a good opportunity to observe pragmatic skills. While not a diagnostic test per se, the Clinical Management of Right Hemisphere Dysfunction[39] provides a good check list and rating scale for pragmatic functions, such as the ability to participate adequately in the conversation by making eye contact and understanding the nature of the exchange.

EMOTIONAL RESPONSIVENESS

Responsiveness to emotional content can be assessed in the interview by judging response to the illness (is he/she excessively jocular, for example, or lacking affective response?). In addition, clients can be asked to explain or evaluate the emotional content in pictures and stories. It is best to begin with straightforward materials and advance to ones in which the emotion is strong, but more implied. One also can use pictures of faces depicting emotions and ask the person to match emotional expression across faces or point to the one that best represents the emotion contained in a brief story.

PROSODIC SKILLS

Control over the prosodic features of speech can be tested using sentences devoid of emotional content (e.g., "The paint was green" or "We ate cake"). RHD individuals can be asked to read aloud or repeat the sentences with varying emotional overlays (happy, sad, angry). The sentences can be taped and played back to neutral judges who are asked to determine the speaker's mood. Receptive capacity can be evaluated by asking patients to judge the mood of a speaker on a prerecorded sentence list of the same type. Prosodic disturbances associated with RHD must be distinguished from the impaired prosody that can accompany dysarthria.

Summary

It is important to remember throughout extralinguistic testing that a person's capacity to explain or define may be within normal limits. That is, he/she may be able to use analytic skills to describe the sequence of steps necessary to a given activity or to define a metaphor. It is the capacity to *perform* that needs to be evaluated. Can the activity be performed that has just been described? Can the interpretation of figurative language and connotative meaning be used? Does emotional content elicit a response? Can contextual features be synthesized into a meaning that is more than the sum of its parts, or are just the parts themselves appreciated? These tasks should be given with the thought in mind that it is not language, but communicative ability that is at issue.

Treatment

The RHD person's communicative impairment manifests itself primarily in *extralinguistic* impairments. Current therapy for deficits in this area almost always involves compensation techniques in which people are asked to adopt alternative modes of processing to overcome their deficits in attention and perception. For example, clients are asked to verbalize procedures, to respond to clinician cues, to verbally self-cue, to sequence what was once synthesized, to analyze when insight fails. If they fail to maintain eye contact or digress from the topic, they are taught to recognize a clinician cue in the hope that external monitoring will be replaced by internal self-monitoring. They are taught to apply feature analysis and step-by-step integration to stimuli that were once synthesized and processed automatically. They are given tasks in categorization, in verbally prioritizing information, and in sequencing in the hope that the ability to verbalize will transfer to the ability to perform.

These compensation strategies are valuable but do not address the cause of the deficits and, perhaps for this reason, fail to generalize to other tasks. They should be used in concert with tasks that stimulate the recovery of impaired processing. RH damage does not compromise the capacity to perform feature analysis or to verbalize information. It does impair the capacity to recognize significant features in the first place, and to integrate them into a pattern of meaning with a speed and ease that defies step-wise analysis or verbalization. Tasks that address nonlinguistic deficits in attention and perception are aimed at stimulating recovery of the cause of extralinguistic impairments. The following discussion on treatment of extralinguistic deficits looks at both compensation strategies and ones that focus on stimulating the recovery of function. *Linguistic* impairments are not included in the discussion since it is assumed clinicians will use techniques similar to those used in aphasia therapy.

Specific Treatment Tasks

Compensation Strategies

INTEGRATION AND INTERPRETATION TASKS

Problems in the interpretation of intended meaning include deficits in recognizing stimulus significance and in seeing the relationships among those significant contextual features. Therapy techniques addressing compensation for these problems require the RHD person to analyze key features for significance and to identify their relationships. The objective is to understand and consciously follow the process involved in interpretation. The technique begins with the clinician explaining what is involved in the process of interpretation using readily interpreted pictures and stories. The clinician then asks the patient to identify the features that led to his or her interpretation and to identify the relationships among those features. For example, an appropriate interpretation of a picture showing a dog standing in front of the ocean shaking water from its coat is that the dog has been swimming. The literal interpretation is that he is shaking water from his coat. The patient can be trained to see that it is the relationship between the ocean and the water on the dog's coat that leads to an accurate conclusion about the intended meaning of the picture. When the client is able to identify the steps involved in interpreting pictures with obvious meaning, more subtle pictures are introduced. If the patient fails, the clinician may give a model, identifying key features and noting their interconnectedness.

This same technique of feature detection and integration can be used with narratives and stories. Accurate assessment of emotional content can be approached in a similar way by training the patient to look for obvious cues, such as intonation, facial expression and body language. Later stages can include stimuli in which the emotional tone of a story or picture depends on a more subtle interplay of contextual cues, such as setting.

Comparison and contrasting exercises also help the discrimination of key features. Tasks may include defining likenesses and differences involving the identification of the most obvious distinguishing characteristics in a set of objects or concepts. The task can begin with simple stimuli that have only a few defining characteristics and progress to those with multiple features.

TOPIC MAINTENANCE, EFFICIENCY OF EXPRESSION,
AND PRAGMATIC TASKS

The clinician can play back taped conversations with clients, identifying digressions and excessive detail for them, and then ask them to do the same. Tasks that call for the organization of salient information can be beneficial in training verbal efficiency as also can requiring clients to alphabetize, sequence steps for common activities, and organize written paragraphs into a coherent whole.

Appreciating the nature of a communicative situation, making eye contact, inhibiting impulsive responses, and maintaining adequate turn taking can be trained in individual treatment through clinician prompting of the sort described above. Group therapy also can be used to help the patient relearn pragmatic skills. Once rapport and trust are developed, group members are frequently the best critics and providers of support for each other. If a person is unable to identify a deficit independently, identification by a group in which other individuals share the same deficit may help the person recognize his or her deficit without feeling threatened. Activities should be structured in such a way as to provide immediate reinforcement or consequences for specific aspects of performance.

Facilitating Recovery of Function

It seems intuitive that stimulation of the recovery of impaired processing in RHD should focus on deficits in perception and directed attention. Unfortunately, we know very little about how to do this. There is some evidence, however, that working directly on the symptoms associated with left-sided neglect can improve cognitive functioning.[40] The techniques described below were designed by the second author and have been used extensively in her clinical practice.

EDGENESS

This technique is in the experimental stages, but our clinical impression is that it appears to aid in recovery of directed attention by presenting clients with a task that requires them to detect the boundaries of relevant space and perform tasks within that space.

The materials consist of a flat board or grid divided into equal blocks or segments and a set of colored cubes (see Figure 9–1). It is important that the grid and its divisions be three-dimensional so that the RHD individual can use tactile cues to establish boundaries.

The purpose of the task is to establish the boundaries of relevant space and explore within the boundaries by asking clients to find colored cubes placed in varying locations on the grid. Entry into the program requires the ability to match colors. The grid is placed in front of the person at midline on a lap board or table.

Stage 1.   The client is asked to trace the edge of the grid with his or her fingers and to follow the tracing with his eyes. While the client looks away, a single cube is placed

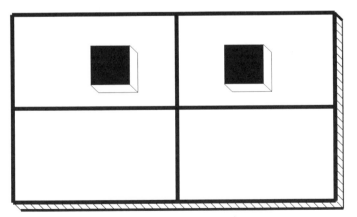

MATERIALS: (SIZES ARE APPROXIMATE)

8"X13" DIVIDED INTO 4 EQUAL SEGMENTS   DLM 1" COLORED CUBES
8"X13" DIVIDED INTO 6 EQUAL SEGMENTS   CONSTRUCTION: 1/2" WHITE PLYWOOD
14"X24" DIVIDED INTO 8 EQUAL SEGMENTS   WITH 1/8" GROVES TO MARK SEGMENTS

Figure 9–1.   4-Segment board with colored cubes in stage two placement.

in the center of the top right segment. The client then looks at the grid and is asked to pick up the cube and hand it to the clinician. This step is repeated by placing the cube in varying locations within the top right segment, then in the lower right, upper left, and lower left segment, in that order. Within segments the cube should be moved systematically from center out and from top to bottom.

Criterion for movement to any subsequent stage is three accurate retrievals out of four per placement. In all stages, clients use both visual and tactile tracing of the edge of the grid before each retrieval until the clinician determines these cues can be faded.

Stage 2.   Two cubes of the same color are placed on either side of the midline in the top segments, one on the right and one on the left. The task is to retrieve both cubes.

Stage 3.   The left cube is placed next to the midline while the right cube is moved progressively farther out to the edge in a horizontal plane. The client retrieves both cubes each time the right cube is moved. These steps are then repeated in the lower segments.

Stage 4.   The entire sequence in Stage 3 in repeated but with the right cube placed close to midline and the left cube moved progressively further out to the edge.

Stage 5.   The order of placement is randomly mixed and the client is asked to retrieve both cubes. More cube pairs (as many as eight) are introduced, and the task continues until all cube pairs are retrieved in all possible position combinations.

Stage 6.   Cube pairs are replaced by random numbers and colors of cubes. At first, random numbers of cubes of the same color are in the same location of either side of the midline. Later, location varies.

Stage 7.   Larger grids with six to eight segments are then introduced and the cube retrieval procedure is continued at the stage required by the client (i.e., random or set number and color). The eight-segment board increases the field beyond the confines of 8 × 11 inches, a size limit usually imposed by the materials available. It is important that left-to-right scanning be introduced along with right-to-left as soon as possible, not only to prepare the person for reading but also to attune them to the exploration of the general boundaries of their immediate environment.

Having worked with the grid, RHD individuals can be encouraged to trace the perimeter of any surface on which they are working (lapboard, table, picture, or book), at any level (table, floor, bed). Their experience in exploring the entire relevant surface to find cubes appears to help them attend to and search for salient visual information in other tasks. For this reason, clinicians are encouraged to begin therapy sessions focused on extralinguistic deficits with a brief warm-up using the grid.

BOOKNESS

"Edgeness" translates readily into a reading technique. It is called "bookness" because the concept of reading is treated as a whole, rather than as a left to right scanning task. The technique begins by placing a thick closed book at the person's midline. Clients are asked to describe everything they know about the physical characteristics of books and to explain how we read (left to right, top to bottom, use of margins). They are then asked to trace the edge of the book, following with their eyes, and to describe what they see. The same tracing and description process continues when the book is open.

Initial reading tasks involve matching a stimulus on the left page with one of four on the right page. Initial stimuli can include shapes and letters until patients can progress to words and sentences. The number of foils can be increased and the space between stimuli decreased as progress is made in the program. Tracing the edge of the book at each new trial should continue until the clinician feels this cue can be faded.

Summary

These tasks have several advantages over asking the client to "look to the left" or verbally self-cue to "look to the left." First, they take into account the fact that an impairment in directed attention resulting in hemispatial neglect can affect the capacity to *explore* space as well as to respond to sensory input within that space. In addition, these techniques are sensitive to the fact that neglect may impair the response to ipsilateral as well as contralateral space.

Second, RHD clients are no longer passive participants relying on external monitoring. The burden of search and discovery is on them and appears to become internalized. For example, clients search for the second cube in a pair, not because the clinician requires it each time, but because it is understood that one more is needed to make a pair. The stimuli are simple enough and meaningless enough to be free of the confounding influence of memory and interpretation. In the "bookness" task clients also know that they cannot match a stimulus without finding it first. Tactile tracing appears to encourage this exploration without external monitoring. The main advantage of these tasks is their apparent capacity to promote generalization. Clients seem to be more aware of their environment and more aroused to key features within it when performing extralinguistic tasks using visual stimuli and even in some tasks using verbal stimuli.

"Edgeness" and "bookness" represents a first step in treating perceptual and attentional impairments in recognizing the boundaries of relevant space, the significant features within that space, and the integration of those features into a meaningful pattern. More tasks of this type need to be developed and empirically verified so that we can help individuals with the puzzling and often devastating sequelae of right hemisphere damage recover or compensate for these impaired processes.

Suggested Readings

Heilman KM: Neglect and related disorders. In Heilman KM, and Valenstein E (eds): *Clinical Neuropsychology.* New York: Oxford University Press, 1979.

Mesulam MM: A cortical network for directed attention and unilateral neglect. *Ann Neurol* 1981; 10:309–321.

Mesulam MM: Attention, confusional states, and neglect. In Mesulam MM (ed): *Principles of Behavioral Neurology.* Philadelphia, FA Davis, 1985.

Myers PS, Linebaugh CW, Mackisack EL: Extracting implicit meaning: Right versus left hemisphere damage, vol 15. In Brookshire RH (ed): *Clinical Aphasiology,* 1985. Minneapolis: BRK Publishers.

Myers PS: Right hemisphere communication impairment. In Chapey R (ed): *Language Disorders in Adults,* ed 2, Baltimore: Williams & Wilkins, 1985.

Perecman E (ed): *Cognitive Processing in the Right Hemisphere.* New York: Academic Press, 1983.

Wapner W, Hamby S, Gardner H: The role of the right hemisphere in the apprehension of complex linguistic materials. *Brain Lang* 1981; 14:15–33.

References

1. Goldberg E, Costa LD: Hemispheric differences in the acquisition and use of descriptive systems. *Brain Lang* 1981; 14:144–173.
2. Semmes J: Hemispheric specialization: A possible clue to mechanism. *Neuropsychologia* 1968; 6:11–26.
3. Mesulam MM: A cortical network for directed attention and unilateral neglect. *Ann Neurol* 1981; 10:309–325.
4. Lavine DN, Finkelstein S: Delayed psychosis after right temperoparietal stroke or trauma: Relation to epilepsy. *Neurology* 1982; 32:267–273.
5. Mesulam MM: Attention, confusional states, and neglect, In Mesulam MM (ed): *Principles of Behavioral Neurology.* Philadelphia, FA Davis, 1985.
6. Lavine DN, Grek A: The anatomic basis of delusions after right cerebral infarction. *Neurology* 1984; 34:577–582.
7. DeRenzi E: Prosopagnosia in two patients with CT scan evidence of damage confined to the right hemisphere. *Neuropsychologia* 1986; 24:385–389.
8. Meadows JC: The anatomical basis of prosopagnosia. *J Neurol Neurosurg Psychiatry* 1974; 37:489–501.
9. Landis T, Cummings JL, Christen L, et al: Are unilateral right posterior cerebral lesions sufficient to cause prosopagnosia? Clinical and radiological findings in six additional patients. *Cortex* 1986; 22:243–252.
10. Damasio AR, Damasio H, Van Hoesen GW: Prosopagnosia: Anatomic basis and behavioral mechanisms. *Neurology* 1982; 32:331–341.
11. Damasiao AR: Disorders of complex visual processing: Agnosias, achromatopsia, Balint's syndrome, and related difficulties of orientation and construction. In Mesulam MM (ed): *Principles of Behavioral Neurology.* Philadelphia, FA Davis, 1985.
12. Benson F, Gardner H, Meadows JC: Reduplicative paramnesia. *Neurology* 1976; 26:147–151.
13. Fisher CM: Disorientation for place. *Arch Neurol* 1982; 39:33–36.
14. Ruff R and Volpe BT: Environmental reduplication associated with right frontal and parietal lobe injury. *J Neurol Neurosurg Psychiatry* 1981; 44:382–386.
15. Heilman KM, Bowers D, Speedie L, et al: Comprehension of affective and non-affective prosody. *Neurology* 1984; 34:917–921.
16. Ross ED: The aprosodias. *Arch Neurol* 1981; 38:561–569.
17. Ross ED: Modulation of affect and nonverbal communication by the right hemisphere. In Mesulam MM (ed): *Principles of Behavioral Neurology.* Philadelphia, FA Davis, 1985.
18. Myers PS: Right hemisphere communication impairment. In R. Chapey (ed): *Language Intervention Strategies in Adult Aphasia,* ed. 2. Baltimore: Williams & Wilkins, 1986.
19. Myers PS: Profiles of communication deficits in patients with right cerebral hemisphere damage. In Brookshire RH (ed): *Clinical Aphasiology Conference Proceedings,* 1979. Minneapolis: BRK Publishers.
20. Myers PS, Linebaugh CW: The perception of contextually conveyed relationships by right brain-damaged patients. Paper presented to the American Speech–Language–Hearing Association Convention. Detroit, 1980.
21. Mackisack EL, Myers PS, Duffy JR: Verbosity and labeling behavior: The performance of right hemisphere and non-brain-damaged adults on an inferential picture description task, vol 17. In Brookshire RH (ed): *Clinical Aphasiology,* 1987. Minneapolis: BRK Publishers.
22. Myers PS, Linebaugh CW, Mackisack EL: Extracting implicit meaning: Right versus left hemisphere damage, vol 15. In Brookshire RH (ed): *Clinical Aphasiology,* 1985. Minneapolis: BRK Publishers.
23. Wapner W, Hamby S, Gardner H: The role of the right hemisphere in the apprehension of complex linguistic materials. *Brain Lang* 1981; 14:15–33.
24. Winner E, Gardner H: The comprehension of metaphor in brain-damaged patients. *Brain* 1977; 100:719–727.
25. Myers PS, Linebaugh CW: Comprehension of idiomatic expressions by right-hemisphere-damaged adults. In Brookshire RH (ed): *Clinical Aphasiology: Conference Proceedings,* 1981. Minneapolis: BRK Publishers.
26. Myers PS, Mackisack EL: Defining single versus dual definition idioms: The performance of right hemisphere and non-brain-damaged adults, vol 16. In Brookshire RH (ed): *Clinical Aphasiology,* 1986. Minneapolis: BRK Publishers.
27. Goodglass H, Kaplan E: *The Boston Diagnostic Aphasia Examination.* Philadelphia: Lea and Febiger, 1983.
28. Mesulam MM: Patterns in behavioral neuroanatomy: Association areas, the limbic system, and hemispheric specialization. In MM Mesulam (ed): *Principles of Behavioral Neurology.* Philadelphia: FA Davis, 1985.

29. Tucker DM, Watson RT, and Heilman KM: Discrimination and evocation of affectively intoned speech in patients with right parietal disease. *Neurology* 1977; 27:947–950.

30. Buck R, Duffy RJ: Nonverbal communication of affect in brain-damaged patients. *Cortex* 1981; 6:351–362.

31. Robinson RG, Kubos KL, Starr LB, et al: Mood disorders in stroke patients: Importance of location of lesion. *Brain* 1984; 107:81–93.

32. Heilman KM, Valenstein E, Watson RT: Neglect and related disorders. *Semin Neurol* 1984; 4:209–219.

33. Moya KL, Benowitz LI, Levine DN, et al: Covarient deficits in visuospatial abilities and story comprehension after right hemisphere stroke. *Cortex* 1986; 22.

34. Albert ML: A simple test of visual neglect. *Neurology* 1973; 23:658–664.

35. Hooper E: *The Hooper Test of Visual Organization*. Los Angeles: Western Psychological Services, 1958.

36. Ravens JC: *Coloured Progressive Matrices*. Los Angeles: Western Psychological Services, 1962.

37. Woodcock RW, Johnson MB: *The Woodcock–Johnson Psycho-Educational Battery*. Allen, Texas, DLM Teaching Resources, 1977.

38. Hammill DD: *Detroit Test of Learning Aptitude*. East Aurora, New York: Slossom Educational Publishers, 1967.

39. Burns MS, Halper AS, Mogil SI: *Clinical Management of Right Hemisphere Dysfunction*. Rockville, Maryland: Aspen, 1985.

40. Weinberg J, Diller L, Gordon WA, et al: Training sensory awareness and spatial organization in people with right brain damage. *Arch Phys Med Rehabil* 1979; 60:491–496.

10

Traumatic Brain Injury

Brenda L.B. Adamovich
Jennifer A. Henderson

Introduction

Each year 200 of every 100,000 persons sustain a traumatic brain injury, or closed head injury, as it is labeled in much of the literature. Approximately 400,000 head injuries occur in the United States each year—about 1 every 16 seconds.[1] The number of rehabilitation programs for head-injured persons has significantly increased during the past 10 years. However, there is a need for a great deal more research and program development in this area.

Pathophysiology

It is now generally acknowledged that acceleration–deceleration injuries are responsible for the predominant pathologic lesion in traumatic closed head injuries. More specifically, the head is accelerated and then suddenly stopped. The forces involved may be translational when movement is in a horizontal plane due to direct impact, or angular when there is a rotational or inertial component, with damage frequently occurring about the diencephalic–midbrain junction. It is generally accepted that the angular acceleration injury is most likely to produce the diffuse injury and the concussion associated with closed head injury.

Direct impact forces usually result in discrete focal lesions. Contusions may be found at the site of direct impact or, as the brain shifts in relation to the skull, contrecoup contusions may be found at sites remote from the point of direct impact. The distribution of these contusions relates to the rotational forces and to contact of the brain surface with certain bony prominences in the skull.

Focal cortical contusions are generally found in the frontal (frontopolar and orbitofrontal) and temporal (anterior temporal, but not necessarily medial temporal) lobes. Diffuse axonal injury of the white matter is associated with high acceleration injuries. The severity of diffuse axonal injury correlates with the severity of the post-traumatic coma and is associated with focal lesions in the corpus callosum and the dorsolateral quadrants of the midbrain.

Nature and Differentiating Features

Two classes of neurobehavorial sequelae occur following closed head injury as a result of discrete, focal, or widespread diffuse brain lesions. Speech, language, voice, hearing, fluency, and/or swallowing deficits may occur secondary to focal lesions most typical of those that occur following cerebrovascular accidents. Specific language problems may be confused with problems due to more general disruptions of attention, information processing, and/or cognition. For example, comprehension deficits may be due to memory disturbances rather than to a linguistic disturbance. The level of cognitive functioning and information processing abilities must be considered when evaluating and treating specific language disorders.

Widespread, diffuse brain damage, which most typically occurs following closed head injury, generally results in communication disorders created by impaired attention, information processing, and cognition. To communicate effectively, an individual must possess attentional skills that allow the manipulation of the focus of attention in three basic ways: (1) initiating and sustaining attention; (2) shifting the focus of attention when appropriate; and (3) inhibiting the inappropriate shifting of attention. Behaviors which may be attributed to attentional disturbances include impulsivity, inappropriate social judgment, lack of insight, literal interpretations, perseveration, stimulus boundedness, disinhibition, and comprehension difficulties.

Information processing refers to those processes generally associated with memory, including the analysis and synthesis of information in sequential steps, or encoding, storage, and retrieval. All information (concrete, abstract, and pragmatic) must be dealt with in an organized, step-by-step fashion if it is to be learned or become meaningful.

Cognition is a complicated and misunderstood term around which an entire subscience in psychology has been formed. Generally, it refers to the knowledge base necessary to comprehend or use specific information. Some cognitive processes include perception, discrimination, organization, recall, and problem-solving, all of which may be integrated with, and difficult to separate from, language.

Evaluation

Clinicians working with closed head injured individuals should be concerned with the identification of focal lesion disorders in addition to the general attention, information processing, and cognitive deficits most characteristic of the closed head injured. Thus, diagnostic batteries should provide for at least a screening of the person's speech, fluency, voice, swallowing ability, visual processing (neglect, discrimination, and organization), hearing, and language. Specific deficits are often difficult to identify as they can be masked by severe cognitive deficits.

A diagnostic/treatment hierarchy of cognitive–communicative processes was designed by Adamovich and Henderson[2] in an attempt to establish (1) an organized approach to cognitive rehabilitation progressing from easy to difficult levels of processing in a gradual, step-by-step fashion and (2) a diagnostic battery that is directly applicable to treatment so that clinicians begin treating at the level in the hierarchy where the individual begins to have difficulty and progress through the hierarchy of processes. However, a division between the levels is somewhat artificial; the most difficult task at one level may be more difficult than the lower level activities at the next level. It may be necessary to move to the next level in the continuum before completing more difficult activities at the previous level. Attention, information processing, and memory skills must continue to improve if the patient is to move through the treatment continuum to higher-level cognitive activities. The treatment continuum includes the processes of perception, discrimination, organization (categorization, closure and sequencing), and high-level problem solving (convergent thinking, deductive reasoning, inductive reasoning, divergent thinking and multiprocess reasoning). These processes will be elaborated upon below.

Perception refers to the process of integration and interpretation of information received at the level of the sense organs with an internal or stored representation of the stimulus.

Discrimination refers to the ability to make a choice between two or more stimuli. Specific skills include the visual discrimination of color, shape, and/or size as well as the aural and visual discrimination of pictures, words, sentences, and situations. In daily activities, multiple aspects of a situation must be discriminated at any moment in time. Relevant, irrelevant, and extraneous stimuli must be identified relying on contextual cues.

Organization refers to the ability to use a learned strategy to deal with discrete actions or components that must be grouped or sequenced according to the priority of each component. General organizational skills include categorization, closure, and sequencing.

Recall is the process of retrieving presumably stored information; recall disturbances occur because of ineffective encoding, inadequate storage, retrieval difficulties, or lack of strategies to deal with interferences. We evaluate immediate recall, delayed recall with a 30-second delay, recall with interference, free recall, the ability to follow directions, and aural and visual recall of short stories.

Head-injured persons tend to experience *problem-solving* difficulties primarily due to a narrow perspective, concrete and incomplete analyses of problems, an impulsive approach that does not allow them to think through the problem, a lack of an organized approach to the problem, and a tendency not to recognize when additional information is needed. When working on problem-solving skills, we provide a demonstration and a description rather than a description alone. Problem-solving or reasoning occurs in several stages: a person must first attempt to understand or analyze the problem; a solution, a strategy, and several alternatives are then formulated based on past experiences stored in long-term memory; next, the solution can be generated or executed; and finally, the solution is evaluated.

Convergent thinking refers to the recognition and analysis of relevant information to identify the central theme or main point. In communicative situations, convergent thinking skills allow an individual to understand and formulate the general theme of a conversation, situation, or written article.

Deductive reasoning refers to problem-solving in a step-by-step fashion in such a way that individuals utilize or eliminate various clues sequentially.

Inductive reasoning refers to the formulation of solutions based on details that lead to, but do not necessarily support, a standard conclusion. This requires an analysis of parts or details to formulate an overall, or whole, concept. In communicative situations, a person must analyze given details and gather additional information in order to assess the situations. For example, in determining whether a call should be placed to the rescue squad, a person must gather information to determine the seriousness of the situation.

Divergent thinking refers to the generation of unique abstract concepts or hypotheses that deviate from or enhance standard concepts or ideas. The hypotheses or concepts must then be tested. Without divergent thinking skills, linguistic and situational paradoxes, abstractions, and subtleties are overlooked and experiences are often viewed incorrectly due to literal or concrete interpretations. Multiprocess reasoning requires the use of two or more reasoning processes.

Treatment

Traditional methods of treatment as outlined in other chapters in this text are used to treat focal lesion deficits, including speech, language, voice, fluency, and swallowing deficits, provided that attention and recall abilities allow the individual to actively participate in therapy. Nonvocal communication devices should be considered for head-injured patients who are unable to communicate verbally, providing patients possess the cognitive and physical abilities necessary to use these devices.

Techniques used to treat diffuse brain damage disturbances in attention, information processing and cognition, which most typically occur following closed head injury, are described in this chapter. Clinicians working with head-injured persons must develop functional treatment programs that focus on behaviors which would make a difference in each person's ability to function in his/her home and community. Behavioral observations to determine the functional consequences of cognitive deficits are made on the rehabilitation unit, in the home, in the community, and on the work-site. Generalization of treatment strategies is best accomplished when the clinical setting and treatment materials are as similar as possible to each person's real-life situation. Simulation of this real-life environment generally occurs first. The book *The Amazing Adventures of Harvey Crumbaker: Skills for Living*[3] is a helpful therapy tool. However, the patient's ability to generalize should be tested by observing the use of compensatory techniques in settings in the home and community.

Specific Treatment Tasks

Attention

1. Limit aural and visual distractions or competing cues in the environment. Gradually add distractions as attentional skills improve.
2. Limit the length and intensity of work periods. Gradually increase the time periods.
3. Use techniques that focus attention, such as addressing the person by name before initiating a task, waiting for eye contact, touching the patient, or using starter phrases, e.g., "Are you ready?"
4. Use pertinent meaningful stimuli. Move gradually from self-related, familiar items to external, less familiar items.

5. Vary treatment concepts, rates, and sequences in an attempt to expand attentional skills. If a person is capable of attending for five minutes, changing tasks at the end of a five-minute period, might help increase attentional duration. Varying the sequence of therapy activities and the therapy concepts themselves creates more novel situations that generally result in improved attention to the situation.

6. Sensory stimulation to activate any response to a stimulus and to gradually increase the frequency, type, and duration of the response.

   a. Auditory stimulation and tracking tasks that progress from the use of gross, nonspeech sounds (bells, buzzers, musical instruments) to more finely discriminate speech sounds. Begin with both live and taped familiar voices of family members and progress to unfamiliar voices, including those on the radio and television.

   b. Oral peripheral stimulation, including passive stretching and the use of facilitative exercises for increasing the range of the articulators, e.g., licking a lollipop or placing food at the corner of the mouth for tongue control or sipping liquid through a straw for lip control.

   c. Verbal stimulation in which gross, reflexive sounds are elicited first; work toward appropriate situation-specific vocalizations, e.g., required vocalization prior to participation in an enjoyable activity such as eating, with gradual shaping toward the naming of the foods before they are given.

   d. Tactile stimulation using hot and cold temperatures and a variety of textures including a feather, sandpaper, tongue blade, cotton swab, oral hygiene swab, and hand. Begin with familiar items: the person's own bathrobe, nightgown, rocking chair, afghan, slippers, and other articles of clothing.

   e. Visual stimulation using bright lights, colors, familiar objects (calendars, clocks, and personal grooming items).

   f. Gustatory stimulation using foods that include bitter, sour, sweet, salty, and bland flavors. Begin with the most liked and disliked foods and drinks.

   g. Olfactory stimulation beginning with strong noxious smells, e.g., ammonia or sulpher, followed by strong pleasant smells, e.g., perfume, coffee, and finally external environmental smells. Familiar items may include an individual's favorite perfume or after shave lotion, or their spouse's usual perfume or after shave lotion, soap, spices, as well as smells associated with foods and drinks, such as coffee brewing or spaghetti sauce cooking.

   h. Vestibular stimulation is best accomplished in physical therapy and occupational therapy sessions using techniques typically used with sensory impaired children such as rocker boards, balancing balls, and other devices used to work with positioning and balance.

Information Processing

1. Begin with meaningful, verbal information to facilitate the registering of sensory information and the progression of that information to short-term storage.

2. Use techniques that allow the person to analyze, organize, and rehearse information in order to facilitate progression of information from short-term to long-term storage.

3. Use cues that are gradually faded to assist the person in the recognition and utilization of feedback, as well as to wean dependence on feedback.

4. Determine the best method of processing information for each person, i.e., simultaneous information processing in which all information, particularly visual, is given simultaneously versus sequential information processing in which information, particularly verbal, is presented one bit at a time.

Cognition

PERCEPTION

One modality, e.g., auditory, visual, etc., should be stimulated at a time in order to assess each person's preferred mode of stimulus presentation. This method can then be used to stimulate more impaired areas. For example, if the most impaired performance is observed in the auditory modality followed by the visual modality with relatively accurate performance by the tactile modality, the clinician presents a stimulus item through the auditory channel in the form of a command first. If the patient fails to respond, the next presentation is an auditory command with a visual model, and finally, the auditory command with the visual model and a tactile cue. Individuals are rated on the type of response given, i.e., prompt, delayed, or cued. Specific perceptual activities include the following:

1. Tracking
   a. Visual: Instruct the person to follow a light with the eyes.
   b. Auditory: Instruct the person to close his or her eyes and listen for sounds, e.g., that of a bell. Once the bell has been rung, the person is to look or point toward the bell.

2. Sound Recognition: Ask the individual to raise his/her hand (or indicate in some agreed upon method) when a specified sound, such as a horn, is identified in a tape recording or in a series of randomized sounds, such as a buzz, telephone ring, and click.

3. Shape Recognition: Ask the person to trace or copy shapes (a vertical line, circle, square, or letter).

4. Work Recognition: Instruct the person to raise his/her hand or respond in some agreed upon manner every time he/she hears a specified word in a paragraph.

DISCRIMINATION

Our treatment focuses on gradually increasing the number and degree of similarity of stimuli that compete with the most pertinent stimuli. Specific discrimination activities include the following:

1. The person is to discriminate color, shape, or size by visually matching geometric forms or by pointing to the forms following an auditory command. Initially, present only two response items which differ by only one feature, e.g., same shape, same size, different colors. Gradually, the number of items and the features per response set are increased.

2. The person is to match objects-to-objects visually, followed by pictures-to-objects, pictures-to-pictures, letters-to-letters, words-to-words, and words-to-objects.

3. The person is required to point to objects, pictures, letters, and words by name.
4. The person is required to match visually a picture to a sentence.
5. The person must discriminate auditorily between words or sentences. When given two visually and/or auditorily similar words, e.g., cat and cot, or sentences, e.g., "She picked up the dog" or "She picked at the dog", the person is to identify correctly the word or sentence given verbally by the clinician.
6. The person is required to respond to questions regarding biographical information. Initially, we require yes/no responses (gestures or words) followed by the provision of the actual information by the patient.

ORGANIZATION

Categorization

1. The patient is to sort visually, or give to the clinician upon request, a group of geometric forms according to sizes, shapes, and colors. We discuss attributes of various geometric shapes, e.g., numbers, sides, angles, horizontal line.
2. We arbitrarily assign nonsense names to several groups of geometric shapes. The features of each group must be analyzed by the patient to assign appropriate names to new stimuli presented by the clinician.
3. The patient is to sort objects followed by pictures of objects according to physical characteristics: size and color, general categories: food or furniture, or by functions: writing implements or eating utensils. Items should then be subdivided into more specific categories. For example, items first sorted into a food category should then be sorted into such categories as fruits, vegetables, and meats.
4. The patient is asked to match items (pictures, letters, and words) that are in the same class but are not identical, e.g., A to a, or different species of birds.
5. The person is asked to identify items that would not be included in particular category or situation. A category exclusion task would be to have the patient name something that he/she would eat that is not hot. A situation exclusion task would be to ask the person to name something that would not be worn skiing.

Closure

1. Nonlinguistic tasks are presented that require the identification of geometric forms with sections missing, for example:

C ⌂

Next, pictures are presented of objects with parts missing and scenes with objects missing.
2. Visual linguistic tasks are presented that require the identification of words with portions of letters missing, e.g., si/; words with letters missing (last letter should be omitted first followed by initial letter, then medial letters), e.g., lak_, _ake, l_ke, b_tt_m; sentences with words missing, e.g., "John ____ to the store"; steps to the completion of task with one or more steps missing; and paragraphs with sentences missing.

3. Auditory linguistic tasks are presented, such as sound blending in which phonemes are individually presented, and the person must identify the word.

Sequencing

1. Nonlinguistic tasks are presented requiring the person to sequence a color from light to dark shades or objects from small to large.

2. Linguistic tasks are presented requiring the person to do the following:

   a. Connect dots in a numerical or alphabetical order.

   b. Reorder (forward and backward) strings of numbers, letters, days of the week, and months of the year.

   c. Visually or auditorially sequence words in which letters or syllables are out of order, sentences in which words are scrambled, and paragraphs in which sentences are scrambled.

   d. Sequence steps of activities of daily living, including washing, eating, shopping.

   e. Match numbers with corresponding letters of a code and then break the code, e.g., "If 1 = A, 2 = B, 3 = C, then what is 3-1-2?"

   f. Follow written directions of increasing complexity, e.g., circle every /e/ in the first and second words of a sentence.

   g. Following and giving directions (written and oral) for filling out forms, following a recipe, and understanding a map.

   h. Sequencing of functional activities in which the patient is asked to list all the steps necessary to make coffee, bake a cake, make a telephone call, and so forth.

RECALL

Our therapy focuses on providing the brain-injured person with strategies to compensate for memory deficits that typically never fully recover. Before we introduce the memory strategies outlined in this section, the patient must achieve competency levels in previous stages of the treatment continuum including the perception, discrimination, and organization of information. Specific recall strategies include the following:

1. Verbal description in which an adequate explanation of items, concepts, etc. to be recalled is provided by the client or clinician in therapy. Visual, auditory, and semantic descriptions are encouraged.

2. Visual imagery in which objects, scenes of a story or situation, and maps of layouts in space are mentally pictured.

3. Chunking activities, in which information is visually or aurally organized into segments that coincide with the patient's memory span, e.g., if the patient can recall only two items, information should be divided into two-item segments.

4. Categorization of information to improve recall of that information, e.g., when required to remember 15 items to be purchased at a grocery store, the patient should group the items into categories: dairy products, frozen foods, meats.

5. Rehearsal, in which information to be recalled is drilled. Verbal repetition is used

in which the information is repeated aloud, subvocally, and finally silently. Visually, the patient can continually review the detail of visual images or written stimuli. Requiring the patient to maintain a daily log of events provides for rehearsal of activities occurring daily and weekly.

6. Associations are generated based on semantic relationships (e.g., cane – crutches and day – night), acoustic relationships (dew – shoe), or visual relationships (desk – dresser).

7. Temporal or spatial ordering, in which events in episodic and semantic memory are recalled by remembering certain landmark events associated with the event to be recalled or those that occurred at a similar point in time. Actions or events can often be recalled if the goals or results of the action are recalled. Initially, we emphasize key events during encoding. Using selective reminding during recall, we question and cue patients regarding key events. Gradually the number of cues are reduced.

8. Primacy and recency benefits are incorporated, in which the first and last items are accented visually using different colors and sizes, or auditorially, using different loudnesses and pitches.

9. PQRST approach: preview, question, read, state, and test.

10. Mnemonic devices, in which specific memory tricks are used to increase associative learning through paired association. During encoding, new words or bits of information are chained or paired to a pre-established set of key words and phrases or a familiar sequence of known locations. Several mnemonic systems are utilized. A peg system links or pegs new items to existing items, e.g., rhyming peg: one = bun; phonetic peg: two = n (2 down strokes), or loci peg: items linked to familiar locations. The substitution word system is based on linking a visual image with word, e.g., "To remember the name Cameron, visualize a camera on his balding head (outstanding facial feature)." The Link system links lists of items together in generally a funny way to facilitate retrieval, e.g., To remember bologna and milk, picture a cow eating bologna as the farmer milks her.

HIGH LEVEL PROBLEM-SOLVING

Convergent Thinking

1. The identification of a common theme in a group of objects, e.g., shoes and bread — both have heels.

2. The identification of one word that could be combined with four other words to form another set of words, e.g., saddle, stroke, track, and show could all be combined with the word side to form the words sidesaddle, sidestroke, and so forth.

3. The identification of relevant information in visually or auditorily presented sentences, paragraphs and conversations with respect to who did what, when and where. The Folkes Sentence Builder series is a helpful resource.[4]

4. The reduction of information to the most salient items by abstracting the main idea of visually and/or auditorily presented sentences, paragraphs, and conversations. Key facts and situations should be identified by considering the intent of the sender and the interpretation of the receiver.

Deductive Reasoning

1. Forward or backward chaining, in which the person is to deal with the relevant information and devise solutions in a progressive (forward) or regressive (backward) step-by-step process until the final solution is reached. Situational pictures can be given that require a backward process of variable elimination, e.g., a picture of an accident involving two cars. The Mind Benders: Deductive Thinking Skills workbook is a useful therapy resource.[5]

2. Missing premise tasks, in which two facts are necessary to reach a conclusion. If given one fact, the person is to choose the second fact that leads to the conclusion, e.g., given "All children must go to school and Bob and Jane are children," the patient is to deduce that Bob and Jane must go to school. The Ross Test of Higher Cognitive Processes is a useful source of specific therapy stimuli.[6]

3. Analysis of sentences and paragraphs to determine punctuation, spelling, and other grammatical errors.

Inductive Reasoning

1. The formulation of antonyms and synonyms. Crossword puzzles are useful in this task.

2. Analogous thinking. Bower[7] suggests that we must first compare one instance to another, (e.g., man to boy and dog to puppy). Next, a list of relationships within each instance must be generated. Finally, lists of relationships are compared.

3. Cause and effect tasks. The person is asked to give the effect if the cause is stated or the cause if the effect is stated, e.g., "Boiling water is spilled on a woman's hand," the patient is to indicate that the woman's hand is burned; or if given "A woman's hand is burned," the patient is to indicate that the woman's hand came in contact with a source of heat such as boiling water, fire, etc.

4. The person is asked to describe what facial expression or emotion would be appropriate in a particular situation.

5. Open-ended problem-solving, including story completion tasks, in which the person is required to complete an unfinished story.

6. Decision-making/problem-solving tasks given problems such as: "John needs money." or "You have a doctor's appointment and your car won't start."

7. Wh-questions in which solutions are to be given to questions such as "Why do cars have wheels? or "Why couldn't you wear shoes swimming?"

Divergent Thinking

1. Multi-meaning stimuli (homographs), in which the patient is required to construct sentences depicting several meanings for each sentence or phrase. Given "shoulder," responses could be: "A shoulder is part of your body," "He drove on the shoulder of the road," or "You don't have to shoulder the burden."

2. Absurdities in which the person is to describe what is absurd about statements and stories, such as, "The temperature rose to 25 degrees, so he chipped through the ice and went for a swim."

3. Idiom interpretation requiring the person to provide explanations of phrases in which the meaning generally cannot be derived from the literal interpretation of its parts, e.g., empty-headed, chicken-hearted, clear as mud, on pins and needles.

4. Proverb interpretations requiring the person to analyze a statement in which true, nonstandard abstract meanings and relationships of items are given. The statements can be satirical and/or paradoxical as well as contraindicatory or nonsensical. These truths are of a general rather than specific sense.

Multiprocess Reasoning

1. The mediation of an argument requiring analysis and synthesis of information. Two points of view in a specific argument should be presented. Using deductive reasoning, the premise or assumptions of each person must be considered in order to arrive at a solution. Once this is accomplished, the solution must be tested by analyzing the truth of the premises. Finally, using complementary reasoning, a compromise must be negotiated based on premises that are accepted and agreed to by both parties.

2. Determining whether or not sufficient, extra, or unnecessary information has been provided in a given problem. If the information is inadequate to solve the problem, the person must use a questioning strategy to gather necessary information regarding the central features of the problem.

3. Responding to questions based on an analysis of syllogisms or arguments consisting of a major and a minor premise and a conclusion. The syllogisms: If-Then Statements Series provides useful stimuli for these tasks.[8]

Use of Computers

Computers can be helpful in the treatment of attention, concentration/persistence, visual localization, visual scanning, visual tracking, reaction time, memory, hand-eye coordination, and specific cognitive tasks including perception, discrimination, and language. Specific benefits of computers include the following: (1) a single stimulus can be presented in a highly controlled manner; (2) the client is required to compete only with himself or herself providing for a sense of control over therapy and progress which leads to increased motivation and feelings of self-worth; (3) accurate, objective, and immediate feedback is received; and (4) people tend to enjoy using computers.

According to Wilson,[9] clinicians should consider the following when selecting computer programs: (1) consistent, controlled levels of difficulty within a task; (2) lesson or file generating capability; (3) concise, easy-to-follow instructions; (4) consistent response format; (5) accurate and age-appropriate content; (6) degree of supervision required; (7) friendly, unambiguous, and informative feedback; (8) control of variables or parameters (i.e., length of time and stimulus is displayed, length of response delay time, task speed, number of trials per set, level of difficulty, type of prompts, size of stimuli, timing, and type of reinforcements); and (9) method of keeping and reporting data.

All computer training should be selected and monitored by professional clinicians as part of a comprehensive treatment program for each individual. Computers should never be used as a substitute for the clinician. Since aides often are used to work with clients during computer treatments, clinicians also should know how to appropriately use aides. Cognitive remediation cannot occur using only a computer and an aide. Computers are merely tools, as are workbooks. All computer treatments designed to assist in the overall cognitive rehabilitation program should be under the direction and supervision of professional rehabilitation specialists.

Group Therapy

Group treatment allows for peer support, peer review, and the sharing of feelings and needs in a communication environment which is more natural than the individual therapy setting. Group therapy provides individuals with opportunities to: (1) increase social interaction and self-monitoring skills in a more natural communication environment; (2) increase self-esteem and self-motivation; (3) increase the ability to develop short- and long-term goals that are meaningful; (4) share feelings and needs; and (5) provide and receive peer review of behaviors.

Group therapy is appropriate at all levels along the treatment continuum. Tasks used at lower and middle cognitive levels are generally similar to tasks used in individual sessions. Group therapy activities that benefit head-injured persons with high level thought-processing and problem-solving deficits are described in the following section.

INTERPERSONAL INTERACTION GROUP

The responsibility for presenting an assigned or selected topic is rotated among group members. A video recording should be made of each presentation. Utilizing the video recording, all group members should evaluate the session using an objective form. Each person should evaluate himself or herself regarding the roles placed as speakers and listeners during the group session. Specific areas to be evaluated include:

Speakers. Presentation of organized, sequential information; conveyance of main point; ability to use abstract information; ability to use feedback; too little or excessive information; irrelevant information; redundant information; observation of rules; appropriate top switching; obscurity or ambiguity; and style of communication.

Listeners. Appropriate questioning strategies; ability to interpret information abstractly; requesting of repetitions when needed; ability to identify missing information; ability to give feedback; ability to identify main point; and content of assertions.

All Group Members (as Appropriate). Pragmatic behaviors: Behavior appropriate to situation; eye contact; turn taking; initiation of conversation; use of gestures; appropriate affect; speed of response; appropriate posture; appropriate rate; appropriate intonation; appropriate social distance; and group support.

Other Behaviors: Ability of profit from cueing; and willingness and ability to modify behaviors.

SOCIAL SKILLS GROUP

The ability of each group member to cooperate and accept group decisions should be evaluated following participation in an assigned social activity. Specific activities include: planning special menus, birthday parties, outings, and family open houses.

The ability of each group member to adjust behavior appropriately with regard to verbal output, dress, gestures, etc., should be evaluated following assigned roleplaying activities. Specific activities could include: a party with friends versus a job interview, or a family dinner versus dinner with a new date.

EMPATHIC ABILITIES GROUP

On a rotating basis, the conflict resolution skills of each group member should be evaluated following the role playing of a dispute between two friends according to a script prepared by the clinician or a subcommittee of group members. Specific abilities to be evaluated include: the ability to determine reasons for the dispute (deductive reasoning); the ability to determine premises or assumptions of each person; the ability to establish compromise; the ability to test solutions, and the ability to negotiate a compromise (complementary reasoning).

PERSONAL AND SOCIAL ADJUSTMENT GROUP

In individual sessions, establish and rehearse various personal statements with each client. For example, a client might be required to make a statement regarding two personal strengths, e.g., "I am a person who . . ." (adapted from Ben-Yishay and Diller[10]). Video recordings should be made of the individual session and should be critiqued by both the client and the clinician. After the client has mastered the individual session, a presentation should be made to the entire group. A self evaluation and group evaluation should be made of the video recording of the group session using a system to score awareness, understanding, assimilation, and acceptance.

LIFE SKILLS GROUP

A list of activities to work on may be generated by the group members themselves. Roleplaying in the group setting should be followed by actual community experiences when appropriate. Activities which might be included are: given and following directions; shopping; using public transportation; emergency skills; meal preparation; household care; management; use of leisure and recreational time; time management; management of personal care attendants; and letter writing skills.

Suggested Readings

Adamovich BB: Treatment of communication and swallowing disorders. Rosenthal M, Griffith E (eds): *Rehabilitation of the Adult and Child with Traumatic Brain Injury.* Philadelphia: FA Davis Company, in press.

Adamovich BB, Henderson JA, Auerback S: *Cognitive Rehabilitation of Closed Head Injured Patients: A Dynamic Approach.* San Diego, California: College-Hill Press, 1985.

Brooks DN: Memory and head injury. *Journal of Nervous Mental Disorders.* 1972; 155(5):350–5.

Geschwind H: Disorders of attention: A frontier in neuropsychology. *Philosophical Transactions of the Royal Society of London,* 1982; 298:173–185.

Levin HS, Benton AL, Grossman RG: *Neurobehavioral Consequences of Closed Head Injury.* New York: Oxford University Press, 1982.

Lezak, MD: (1979) Recovery of memory and learning functions following traumatic brain injury. *Cortex,* 1979; 15:63–72.

Rosenthal M, Griffith ER, Bond MR, et al: *Rehabilitation of the Head Injured Adult.* Philadelphia: FA Davis, 1983.

Wilson BA, Moffat N (eds) *Clinical Management of Memory Problems.* Rockville, Maryland: Aspen Systems Corporation, 1984.

References

1. Friedman SG (ed): *National Head Injury Foundation* Informational Pamphlet. Southborough, Massachusetts: National Head Injury Foundation, 1988.
2. Adamovich BB, Henderson JA, Auerback S: *Cognitive Rehabilitation of Closed Head Injured Patients: A Dynamic Approach.* San Diego, California: College-Hill Press, 1985.
3. Klasky C: *The Amazing Adventures of Harvey Crumbaker: Skills for Living.* Carson, California: Lake Shore Curriculum Materials Company, 1980.
4. Folkes J: *The Folkes Sentence Builder.* Hingham, Massachusetts: Teaching Resources Corporation, 1981.
5. Hernadek A: *Mind Benders: Deductive Thinking Skills.* Pacific Grove, California: Lakeshore Curriculum Materials Company, 1978.
6. Ross J, Ross C: *Ross Test of Higher Cognitive Processes.* New York: Slossen Educational Publications, 1986.
7. Bower Gordon H: Contracts of cognitive psychology with social learning theory. *Cognitive Therapy and Research,* Vol 2, No 2, pp 123–146.
8. Baker M: *Syllogisms: If-Then Statements.* Pacific Grove, California: Midwest Publications, 1981.
9. Wilson BA, Moffat N: (eds) *Clinical Management of Memory Problems.* Rockville, Maryland: Aspen Systems Corporation; 1984.
10. Ben-Yishay Y, Diller L: *Rehabilitation of the Head Injured Adult,* (Rosenthal M, Griffith E, Bond M, Miller J, eds). Philadelphia, Pennsylvania: FA Davis, 1983.

11

Dementia

Lana O. Shekim

Introduction

Dementia refers to an acquired syndrome characterized by persistent intellectual decline which is due to neurogenic causes. The nature and course of the dementia will vary depending upon the etiology. Most dementias are progressive, but some are static and, contrary to widely held belief regarding the disorders, still others are mercifully reversible.[1,2] Hutton reported that from 10% to 20% of the dementias were found to have reversible causes. In addition to injecting a ray of optimism into a generally bleak set of expectations, this finding stresses the need for careful differential diagnosis of the dementias.

The Diagnostic and Statistical Manual[3] states that the essential feature in dementia is impairment in short- and long-term memory. This deficit in memory may be also associated with one or more of the following (1) impairment in abstract thinking, (2) impaired judgment, (3) disturbances in higher cortical function, (4) personality changes.

The language disturbances in dementia long have been reported.[4-7] Interest in the dementias has increased in the past decade resulting in more systematic study of the nature of the communication deficits.[8-10] This systematic description of the effects of dementia on communication should produce not only a more fundamental understanding of the disorder, but improved avenues of management. Both epidemiologists and the popular press have reported the "graying of America," and the increase in the population segment of those more than 65 years of age. By the year 2030, approximately 20% of the U.S. population is expected to be more than 65 years.[11,12] Since dementing illnesses are associated with the elderly, the expectation and unavoidable conclusion is that the prevalence of dementia will increase.

The numbers reported for the prevalence of dementia have varied reflecting differences in methods of study and variations in definition of dementia. Most studies, however, have found severe dementia to affect between 1% and 6% of those over 65, while mild to moderate dementia is found to involve between 2% to 15% of individuals over 65 years.[13] Wang[14] reported that 1 in every 100 persons older than 65 suffers from severe dementia and 10 in 100 suffer mild dementia.

Since some of the prevalence studies failed to include Parkinson's dementia, the number of demented individuals is probably greater than many estimations.

Dementia can be caused by a variety of conditions: diseases, infections, or infarcts. The most commonly occurring cause is Alzheimer's disease accounting for 50% to 60% of all patients with dementia.[15] Vascular dementias (dementias caused by multiple infarcts) are seen in 20% of the dementia patients.

Alzheimer's dementia and vascular dementia co-occur in approximately 15% of this sample, and other conditions, such as Pick's disease, Parkinson's disease, progressive supranuclear palsy, and Creutzfeldt–Jacob disease, account for the remainder of the irreversible dementias.

Pathophysiology

The pathophysiology of Alzheimer's Disease (AD), sometimes called dementia of the Alzheimer's type (DAT), multi-infarct dementia (MID), Parkinson's disease (PD) and Huntington's disease is reviewed in the following section.

Alzheimer's Disease

Alzheimer's disease is characterized by a variety of pathologic changes that occur in specific topographic patterns. These changes are concentrated in the association areas of the parietal, temporal, and frontal lobes and in the hippocampus. On gross inspection, the brains are atrophic.[16,17] During histological study with microscopic enlargement, neuronal loss is evident along with the presence of neurofibrillary tangles, senile plaques, and granulovacuolar degeneration. Tomlinson[18] noted that similar anatomic changes occur in the undemented aging brain, however, to a lesser degree. Neurofibrillary tangles are filaments that pair together in a helical fashion within the cell body. These tangles have been noted in a variety of neuropathologic conditions, most notably in elderly patients with Down's syndrome. Senile plaques are minute areas of tissue degeneration. They are concentrated in the cerebral cortex and hippocampus but also are seen in the corpus striatum, amygdala, and thalamus.[17] The third histologic feature is granulovacuolar degeneration. This change is noted mostly in the pyramidal neurons of the hippocampus.

A number of neurochemical changes also have been reported in Alzheimer's disease in addition to the morphologic changes. Reduction in the cholinergic and noradrenergic systems as well as in neuropeptides have been reported,[19–21] and these changes, coupled with the triad of anatomic degenerative changes, account for the reduced efficiency of nervous system function.

The etiology of AD is still unknown, though a number of theories have been postulated. Aluminum intoxication, disordered immune function, and viral infection all have been offered as possible causes.[1] Equivocal results have been reported for most theories, and etiologic hypotheses continue to be proposed and explored. The association of Alzheimer's disease with Down's syndrome has occurred because the morphologic changes in AD have been observed in individuals with Down's who have survived into their 40s.[22] Others have reported an increased incidence of Down's syndrome in families with a history of AD.[23] Such findings are intensifying the search for possible genetic causes of AD.

Multiple Infarct Dementia

Just as strokes can be responsible for the focal left hemisphere damage that causes aphasia, multiple cerebral infarcts throughout the brain can lead to dementia.[24] Hachinski and colleagues first introduced the term multiple infarct dementia (MID), and a number of clinical features have been identified that indicate the presence of a multi-infarct process.

These features include many of the characteristics indicative of cerebrovascular disease, such as hypertension, previous strokes, abrupt onset, stepwise deterioration, and focal neurologic signs and symptoms. The characteristics of the dementia depend on the exact location of the infarct as well as the total amount of tissue involved.[16] MID can occur with either widespread thrombotic or embolic cerebrovascular disease,[1] and three major subgroups of MID have been identified.[25] The first type is related to large cerebral infarcts and ischemia. The second is associated with many small deep lacunar infarcts, and the third group has Binswanger's disease, a disease of atherosclerosis of the penetrating cerebral arteries.

Parkinson's Disease

Parkinson's disease (PD) is a degenerative disorder presenting as a complex motor symptom disturbance. The classic signs of the condition are bradykinesia (slowed movement), a type of alternating muscular contraction and release called cogwheel rigidity, tremor, a masklike expressionless face, loss of associated movements, and disturbances of gait, posture, and equilibrium.

There are several variants of Parkinson's disease: idiopathic, drug induced, post-encephalitic, and arterosclerotic. The idiopathic form, the most common variant, accounts for 86% of cases.[26] The etiology of idiopathic PD is unknown. At autopsy, horizontal sections of the brain stem reveal significant depigmentation of a deep subcortical structure, the substantia nigra, with extensive neuron loss in an area known as pars compacta.[27] Neurochemical analysis of the basal ganglia in PD reveals that the dopamine content is significantly diminished.[27] This leads to a disruption in the activity of the basal ganglia in coordinating movement[28] and also has led to a form of pharmacologic treatment with the objective of restoring dopamine levels.

Huntington's Dementia

Huntington's disease is a devastating degenerative disorder of the nervous system. Its clinical features are a movement abnormality known as chorea, dementia, and a history of familial occurrence. The disease has been associated with a great American balladeer, Woody Guthrie, who, prior to contracting Huntington's disease, provided a rich legacy of more than 1,000 songs. The caudate nucleus, putamen, and substantia nigra suffer the most atrophic changes; noted as neuronal loss.[29]

Neurochemical alterations also have been described in Huntington's disease. Reduction in gamma-amino-butyric acid and glutamic acid decarboxylase have been found in the striatum, pallidum, and substantia nigra.[28,30] Examination of neurochemical changes in the cortex reveals normal levels or less severe depletions than found in the basal ganglia.[31,32] The pathophysiology of the dementia in HD is a topic that generates rich disagreement. However because of the presence of normal cortical glucose metabolism on positron emission tomography studies, the cause of the dementia is becoming accepted as subcortical.

Nature and Differentiating Features

The deficits in dementia extend beyond communication deficits, as a range of cognitive functions are impaired. Comprehensive neuropsychological assessment usually reveals decline in general intelligence, memory, attention, perception, and purposeful movement or praxis. Careful assessment of communication status reveals deficits in all individuals with dementia.[10,33] Most people with dementia are identified after the disease has progressed well into its course.[34,35] The earliest presenting symptom is a memory problem.[36] (Chenoweth & Spencer, 1986). The person may forget where things are placed, forget peoples' names, and forget appointments. A family member or a friend is usually the first to suspect a dementing illness and then seeks medical attention.

Diagnosis

The identification of moderate or severe dementia is relatively easy, as the deficits are marked. However difficulty exists in the diagnosis when dementia is mild and relatively early in its course. One diagnostic challenge is the differentiation of mild dementia from pseudodementia: a condition characterized by cognitive decline to depression. The diagnosis of dementia is based on clinical examination, CT scanning, various laboratory tests, communication, and neuropsychological assessment. As in any condition, accuracy of diagnosis is crucial for appropriate management. Studies examining the accuracy of diagnosis in dementia have discovered misdiagnosis to be all too common.[37,38] Comprehensive evaluation is vital, and hasty conclusions must be avoided.

The need to refine diagnostic criteria for various dementing conditions has been acknowledged for a long time by various practitioners. In 1983, a work group was established by the National Institute of Neurological and Communicative Disorders and Stroke (NINCDS) and the Alzheimer's Disease and Related Disorders Association (ADRDA). The work group proposed various criteria for diagnosing "probable Alzheimer's disease," "possible Alzheimer's disease," and "definite Alzheimer's disease." It identified features that support the presence of AD and features that make the diagnosis unlikely. The report stated that, for classification of Alzheimer's disease for research purposes, one should specify features that may differentiate subtypes of disorders such as: familial occurrence, onset before 65 years of age, presence of the genetic factor of trisomy-21, and coexistence of the other relevant conditions, such as Parkinson's disease. The report also stated that dementia is a diagnosis based on behavior and cannot be determined by computerized tomography, electroencephalography, or other laboratory instruments, although specific causes of the dementia may be identified by these means.[39]

Stages of Progression

Alzheimer's dementia progresses gradually and does not occur in discrete stages. On the other hand, MID may show abrupt changes with recent infarction. Nevertheless, identifying the course of dementia in stages or phases has been found helpful in understanding the evolution of the condition.[40]

Reisberg[41] has plotted the course of dementia into seven clinical phases with corresponding global deterioration stages. The stages range from no cognitive decline to very severe decline. The clinical stages are characterized as normal, forgetful, confused, and demented.

EARLY DEMENTIA

In early dementia, the individual's behavior is characterized by moderate cognitive decline. Deficits may be noted during assessment of the mental status as well as in daily life. The patient may be disoriented to time and place (e.g., "What year is it?" . . . "1942." "Where are you?" . . . "In a Mackintosh motel.") and may be unable to recall personal information such address or telephone number. An educated person may have difficulty in counting backwards in 2s from 20. The patient may need assistance in activities of daily living (ADL), such as getting dressed or grooming. Communication deficits are present and characterized by disjointed conversation that is reduced in its cohesion and information content.

MIDDLE DEMENTIA

Middle dementia is characterized by severe cognitive decline. The dementing individual may forget a spouse's name and be unaware of recent events. Knowledge of the remote past is better preserved but is impaired. More assistance is needed with daily living activities. Communication skills become increasingly impaired, and verbal output becomes less informative with frequent word finding problems. Personality and emotional changes are seen in this stage. These may include delusional behavior, such as talking to imaginery figures; obsessive symptoms, anxiety or agitation, and cognitive abulia (impaired volition and lack of decisiveness).

LATE DEMENTIA

Very severe cognitive decline is seen in late dementia. In this phase all verbal abilities are reported to be lost. Patients may be mute, perseverative, echolalic, or palilalic (with excessive reiterative utterances).

Communication Deficits

Early study of dementia identified the presence of communication deficits. In fact, early writers listed "aphasia" as the presenting symptom in dementia.[5] Reports on language in dementia stated that patients were anomic, perseverative, disorganized in output, having fluent yet empty speech. Demunting patients were likened to individuals with Wernicke's or posterior aphasia.

Irigaray[7] studied a group of dementing patients and found that the semantic system was more vulnerable than the phonologic or syntactic system. Her finding was later supported by single subject analysis.[42,43] Functions that were overlearned and automatic, such as application of syntactic and phonologic rules, were better preserved. Tasks that were dependent on memory, such as semantics and pragmatics, were found to be more vulnerable. Dementing individuals do exhibit some of the linguistic behaviors exhibited by aphasic persons. This has lead some to describe language in dementia as aphasia. Speech–language pathologists differentiate the language disorder seen in dementia from aphasia.

Halpern used the term Language of Generalized Intellectual Impairment (GII) to distinguish the linguistic profile of dementia from aphasia.[44]

Wertz[45] addressed whether language deficits seen in dementing individuals are best described as aphasia or some other label. He concluded that while the language behaviors may be similar, they were far from identical, and cautioned that talking about aphasia in dementia was not useful.

The communication profile of the dementing patient will vary in relation to both the location and cause of the neuropathology. Dementing patients with cortical pathology may show language disturbances more clearly than patients with subcortical pathology. Individuals with subcortical pathology may be less fluent than those with the cortical dementias because of motor system involvement.

Different behavioral profiles have been identified within the cortical dementias and more recently within Alzheimer's disease. Studies utilizing neurobehavioral as well as cerebral glucose metabolic profiles have suggested the possibility of the existence of distinct subgroups of patients with AD. One subgroup is noted to have mostly visuospatial deficits of a focal nature, but language skills are relatively preserved. In another subgroup, disproportionate difficulty with language was noted.[46-48] One report associated mortality in presenile and senile dementia with communication status. It stated that individuals with AD and a deficit in expressive language have had a poor prognosis for surviving after one year of examination,[49] although a prediction with this grave a consequence must stand the test of reliable replication before it is ever translated into counseling advice passed on to families.

The classic features of language breakdown in dementia are anomia, and reduced efficiency in verbal formulation, and circumlocution. Testing generative naming will reveal significantly reduced output. Confrontation naming is also impaired but not as severely as generative naming.[50] Connected discourse lacks cohesion and is characterized by incomplete phrases, reduced phrase length, concepts, or ideas. Word and phrase repetitions, stereotypic utterances, and irrelevant intrusions are frequent.[10,33,51,52] Discourse may have a disproportionate number of vague referents. Word-finding problems are noted, and the demented person will circumlocute in an attempt either to access the desired word or to compensate for inability to retrieve it. As noted previously, the worsening of the dementia leads to an increase in perseveration and the appearance of increased jargon. Eventually reduced memory will make conversation more disjointed.

Evaluation

The differential diagnosis of dementia requires the assessment of linguistic and nonlinguistic abilities. The clinician must explore the dementing patient's verbal and nonverbal memory, visuospatial construction, and linguistic reasoning in addition to all the parameters usually used in testing language in neurogenic communicative disorders.

The NINCDS – ADRDA workshop (see Diagnosis section) suggested some recommended tests for examining language in dementia. They recommended testing verbal fluency of the semantic or category type and testing confrontation naming with an abbreviated form of the Boston Naming Test.[53] They also suggested administration of any of the standard aphasia batteries such as the Boston Diagnostic Aphasia Examination[54] or the Western Aphasia Battery.[55] The Token Test[56] and the Reporter's Test also were recommended for gaining more insight into specific modality function.

Assessing language through administration of standard aphasia batteries can be useful and informative, but aphasia tests were not designed to assess language in dementia, and clinicians should be aware of their limitations. Currently, standardized tests designed to assess communication function in dementia are not commercially available.

Bayles and colleagues have developed *The Arizona Battery for Communication (ABC) Disorders in Dementia:* a comprehensive battery for the assessment of dementia, which is in the process of being standardized. The ABC assesses receptive and expressive language, orientation, and memory. An auditory discrimination test is included to ensure the presence of adequate hearing sensitivity for conversation. Expressive language is assessed through oral description of objects, pantomime expression, drawing, generative naming, oral sentence disambiguation, and oral and written discourse. Receptive language is assessed through administration of the Peabody Picture Vocabulary Test, reading comprehension of words, sentences and paragraphs, and nonoral sentence disambiguation. Bayles and colleagues have obtained considerable data regarding performance of normal elderly and individuals with dementia on the *ABC.*

The initial step in quantifying an individual's performance is to assess his/her mental status. A number of short measures are available that screen such areas as attention, orientation, concentration, language, and memory. Two of the most commonly used measures are (1) Fuld's modification[57] of the Blessed, Tomlinson, and Roth[58] scale and (2) the Mini-Mental Status (MMS) by Folstein, Folstein, and McHugh.[59] Both are brief examinations that have adequate test-retest reliability. These examinations have demonstrated valid discrimination of individuals with dementia from normal older persons. They can be readministered during longitudinal study and thus can document progressive change with time. The Blessed and the MMS are screening tests, however, and should not be used to diagnose dementia to the exclusion of other tests.

When assessing communicative function in dementia, it is important to assess those linguistic areas found to be most vulnerable to a dementing process: verbal formulation and generative naming. Bayles offers a number of guidelines that are useful in formulating a battery for assessing dementia. These are to (1) assess the integrity of the content of semantic memory, (2) assess the process of semantic memory, (3) analyze communicative skills beyond the sentence level, (4) adopt ecologically valid test paradigms, and (5) assess generative and creative communicative abilities (Ref. 10, pp 176 ff).

Treatment

The focus of treatment of communication is not the dementing individual per se but rather the individuals and the environment surrounding the person with the dementia. The goal of treatment is to preserve communication and compensate for progressive loss. Golper and Rau[60] state that clinicians can maximize the communicative exchange between people with dementia and family members with the manipulation of linguistic and environmental variables. Environmental factors, such as communicating about "here and now" objects/topics, eliminating sources of distraction, and reducing the number of individuals participating in a conversation can aid optimal communication. Manipulating linguistic variables such as speaking directly, concretely, and using common and familiar vocabulary and structure facilitate improved communication. Care-givers must simplify their verbal output in length and in structure. Rate of speech should be reduced to allow the person ample time to understand and respond.

Communication between the individual and care-giver may be ineffective because of problems exhibited by the care-giver such as speaking too softly or using too few coverbal behaviors, such as head nodding, head shaking, or other facial expressions or movements that accompany speech. An evaluation of the care-giver's skills and suggestions for improvement can be instructive and useful. If the person resides in an institution or attends a day care center, the staff must be informed of strategies to maximize communicative effectiveness.

Since dementia is a progressive condition, the treatment must be dynamic with periodic reassessment. Subsequent modification of communicative strategies may be needed.

The decline in dementia is inevitable; this may have discouraged clinicians from undertaking efforts addressing restoration of function. Obler and colleagues[61] found that combining written and verbal input modalities facilitated comprehension in dementia. Sometimes a trial of behavioral intervention may be beneficial when the dementia is mild. The results obtained may be useful to families in their efforts to maximize communication with the dementing person. Further experimental study is sorely needed in the area of appropriate and efficacious intervention strategies.

Dementia is a condition that frequently overwhelms the family and friends of the person with the condition. Emotional support and respite care are integral components of its management. Many times the family can summon the effort and motivation to continue if it is clear that periods of respite are part of the management plan. The speech–language pathologist may act as a resource person linking the family with local chapters of the ADRDA, or to a local support group. The ultimate hope is that with time family members will learn to cope and find their own creative ways of maximizing communication with continued love.

The dementias and the communication disorders that accompany them cause some of the most challenging and frustrating clinical decisions that face both clinicians and families. We are well beyond the point, however, where persons with these disorders are neglected or abandoned. The future will no doubt see increased understanding, explanation, and compassionate and effective treatment strategies for the people affected by these afflictions. We shall continue our efforts to manage the dementias with all of the means at our disposal and expand every effort to advance the clinical science.

Specific Recommendations for Care-Givers

1. Approach slowly: Dementing patients may get apprehensive or agitated with sudden occurrences. Try to be visible while approaching.
2. Establish eye contact: This enhances readiness to listen and will help in comprehension through reception of visual cues.

3. Be pleasant, monitor, and maximize your coverbal behaviors, such as use of smile, gesture, and posture. Dementing individuals like most people respond better to pleasant people.
4. Speak clearly and directly; avoid complex directions.
5. Use referents frequently and avoid pronouns.
6. Speak in short sentences to aid in comprehension and memory.
7. Ask yes/no questions rather than open ended questions.
8. Be redundant; restate critical facts to compensate for memory loss.
9. Keep topics familiar and observable.
10. Use touch.
11. Maintain structure or a routine.
12. Always say goodbye or some other form of departure signal.

Following are samples from patients with mild Alzheimer's dementia describing the "Cookie Theft" Picture from the Boston Diagnostic Aphasia Examination: (/ indicate pause boundaries)

1. Well/let's see/over that way/well it looks to me like uh/the/like here/there's a couple of 'em/but uh/but by the time they really/use you know use them or something/they probably run down already some/but then again/the it's not that bad/now this/this woman here/she's/got/that's her hand I know there/ and she's got a little/a little here/yes/there's a lot to it/to keep you going/and keep things straight.

2. I would say/this is a little girl/she's gonna go with the cookies/and then after that/they'll come out/and they'll come/have something for/um/she's doing the dishes/she's gotta clean them off good/or her mother will spank her/maybe it's like a/or maybe it's a piece of something/I don't know/oh boy/what's this one?/

3. Well uh/somebody was is want to get into the cookie jar/um and/while the mother/I don't know that the the daughter/the daughter is getting cookies out of the/cookie jar/and with the help of his his brother/and I guess uh/then there is a/they have a/apparently her mother wasn't uh/uh paying attention to what she was doing/probably her mind was wondering while all this was going going on/and so this why/this is why you got all the water on the floor/and uh/the kids eating the cookies.

Suggested Readings

Bayles KA, Kaszniak AW: Communication and Cognition in Normal Aging and Dementia. Boston: Little, Brown, 1987.
Cummings JL, Benson DF: Dementia: A Clinical Approach. Boston: Butterworth, 1983.
Mace NL, Rabins PV: The 36 Hour Day. Baltimore: Johns Hopkins University Press, 1981.

References

1. Cummings JL, Benson DF: Dementia: A Clinical Approach. Boston: Butterworths, 1983.
2. Hutton JT: Clinical nosology of the dementing illnesses. In Pirozzolo FJ, Maletta GJ (eds): Advances in Neurogerontology: The Ageing Nervous System. New York: Praeger, 1980, pp 149–174.

3. American Psychiatric Association: *Diagnostic and Statistical Manual of Mental Disorders:* DSM-III-R, 3rd ed. Washington: APA, 1987.

4. Sjogren T, Sjogren H, Lindgren AGH: Morbus Alzheimer and morbus Pick. A genetic, clinical and patho-anatomical study. *Acta Psychiatrica Scandanavica.* (Suppl 82), 1952.

5. Critchley M: The neurology of psychotic speech. *British Journal of Psychiatry* 1964; 110:353-364.

6. Stengel E: Speech disorders and mental disorders. In Reuch AD, O'Conner M (eds), *Symposium on Disorders of Language.* Boston: Little Brown, 1964.

7. Irigaray L: *Le Langage de Dements.* The Hague: Mouton, 1973.

8. Appell J, Kertesz A, Fishman M: A study of language functioning in Alzheimer patients. *Brain and Language.* 1982; 17:73–91.

9. Obler LK: Language and brain dysfunction in dementia. Segalowitz SJ (ed): *Language Functions and Brain Organization.* New York: Academic Press, 1983, pp 267–282.

10. Bayles KA, Kaszniak AW: *Communication and Cognition in Normal Aging and Dementia.* Boston: Little, Brown, 1987.

11. Brody JA: An epidemiologist's view of the senile dementias—Pieces of the puzzle. In Wertheimer J, Marois M (eds): *Senile Dementia: Outlook for the Future.* New York: Alan R. Liss, 1984, pp 383–393.

12. Plum F: Dementia: an approaching epidemic. *Nature* 1984; 279:372–373.

13. Mortimer JA: Alzheimer's disease and senile dementia: Prevalence and incidence. In Reisberg B: *Alzheimer's Disease.* New York: Free Press, 1983, pp 141–148.

14. Wang HS: Neuropsychiatric procedures for the assessment of Alzheimer's disease, senile dementia and related disorders. In Miller NE, Cohen GD (eds): *Clinical aspects of Alzheimer's disease and senile dementia.* New York: Raven Press, 1981.

15. Jellinger K: Neuropathological aspects of dementias resulting from abnormal blood and cerebrospinal fluid dynamics. *Acta Neurologica Belgica* 1976; 76:83–102, 1976.

16. Tomlinson BE, Blessed G, Roth M. Observations on the brains of demented old people. *Journal of Neurological Sciences,* 1970; 11:205–242.

17. Corsellis J: Ageing and the dementias. In Blackwood W, Corsellis J (eds): *Greenfield's Neuropathology.* Chicago: Year Book Medical Publishers, 1976, 796–848.

18. Tomlinson BE: The pathology of dementia. In Wells CE (ed): *Dementia.* Philadelphia: FA Davis, 1977, pp 113–153.

19. Coyle JT, Price DL, DeLong MR: Alzheimer's disease: A disorder of cortical cholinergic innervation. *Science* 1983; 219:1184–1190.

20. Berger B, Tassin JP, Rancurel G, et al: Catecholaminergic innervation of the human cerebral cortex in presenile and senile dementia: Histochemical and biochemical studies. In Usdin E, Sourkes TL, Youdin MBH (Eds): *Enzymes and Neurotransmitters in Mental Disease.* New York: John Wiley, 1980, pp 317–322.

21. Davies P, Katz DA, Crystal HA: Choline acetyltransferase, somatostatin, and substance P in selected cases of Alzheimer's disease. In Corkin S, Davis KL, Growdon JH, et al: (eds): *Aging: vol 19, Alzheimer's disease: Report of Progress in Research.* New York: Raven, 1982, 9–14.

22. Burger PC, Vogel FS: The development of the pathologic changes of Alzheimer's disease and senile dementia in patients with Down's syndrome. *American Journal of Pathology* 1973; 73:457–476.

23. Wisniewski K, Howe J, Williams DG, et al: Precocious aging and dementia in patients with Down's syndrome. *Biological Psychiatry* 1978; 13:619–627.

24. Hachinski VC, Lassen NA, Marshall J: Multi-infarct dementia. A cause of mental deterioration in the elderly. *Lancet* 1974; 2:207–210.

25. Rogers RL, Meyer JS, Mortel KF, et al: Decreased cerebral blood flow precedes multi-infarct dementia, but follows senile dementia of the Alzheimer's type. *Neurology* 1986; 36:1–6.

26. Rajput AH, Offord KP, Beard M, et al: Epidemiology of parkinsonism: Incidence, classification and mortality. *Annals of Neurology, 16,* 278–282, 1984.

27. McDowell FH, Lee JE, Sweet RD: Extrapyramidal disease. In Baker AB, Baker LH, (eds): *Clinical Neurology.* New York: Harper and Row, 1978, pp 1–67.

28. Sourkes TL: Parkinson's disease and other disorders of the basal ganglia. In Siegel GJ, Albers RW, Katzman R, (eds): *Basic Neurochemistry,* 2nd ed. Boston: Little, Brown, 1976, pp 668–684.

29. Lange HW: Quantitative changes of telencephalon, diencephalon, and mesencephalon in Huntington's chorea, post-encephalitic, and idiopathic parkinsonism. *Verhandlungen Der Anatomischen Gesellschaft* 1981; 75:923–925.

30. Bird ED, Iverson LL: Huntington's chorea. Post mortem measurement of glutamic acid, decarboxylase, choline acetyltransferase and dopamine in basal ganglia. *Brain* 1974; 97:457–472.

31. Kremzner LT, Berl S, Stellar S, et al: Amino acids, peptides, and polyamines in cortical biopsies and ventricular fluid in patients with Huntington's disease. *Advances in Neurology,* 1979; 23:537–46.

32. Wu J-Y, Bird ED, Chen MS, et al: Studies of neurotransmitter enzymes in Huntington's chorea. *Advances in Neurology* 1979; 23:527–536.

33. Obler LK, Albert ML: Language and aging: A neurobehavioral analysis. In Beasley DS, Davis GA

(eds): *Aging: Communication Processes and Disorders.* New York: Grune and Stratton, 1981, pp 107–121.

34. Pfeffer RI, Kurosaki TT, Harrah CH, Chance JMR & Filos S. Measurement of Functional activities in older adults in the community. *Journal of Gerontology* 1981; 37:323–329.

35. Roth M: Senile dementia and its borderlands. In Cole JO, Barret JE (eds): *Psychopathology in the Aged.* 205–232, New York: Raven, 1980, pp 205–232.

36. Chenoweth B, Spencer B: Dementia: The experience of family caregivers. *The Gerontologist* 1986; 26:267–272.

37. Ron MA, Toone BK, Garralda ME, et al: Diagnostic accuracy in presenile dementia. *British Journal of Psychiatry* 1979; 134,161–168.

38. Garcia CA, Reding MJ, Blass JP: Overdiagnosis of dementia. *Journal of the American Geriatrics Society* 1981; 29:407–410.

39. McKahnn G, Drachman D, Folstein M, et al: Clinical diagnosis of Alzheimer's disease: Report of the NINCDS–ADRDA work group under the auspices of the Department of Health and Human Services Task Force on Alzheimer's disease. *Neurology* 1984; 34:939–944.

40. Schneck MK, Reisberg B, Ferris S: An overview of current concepts of Alzheimer's disease. *American Journal of Psychiatry* 1982; 139:165–173.

41. Reisberg B, Ferris SH: Diagnosis and assessment of the older patient. *Hospital and Community Psychiatry* 1982; 33:104–110.

42. Whitaker HA: A case of isolation of the language function. In Whitaker H, Whitaker HA (eds): *Perspectives in Neurolinguistics.* New York: Academic Press, 1976, pp 1–58.

43. Schwartz MF, Marin OSM, Saffran EM: Dissociations of language function in dementia: A case study. *Brain and Language* 1979; 7:277–306.

44. Halpern H, Darley FL, Brown JR: Differential language and neurological characteristics in cerebral involvement. *Journal of Speech and Hearing Disorders.* 1973; 38:162–173.

45. Wertz RT: Language deficit in aphasia and dementia: The same as, different from, or both. In Brookshire R (ed): *Proceedings of the Clinical Aphasiology Conference,* 1982. Minneapolis: BRK Publishers, pp 350–359.

46. Chase TN, Fedio P, Foster NL, et al: Wechsler adult intelligence scale performance: Cortical localization by fluorodeoxyglucose F 18-positron emission tomography. *Archives sof Neurology* 1984; 41:1244–1247.

47. Martin A, Brouwers P, LaLonde F, et al: Towards a behavior typology of Alzheimer's patients. *Journal of Clinical and Experimental Neuropsychology* 1986; 8:594–610.

48. Becker JT, Huff J, Nebes RD: Neuropsychological function in Alzheimer's disease. *Archives of Neurology* 1988; 45:263–268.

49. Kaszniak AW, Fox J, Gandell DL, et al: Predictors of mortality in presenile and senile dementia. *Annals of Neurology* 1978; 3:246–252.

50. Bayles KA, Tomoeda C: Confrontation naming impairment in dementia. *Brain and Language* 1983; 19:98–114.

51. Horner J, Heyman A: *Aphasia associated with Alzheimer's dementia.* Paper presented at the International Neuropsychological Society meeting, Pittsburgh, Pennsylvania, 1982.

52. Shekim LO, LaPointe LL: *Production of discourse in patients with Alzheimer's dementia.* Paper presented at the International Neuropsychological Society meeting, Houston, Texas, 1984.

53. Goodglass H, Kaplan E, Weintraub S: *The Boston Naming Test,* 2nd ed. Philadelphia: Lea and Febiger, 1983.

54. Goodglass H, Kaplan H: *The assessment of Aphasia and Related Disorders,* Philadelphia: Lea and Febiger, 1972.

55. Kertesz A: *Western Aphasia Battery.* New York: Grune & Stratton, 1982.

56. DeRenzi E, Vignolo LA: The token test: A sensitive test to detect receptive disturbances in aphasics. *Brain* 1962; 85:665–678.

57. Fuld PA: Psychological testing in the differential diagnosis of the dementias. In Katzman R, Terry RD, Bick KL (eds): *Alzheimer's Disease: Senile Dementia and Related Disorders.* New York: Raven, 1978, pp 87–93.

58. Blessed G, Tomlinson BE, Roth M: The association between quantitative measures and of senile change in the cerebral gray matter of elderly subjects. *Journal of Psychiatary* 1968; 114:797–811.

59. Folstein MF, Folstein SE, McHugh PR: Mini-mental state: A practical method for grading the cognitive state of patients for the clinician. *Journal of Psychiatric Research* 1875; 12:189–198.

60. Golper LAC, Rau MT: Treatment of communication disorders associated with generalized intellectual deficits in adults. In Perkins W (Ed): *Language Handicaps in Adults,* New York: Thieme-Stratton, 1983, pp 119–129.

61. Obler LK, Oberman L, Samuels I, et al: *Written input to enhance comprehension in Alzheimer's dementia.* Paper presented to the American Speech–Language Hearing Association, Washington, DC, 1985.

12

Impairments in Pragmatics

Marilyn Newhoff
Kenn Apel

Introduction

A longstanding assumption in the provision of clinical services to the brain-damaged population has been that the unit of measurement for language abilities is the sentence. Thus, traditional assessment and intervention procedures did not consider how language is *used* within specific contexts (i.e., the pragmatic aspect of language). Instead, the evaluation and treatment of language focused on the content (i.e., semantics) and form (i.e., syntax) of a person's language comprehension and production abilities. This approach, unfortunately, while offering valuable information, ignored many variables that would have allowed for richer descriptions of the language and communication systems.

In the past 10 years, however, a steadily growing number of researchers and clinicians has been concerned with the overall communicative abilities of their brain-damaged subjects.[1-4] These concerns have led to a realization that communication is inherently interactive and that nonlinguistic information impinges greatly on the perceived meaning of a message. Communication competence, therefore, has evolved slowly as the composite of behaviors to be measured. As this shift in thinking has emerged, researchers and clinicians have begun to examine the comprehension and production of language in social and conversational contexts.[2,5,6] They are not only concerned with knowing the linguistic structures that a brain-damaged person is capable of producing and understanding, but also how these linguistic structures are influenced by, and implemented in, communicative settings. The analysis and treatment of pragmatic impairments, then, has become a viable and important element in the clinical services provided to the brain-damaged population. By pushing assessment of language skills beyond the sentence level to the level of discourse, clinicians have begun to identify and remediate pragmatic deficits that considerably affect the communicative interactions of their clients.

The purpose of this chapter is to discuss the pragmatic impairments of brain-damaged individuals, as well as the assessment and intervention procedures that have as their focus the identification and remediation of these pragmatic impairments. The intent herein is to look beyond the word and sentence level to the level of conversation or discourse. To achieve this purpose, those behaviors that often are identified as pragmatic skills will be discussed first. Following this, literature that reflects both pragmatic strengths and weaknesses of brain-damaged individuals will be reviewed. Finally, the remaining sections will focus on general considerations and specific suggestions for the assessment and intervention of pragmatic impairments in the brain-damaged population.

Pathophysiology

The focus of this chapter differs from that of the previous eleven chapters. The preceding chapters have dealt with particular syndromes of brain damage and the resulting functional changes in speech and language abilities. In this chapter, the emphasis changes from an etiological focus on disruption of the nervous system to a focus on disruption of one specific area of the language system, pragmatics, and the resulting affects on the communicative competency of brain-damaged individuals.

Nature and Differentiating Features

Definition of Pragmatics

Before the pragmatic impairments evidenced by brain-damaged individuals will be discussed, a description of the types of skills involved is in order. Pragmatics is the set of rules that govern the use of language in context.[7] Pragmatics includes the ability to use language for a variety of functions, such as to comment, warn, request, protest, and acknowledge. Other pragmatic uses of language include the ability to use linguistic and nonlinguistic devices to regulate conversations, repair conversations, request clarifications, initiate and maintain topics, take conversational turns, and use appropriate eye gaze and facial expressions. The pragmatic dimension of language, then, determines why a speaker says something, when the speaker says it, to whom the speaker says it and how it is said.

Since the surge of interest in the pragmatic aspect of language in the 1970s, a number of authors have presented taxonomies that depict a wide range of pragmatic skills.[8-12] Although considerable agreement exists on the type of skills in question, authors often differ in how they organize or categorize these skills. In a very general sense, pragmatic skills can be categorized into two major divisions. The first division involves those skills that have as their basis the linguistic aspect of language. For example, pragmatic adaptations to a listener (i.e., changing the content or topic of a message depending on the listener) are often accomplished via specific syntactic forms (e.g., definite and indefinite articles, anaphoric pronouns) and specific lexical choices. Second, pragmatic skills can be classified as nonlinguistic. For example, changes in the suprasegmental aspects of speech or eye gaze can provide information to the listener regarding the intent of the speaker to maintain or relinquish his or her conversational turn. (See Table 12 – 1, for a list of commonly identified pragmatic skills).

Table 12–1.   Pragmatic Skills

I. Linguistic Conversational Skills
   A. Speech act use (e.g., comment, request, warn, assert, promise, direct, acknowledge)
   B. Topic skills (e.g., initiation, maintenance, shift)
   C. Turn-taking skills (e.g., initiating, responding, interrupting, pausing)
   D. Conversational repair skills (e.g., requesting clarification, revising utterances)
   E. Adaptations to listener (e.g., contingent responses, lexical selection, quantity and conciseness of information, changing register of voice)

II. Nonlinguistic Conversational Skills
   A. Paralinguistic aspects of communication (e.g., pitch and intensity, fluency, intelligibility)
   B. Extralinguistic aspects of communication (e.g., eye gaze, proximity to conversational partner)

Differentiating Features of Pragmatic Impairments

During the past 10 years, as researchers have studied the pragmatic skills of brain-damaged individuals, a variety of findings regarding pragmatic impairments have been reported.[2,13] Type of pragmatic impairment seems to depend on the site of brain damage.[6,9] Left hemisphere-damaged persons often demonstrate impairments in the production and/or comprehension of linguistic units (semantics, syntax, morphology) with relatively intact pragmatic skills.[1–5,14] Most researchers comment that these subjects demonstrate less deficient pragmatic skills than might be expected from their linguistic deficits. In contrast, many researchers have offered an opposite profile regarding right hemisphere-damaged individuals.[4,15–17] Right hemisphere-damaged subjects often are reported to be competent in their production and understanding of the semantic content and syntactic forms of language; however, they evidence deficits in pragmatics.

Conclusions regarding pragmatic skills of brain-damaged individuals may serve to oversimplify their communicative strengths and weaknesses. There is growing evidence that all brain-damaged persons demonstrate some impairments in the pragmatic use of language while they maintain a number of appropriate pragmatic abilities.[9,18] The following sections, then, will summarize the findings from investigations of the pragmatic skills of brain-damaged individuals. In varying degrees, previous chapters have considered the pragmatic abilities following brain damage. Therefore, the focus of the following sections will be to emphasize two notions. First, any person who has suffered brain damage may demonstrate a pragmatic impairment. Second, the pragmatic impairments after brain damage may be manifestations of primary or general linguistic or metalinguistic deficits. These two premises will serve as springboards for the advocacy of pragmatically oriented assessment and intervention for all brain-damaged persons.

Pragmatic Skills of Right Hemisphere-Damaged Individuals

In an earlier chapter, Myers and Mackisack provide a review of research on pragmatically inappropriate behaviors of right hemisphere-damaged persons. These investigations suggested a number of areas of impairment.[15,19,20] For example, right hemisphere-damaged persons often do not comprehend indirect requests, such as "Can you open the box?" They tend to interpret indirect requests in a literal sense and seem to miss the purpose for which they are intended.[4,6,13] Similarly, those with right hemisphere damage often misinterpret figurative language (e.g., metaphors, idioms, proverbs) and humor, and they seem to respond to the literal, or surface form, of a message.[4,16,17] They also demonstrate difficulty in relating logically ordered actions or events to their listener.[4,13] Finally, some reports suggest that suprasegmental or prosodic aspects of speech are inappropriate to the situation.[4,15]

The pragmatic deficits caused by right hemisphere damage appear to be due to an inability to integrate available nonlinguistic and linguistic information to develop a unified or wholistic understanding of the intent underlying an utterance. These individuals often are unable to divorce the form of an utterance from its literal or common meaning in order to interpret figurative, humorous, or indirect meanings. They often are characterized as rigid in their inability to consider the gestalt or general notion of specific aspects of discourse.[4,20] This suggests a metalinguistic deficit; that is, a lack of ability to use available linguistic and nonlinguistic contexts to reflect on the nature and properties of language.

Although several reports suggest pragmatic deficits, right hemisphere-damaged individuals demonstrate a number of appropriate pragmatic skills,[9,18] and the pragmatic skills left intact appear to be those that tap less into metalinguistic knowledge. A recent report by Prutting and Kirchner[9] suggests that the majority of right hemisphere-damaged subjects' pragmatic skills are appropriate. These authors examined conversational abilities within a normal, conversational setting. The emphasis of the interaction was not on specific comprehension and/or production of linguistic information that required metalinguistic abilities; rather, subjects were observed in conversations with familiar listeners during which linguistic and nonlinguistic context could be used. Prutting and Kirchner found that their subjects experienced some difficulty in maintaining a topic, providing enough information for their listener, providing appropriate eye gaze, and using appropriate intonational patterns. However, overall, 84% of the right hemisphere-damaged subjects' pragmatic skills were judged to be appropriate.

In summary, damage to the right hemisphere does not appear to affect all pragmatic use of language. Instead, the damage appears to affect abilities to interpret language used in nonliteral ways. Thus, many of the pragmatic deficits of right hemisphere-damaged persons seem to stem from metalinguistic impairment.

Pragmatic Skills of Left Hemisphere-Damaged Individuals

Several years ago, Holland[21] remarked that left hemisphere-damaged people often remained communicatively competent in the face of semantic and syntactic deficits. A number of investigative findings support her statement.[1,2,5] In general, the left hemisphere-damaged tend to retain far greater ability to use specific pragmatic skills than they do for the linguistic aspects of language. For example, in situations of communication failure, these individuals demonstrate some skills in requesting clarification of their listener in order to continue the conversation. They also have been observed to respond to requests for clarification of their own messages. Specific subgroups of left hemisphere-damaged individuals have demonstrated adequate turn-taking abilities and other nonverbal pragmatic behaviors, such as the use of eye gaze and head nods.[3,9,22] Left hemisphere-damaged subjects also tend to retain their ability to relate logically ordered actions or events to their listener.[23,24] Finally, they have demonstrated the ability to comprehend indirect requests.[6,25]

These findings suggest that the pragmatic skills of left hemisphere-damaged subjects are less deficient than the linguistic aspect of their language. However, these results should be tempered with other reports of pragmatic deficits in this population. For example, the left hemisphere-damaged experience some difficulty in their ability to use a wide variety of speech acts,[26] topic initiations,[27] and recognition of shared versus new information in cohesion devices.[28] In the previously mentioned Prutting and Kirchner[9] report, left hemisphere-damaged subjects were judged to demonstrate inappropriate pause during conversational turn-taking, provide less informative messages, choose ambiguous words, and, to a somewhat lesser extent, produce a narrow range of speech acts. However, similarly to the right hemisphere-damaged subjects, 82% of the pragmatic behaviors demonstrated by the left hemisphere-damaged were judged to be appropriate.

The above studies suggest that both right and left hemisphere-damaged subjects seem to perform appropriately across a large number of pragmatic skills. Both also exhibit some pragmatic impairments. Although the two groups do not seem to differ in the *amount* of inappropriate behaviors they exhibit, they do seem to differ on the *types* of impaired skills, as well as on possible contributing sources. Although the impaired pragmatic skills of right hemisphere-damaged subjects seem to be related to the more general problem of integrating the available contexts to determine alternative interpretations of a message, the left hemisphere-damaged subjects' pragmatic deficits seem to stem from two possible sources. First, the linguistic deficits of these subjects interfere with their ability to use language (e.g., inappropriate lexical choices, less than informative utterances). Second, their reduced pragmatic abilities may be a result of compensatory mechanisms or adaptations for dealing with reduced linguistic abilities. Several anecdotal comments from the literature suggest that pragmatic impairments may arise from adaptations of speakers to their perceived linguistic inadequacies.[1,5,27,28] For example, Newhoff and her colleagues[1] suggested that their subjects' revisions of immediately preceding utterances seemed to be based more on the assumption that their message was unclear than on the assumption that the problem was in the ear of their listener. They posited that their subjects may have become accustomed to communicative failure and, therefore, assumed that the error or breakdown in communication was theirs.

Summary

The findings from investigations of the pragmatic skills of brain-damaged individuals lead to two conclusions. First, the presence of pragmatic impairments in brain-damaged individuals does not appear to be easily localized to a specific area of the brain. Second, both right and left hemisphere-damaged persons demonstrate pragmatic strengths as well as pragmatic weaknesses. Often, however, assessment and intervention paradigms fail to include these skills. Further, the pragmatic strengths retained by these brain-damaged individuals may not be utilized. The purpose of the remainder of this chapter, therefore, is to provide considerations for assessment and intervention of pragmatic impairments and to advocate the incorporation of functional approaches during all clinical interactions with brain-damaged persons.

Evaluation

Pragmatics involves the use of language in context.[7] Given this definition, pragmatic skills must be evaluated within conversational contexts. The wealth of available linguistic and nonlinguistic information found in conversational settings may have a marked impact on comprehension and production capabilities of brain-damaged speakers.[2] One of the most valid measures of a person's pragmatic skills can be obtained by sampling language abilities in a naturalistic communicative setting. In the following section, the process of language sampling and the factors that appear to affect the pragmatic skills of the brain-damaged will be reviewed.

Language Sampling

Language sampling allows clinicians to obtain a representative sample of language within a natural conversational setting. Although language sampling is typically discussed in regard to the assessment of language-impaired children,[8,29] it is an equally successful means of measuring the pragmatic skills of brain-damaged adults.[9,30] When collecting a language sample, clinicians engage clients in conversation in order to determine their pragmatic use of language. Although there is no agreed upon sample "size," the goal of the procedure should be to obtain a large enough sample so that a representative amount of communicative interaction is available for analysis. A sample of approximately 15 to 30 minutes in length is generally suggested as sufficient to yield information to judge appropriateness of pragmatic abilities.[9]

In addition to obtaining a large enough sample, it is important to consider several other factors that researchers have found to influence pragmatic use of language. These factors include the effect of context, listener, and topic on communicative abilities.

Effect of Context on Language Sampling

The quality of the information obtained during a language sample is highly dependent on context. Both comprehension and production abilities of brain-damaged subjects have been shown to be aided by linguistic and nonlinguistic contextual support.[2,31,32] For example, listeners are more likely to comprehend complex syntactic structures when they are provided with concurrent or prior pictorial, sentential, or narrative contextual information. Traditional clinical settings often do not make available these types of contexts to the client. In most clinics, little linguistic or nonlinguistic contextual support is available. For example, a typical language-eliciting technique used with the brain-damaged requires description of a picture that is in full view of the clinician. This technique violates a basic principle of communication; that speakers rarely communicate information that is completely known to their listener. The traditional setting for clinical assessment is not suitable for obtaining a representative measure of pragmatic abilities.[21,27,30] To assess pragmatic skills adequately, the clinician must ensure that the sample is obtained within a naturalistic communicative setting which involves the exchange of new information by both participants.

Effect of the Listener on Language Sampling

In some instances, when an individual suffers brain damage, his or her role as a communicator may change.[34-36] The brain-damaged person may be assigned a role by others (e.g., family members) as the "identified patient."[35,36] In these cases, the "patient" may be considered solely as a listener or a responder to simple questions, rather than as an active communicator. The consequences of such an assignment may be that the aphasic "patient" takes on the role of an inadequate communicator and generalizes that role to all communicative settings. Thus, though adequate communication skills exist to engage in some kind of meaningful dialogue, the individual refrains from initiating or maintaining conversation because of the perceived role of self as an inadequate language user.

The clinician, then, must consider his or her role as the client's listener during the assessment of pragmatic skills. The burden of maintaining a conversation may be placed more on the shoulders of the client's listener. Unfortunately, due to the often didactic nature of clinical interactions, the assessment setting can sustain this image. Restrictions are placed on the interaction, and the client is forced into the role of being a passive communicator, relegated to responding only to clinician requests.[36] The clinician must ensure that the client receives adequate time to participate in conversations.

Effect of Topics on Language Sampling

Finally, topics of conversations for the language sample should be varied and relevant. For example, the clinician may generate a dialogue regarding important events in the client's life.[37] Pictures may be used to elicit discourse; however, in order to simulate the natural exchange of new information normally present in conversation, picture description tasks should be conducted in such a way that the picture is not visible to the clinician. This preserves a reason for the client to convey a message. Additionally, clients can be asked to retell or create stories that contain either familiar or unfamiliar story content. By generating conversations involving a variety of topics, insight can be gained regarding the facility for discussing topics that range from concrete to abstract, personal to nonpersonal, and familiar to unfamiliar.

Analysis of Pragmatic Abilities

After a representative sample of language is collected, the clinician can begin to judge the appropriateness of pragmatic skills. Prutting and Kirchner[9] have published a taxonomy of pragmatic skills suitable for identifying abilities of neurologically impaired adults. Their Pragmatic Protocol provides a range of 30 pragmatic skills thought to be important for communicative competence. These 30 skills are divided into three general headings: verbal aspects, paralinguistic aspects, and nonverbal aspects. Verbal aspects involve such skills as topic selection, initiation, maintenance, turn-taking, specificity of the message, and use of cohesive devices (e.g., anaphoric pronouns). Paralinguistic aspects include speech intelligibility, prosody, and vocal quality and intensity. Finally, nonverbal aspects include eye gaze, facial expressions, and physical proximity of the speaker and listener.

The Pragmatic Protocol is a general measure of pragmatic skills. The pragmatic behaviors exhibited during a 15-minute conversation are judged by the clinician as either appropriate or inappropriate. The frequency of the occurrence of an inappropriate behavior is irrelevant. If the client demonstrates one instance of a behavior which interferes with communication, that behavior is considered to be a possible impairment. Those behaviors judged to be inappropriate should be probed further to determine the extent that they contribute to inadequate communication.

Standardized Measurement of Pragmatic Abilities

Although a language sample can provide information regarding pragmatic skills, there is one standardized measurement tool specifically designed to assess real-life communicative abilities. In 1980, Holland[38] published the assessment battery, Communicative Abilities in Daily Living (CADL), to help clinicians better identify their clients' functional communicative abilities. The focus of this assessment tool is on communicative adequacy, not linguistic accuracy. The CADL was constructed to incorporate daily language contexts and natural communicative style in an effort to approximate more validly the communicative skills of the client. The test examines a wide variety of behaviors, including speech acts, humor and metaphor, numeric estimates and calculations, integration of verbal and nonverbal contexts to understand and relate information, roleplaying, and the use of social language. The CADL allows examination of a number of linguistic and nonlinguistic pragmatic behaviors not normally assessed in traditional diagnostic batteries.

Summary

The context of assessment should be expanded to include interactions that comprise a wide variety of speech acts within a conversational setting. By simulating a conversational context, the clinician will be able to identify a brain-damaged person's pragmatic strengths and weaknesses.

Treatment

Intervention for pragmatic impairments can be successfully accomplished when the therapeutic activities include all of the conversational functions and rules that normally underlie communicative interactions. Generally, the most efficient strategy for targeting pragmatic impairments in intervention involves two simple steps. First, the clinician should determine situations or contexts in which the impaired skills are normally used in a client's daily conversations. Second, similar settings should be constructed in intervention in order to approximate the same context(s). For example, if a person has shown an impairment in the ability to produce comments that are contingent on the listener's utterances, then the first step in intervention would be to determine contexts in which most speakers provide contingent responses. Examples of contexts in which this skill is used include generating information about an episode of a recent television program or requesting information about a speaker's description of photographs from a vacation. Once a number of contexts are determined, the clinician can begin to incorporate and/or simulate these same contexts for interventional purposes. Not only will the intervention be pragmatic in the sense of incorporating the linguistic and nonlinguistic aspects of communication, but it will be pragmatic in that the activities will be of functional use.

In the following section, three techniques that have been used successfully in creating a naturalistic communicative setting in intervention will be reviewed.

Specific Treatment Tasks

PROMOTING APHASICS' COMMUNICATIVE EFFECTIVENESS

The notion of a naturalistic intervention setting serves as a theoretical basis for the intervention protocol devised by Wilcox and Davis entitled Promoting Aphasics' Communicative Effectiveness (PACE).[30] This strategy has been introduced and briefly reviewed in previous chapters. PACE was developed from the recognition that traditional intervention techniques do not replicate the structure of natural conversation. PACE focuses the client and the clinician on ideas to be conveyed rather than on the struggle for linguistic accuracy; divergent linguistic behavior is inherent in the interaction; and the active listening (i.e., listening for the intent of the speaker) is required by both conversational partners. The four principles of PACE[30] are:

1. The clinician and client participate equally as senders and receivers of messages.
2. There is an exchange of new information between the clinician and the client.
3. The speaker has free choice as to which modality is used to convey a message.
4. Feedback to the listener focuses on the adequacy of the message.

PACE intervention frequently centers on the process of the clinician and the client taking turns describing unknown pictures to each other. Typically, the clinician and client sit across from each other. A stack of picture cards is placed face down on a table between them. The clinician and client then take turns choosing a card and describing the contents. For example, clients with problems in providing informative messages may describe pictures of simple objects or actions. If a client has difficulty in providing information in a logically ordered sequence of actions or events, the card may contain a series of pictures that represent a simple storyline or common event or procedure. The goal of the activity is to convey adequate information to the listener. The client's message is judged on how well the clinician is able to understand and visualize the card being described. As a speaker, the clinician models the type of appropriate pragmatic behaviors that are being targeted for change in the activity. The important feature of this intervention protocol is that the use of conversational functions and rules are required of the client and modeled by the clinician.

BARRIER ACTIVITIES

The principles underlying PACE can easily be incorporated into almost any intervention activity. Barrier activities, which were originally devised by researchers to examine children's ability to convey new versus old information,[39] share with PACE protocol the same underlying principle of creating a functional communicative setting. Barrier activities, as the name implies, involve placing an opaque barrier between the clinician and the client so as to create a need for each individual to communicate. For many barrier activities, each participant has the same materials on his side of the barrier. The task usually requires each conversational partner to take a turn describing a move or change in the materials, requesting additional information about the materials, and/or commanding the other partner to move the materials. After a message is conveyed, the barrier is removed so that the two participants may judge the effectiveness of the speaker's message. As does PACE, these activities stress the importance of conveying new information adequately to a conversational partner, a principle often ignored in typical clinical intervention.

Barrier activities are general enough to use in remediation for a variety of pragmatic impairments. These activities provide numerous avenues for comprehending and producing a variety of speech acts as well as conversational devices that serve to maintain the communicative interaction. For example, in the manipulation of common objects on each side of the barrier, a client practices making and understanding requests for information, indirect requests for action, comments on actions, requests for clarification, and revisions of prior utterances. Other pragmatic goals can be targeted and accomplished by changes in the materials. For example, one commonly used barrier activity involves giving directions from one destination to another along a simple map. Clinicians can use this activity to work on procedural discourse skills in a functional communicative setting. To increase the quality and quantity of a client's conversational turn, a barrier activity might involve description of the arrangement of similarly shaped objects that vary in size or color. This type of activity increases the need to provide more descriptive information to a listener. Whatever the activity, the use of a barrier between the speaker and the listener forces a conversational dialogue. These activities also remove emphasis from the clinician as the "teacher" and places more emphasis on the role of an equal partner in the communication event. This minimizes some of the problems inherent in a traditional didactic format.

ROLEPLAYING

A third useful intervention technique that can be utilized is roleplaying. Roleplaying provides opportunities to practice communication in situations that arise in everyday experiences, and enables the clinician to discuss and implement possible strategies useful outside the clinic environment. Finally, roleplaying allows for a free exchange of information between the participants, thus emphasizing the use of language in context.

A roleplaying activity typically involves three phases.[35] During the first phase, the clinician and the client discuss the goal of the roleplay activity as well as possible responses and behaviors that can be used during the activity. For example, if the goal is to initiate and maintain a topic across several conversational turns, one possible roleplay situation might be the meeting of an old friend for the first time in several years. The clinician and the client first discuss possible "opening lines" that the client might use as well as possible statements or questions that can serve to continue the topic.

After the clinician and the client have discussed the situation, roleplaying commences. The emphasis during this second phase of roleplaying changes from practice and discussion of target pragmatic behaviors to use of these skills in a "spontaneous" conversational setting. It is essential that the clinician retain his or her role throughout the roleplay, so as to best represent a situation in which the client must use the target skills. When the clinician steps out of his or her role during this phase, he or she risks the chance of turning a functional, communicative setting into a nonfunctional, instructional setting.

The third intervention phase follows completion of the roleplay. After the roleplaying is completed, the clinician and client discuss and evaluate the adequacy of the information exchanged. This last phase is particularly important since it enables the clinician and the client to reflect on specific communicative behaviors. Additionally, it allows the clinician to reinforce those behaviors that contributed to the adequacy of the message conveyed, while providing possible alternative strategies for remediating inappropriate pragmatic skills. Although not a requirement, videotape playback enhances the evaluation of those communicative behaviors that have been targeted.

Situations for roleplaying are many and varied and should be guided by the specific pragmatic goal of remediation, as well as by the usefulness of the content of the roleplay for the client's everyday living. Roleplaying may be used to develop a number of pragmatic skills including providing unambiguous messages, producing different speech acts, and practicing appropriate eye gaze and proxemics. The main point is that roleplaying is a viable activity not only for encouraging spontaneous communication, but also for providing a means of discussing and building pragmatic skills for effective communication.

Summary

Brain-damaged individuals demonstrate both intact and impaired pragmatic skills. The assessment and intervention of pragmatic impairments necessitates evaluation and treatment in as naturalistic a setting as possible. The most opportune settings for examining pragmatic skills are the person's real-life environments (e.g., social clubs, home). Realistically, however, many clinicians have neither the time nor the resources to evaluate pragmatic skills in the natural environment. The most likely alternative is stimulation of a natural conversational setting within the clinic itself. Either way, the use of functional, communicative procedures that have been overlooked in traditional management paradigms, allow real communication to be experienced in a clinical setting. If a setting is created that fosters genuine communication, then clients have the chance to improve their communicative effectiveness through conversational reinforcement of their pragmatic strengths and through opportunities to develop skills and strategies that compensate for their weaknesses.

Acknowledgment

We would like to express our warmest appreciation to Melanie Teal, the senior author's office manager, for her typing and proofing efforts leading to the completion of this chapter.

Suggested Readings

Davis GA, Wilcox MJ: *Adult Aphasia Rehabilitation: Applied Pragmatics.* San Diego: College-Hill Press, 1985.

Foldi NS, Cicone M, Gardner H: Pragmatic aspects of communication if brain-damaged patients. In Segalowitz SJ (ed): *Language Functions and Brain Organization.* New York: Academic Press, 1983; pp 51–86.

Prutting CA, Kirchner DM: A clinical appraisal of the pragmatic aspects of language. *Journal of Speech and Hearing Disorders* 1987; 52:105–119.

Weylman ST, Brownell HH, Gardner H: "It's what you mean, not what you say": Pragmatic language use in brain-damaged patients. In Plum F (ed): *Language, Communication and the Brain.* New York: Raven Press, 1988; pp 229–243.

References

1. Newhoff M, Tonkovich JD, Schwartz SL, Burgess EK: Revision Strategies in Aphasia. *Journal of Neurological Communication Disorders* 1985; 2:2–7.
2. Pierce RS, Beekman LA: Effects of Linguistic and Extralinguistic Context on Semantic and Syntactic Processing in Aphasia. *Journal of Speech and Hearing Disorders* 1985; 28:250–254.
3. Schienberg S, Holland A: Conversational turn-taking in Wernicke's aphasia. In Brookshire R (ed): *Clinical Aphasiology Conference Proceedings,* 1980. Minneapolis: BRK Publishers, pp 106–110.
4. Weylman ST, Brownell HH, Gardner H: "It's what you mean, not what you say": Pragmatic language use in brain-damaged patients. In Plum F (ed): *Language, Communication and the Brain.* New York: Raven Press, 1988, pp 229–243.
5. Apel K, Browning-Hall J, Newhoff M: *Contingent queries in Broca's Aphasia* Paper presented to the American Speech–Language–Hearing Association, Toronto, 1981.
6. Foldi NS: Appreciation of pragmatic interpretations of indirect commands: Comparison of right and left hemisphere brain-damaged patients. *Brain and Language* 1987; 31:88–108.
7. Bates E: *Language in Context.* New York: Academic Press, 1976.
8. Lahey M: *Language Disorders and Language Development.* New York: Macmillan, 1988.
9. Prutting CA, Kirchner DM: A clinicl appraisal of the pragmatic aspects of language. *J Speech Hear Disord* 1987; 52:105–119.
10. Wollner S, Geller E: Methods of assessing pragmatic abilities. In Irwin JV (ed): *Pragmatics: The Role in Language Development.* La Verne, California: Fox Point Publishing, 1982, pp 135–160.
11. Rees N: An overview of pragmatics of what is in the box? In Irwin JV (ed): *Pragmatics: The Role in Language Development.* La Verne, California: Fox Point Publishing, 1982, pp 1–14.
12. Roth F, Spekman N: Assessing the pragmatic abilities of children: Part 1. Organizational framework and assessment parameters. *Journal of Speech and Hearing Disorders* 1984; 49:2–11.
13. Brownell HH, Potter HH, Bihrle AM, et al: Inference deficits in right brain-damaged patients. *Brain and Language* 1986; 27:310–321.
14. Hirst W, LeDoux J, Stein S: Constraints on the processing of indirect speech acts: Evidence from aphasiology. *Brain and Language* 1984; 23:26–33.
15. Buck R, Duffy R: Nonverbal communication of affect in brain-damaged patients. *Cortex* 1980; 16:351–362.
16. Myers PS, Linebaugh CW: Comprehension of idiomatic expressions by right hemisphere-damaged adults. In Brookshire R (ed): *Clinical Aphasiology Conference Proceedings,* 1981. Minneapolis: BRK Publishers.
17. Brownell HH, Michel D, Powelson J, et al: Surprise but not coherence: Sensitivity to verbal humor in right-hemisphere patients. *Brain and Language* 1983; 18:20–27.
18. Behrens S: The role of the right hemisphere in the production of linguistic stress. *Brain and Language* 1988; 33:104–127.
19. Weintraub S, Mesulam H, Kramer L: Disturbances in prosody: A right hemisphere contribution to language. *Archives of Neurology* 1981; 38:742–744.
20. Schneiderman EI, Saddy JD: A linguistic deficit resulting from right-hemisphere damage. *Brain and Language* 1988:38–53.
21. Holland A: *Aphasics as communicators: A model and its implications.* Paper presented to the American Speech–Language–Hearing Association, Washington, DC, 1981.
22. Katz RC, LaPointe LL, Markel NN: Coverbal behavior and aphasic speakers. In Brookshire R (ed): *Clinical Aphasiology Conference Proceedings,* 1978. Minneapolis: BRK Publishers.
23. Ulatowska H, Doyel A, Stern R, et al: Production of procedural discourse in aphasia. *Brain and Language* 1983; 18:315–341.

24. Ulatowska H, Freedman-Sterne R, Doyel A, et al: Production of narrative discourse in aphasia. *Brain and Language* 1983; 19:317–334.
25. Wilcox MJ, Davis GA, Leonard LB: Aphasics' comprehension of contextually conveyed meaning. *Brain and Language* 1978; 6:363–377.
26. Wilcox MJ, Davis AG: Speech act analysis of aphasic communication in individual and group settings, in Brookshire R (ed): *Clinical Aphasiology Conference Proceedings,* 1977. Minneapolis: BRK Publishers, pp 166–174.
27. Linebaugh C, Kryzer K, Oden S, et al: Reapportionment of communicative burden in aphasia: A study of narrative instructions. In Brookshire R (ed): *Clinical Aphasiology Conference Proceedings,* 1982. Minneapolis: BRK Publishers, pp 4–9.
28. Bates E, Hamby S, Zurif E: The effects of focal brain damage on pragmatic expression. *Canadian Journal of Psychology* 1983; 37:59–84.
29. Lund NJ, Duchan JF: *Assessing Children's Language in Naturalistic Contexts,* ed 2. Englewood Cliffs, New Jersey: Prentice-Hall, 1988.
30. Davis GA, Wilcox MJ: *Adult Aphasia Rehabilitation: Applied Pragmatics,* San Diego: College-Hill Press, 1985.
31. Kimbarrow M, Brookshire R: The influence of communicative context on aphasic speaker's use of pronouns, in Brookshire R (ed): *Clinical Aphasiology Conference Proceedings.* Minneapolis: BRK Publishers, 1983, pp 195–201.
32. Kudo T, Segawa N, Ihjima A, et al: The effect of pictorial context on sentence memory in Broca's and Wernicke's aphasia. *Brain and Language* 1988; 34:1–12.
33. Williams SE, Canter GJ: The influence of situational context on naming performance in aphasic syndromes. *Brain and Language* 1982; 17:92–106.
34. Webster E, Newhoff M: Intervention with families of communicatively impaired adults. In Beasley D, Davis GA (eds): *Aging: Communication Processes and Disorders.* New York: Grune and Stratton, 1981; pp 229–240.
35. Webster E: *Counseling with Parents of Handicapped Children,* New York: Grune and Stratton, 1977.
36. Lubinski R: Environmental language intervention. In Chapey R (ed): *Language Intervention Strategies in Adult Aphasia.* Baltimore: Williams & Wilkins, 1981, pp. 223–245.
37. Wallace-Hunter G, Canter GJ: *Comparative performance of severe aphasics with personally relevant versus extrapersonal language.* Paper presented to the American Speech–Language–Hearing Association, Toronto, 1982.
38. Holland A: *Communicative Abilities in Daily Living.* Baltimore: University Park Press, 1980.
39. Glucksberg S, Krauss R: What do people say after they have learned to talk? Studies of the development of referential communication. *Merrill-Palmer Quarterly* 1967; 13:309–316.

Index